FUNCTIONAL MEDICINE UNLOCKED

Root-Cause Protocols + Profit Strategies
for Purpose-Driven Practitioners

LAUREN DUROY
DNP, APRN, FNP-C, FIM-P

Functional Medicine Unlocked

Root-Cause Protocols + Profit Strategies for Purpose-Driven Practitioners

Lauren Duroy, DNP, APRN, FNP-C, FIM-P

Published by Game Changer Publishing

Paperback ISBN: 979-8-90158-084-4

Hardcover ISBN: 979-8-90158-085-1

Digital ISBN: 979-8-90158-086-8

GAME CHANGER PUBLISHING

www.GameChangerPublishing.com

This book is dedicated to the people who make my life worth living.

To my boys, you transformed me in ways no one could imagine. Knowing the love I have for you, Gauge and Drake, gives me a strength I never knew possible. Gauge, my first baby boy, without you I would have never understood the true meaning of life—or what it means to love at a depth I didn't know existed. Drake, without you, I would have never found the courage and power I needed to chase our dreams of being a family with a Mom at home, through entrepreneurship. When you were born, I learned what it meant for a heart to grow in size. From the moment I knew you were coming into our lives, it became my deepest desire to stop working nonstop so that neither of you would ever have to go without your momma. I need you both more than the air I breathe.

To my husband, my ride or die. We are living proof of the amazing grace and power of our Lord Jesus Christ, which I love so much and am so proud of. One of my favorite things in life—if not my very favorite—is laughing with you about this crazy journey we call life. In those rare moments when it's just the two of us, it feels like we're kids again (just a little more sleep-deprived), watching the world go by while we stay in our own little bubble. I remember on our wedding weekend thanking God for giving me the man of my dreams, and fourteen years later, I'm still saying the same prayer of gratitude—only now with even more love than I had back then.

To my mom, my bestie—we are like two Tamagotchi peas in a pod, bouncing around this world and making everyone's head spin (for better or worse). I'm so glad that I was gifted a mom who taught me to think for myself. This book would have never happened without that life skill. I can't imagine where I'd be without you teaching me resilience, empathy, and how to follow my heart by trusting my intuition and God.

To my dad, who taught me the value of hard work and what it means to keep my word—not only to others but to myself. You showed me never to give up on what I start, and that giving your very best is one of the most rewarding things a person can do. At the same time, your humor, quick wit, and family inside jokes bring me a joy I will always cherish.

Watching both of you step into your roles as Papa and Nana, loving on our boys, has been one of the most fulfilling and beautiful gifts of my life.

I thank God every day that you are all in my life. Most importantly, I thank the Lord Almighty for being in my life. His loving grace and the gift of the Holy Spirit have, without a doubt, been the driving force that allowed me to lead with passion and make dreams of healing and freedom come true—not only for myself, but for patients and my students, many of whom have become close friends.

Which brings me to this last part of my dedication: to my students. Thank you. Thank you to those who trusted me when I was just getting started, and thank you to those who suspended disbelief and went all in on a mission to heal, even when others said it couldn't be done. I write these words with tears in my eyes, grateful that God brought you to me. I have been blessed with the most incredible people to work alongside, and helping you build your passions and missions in life has been one of the greatest honors I have ever been given.

Thank you for trusting me and for having the courage to go forward in a world often rigged by large organizations, and for standing with me in our mission to heal people and give voice to unheard pain. None of this would be possible without you. Your courage matters. Your impact matters. And you deserve credit for this book being written—to help even more people discover the healing power of functional medicine and the freedom of self-owned practices that lead with results over numbers.

If I could, I would place each one of your names in this book. You deserve the recognition. Thank you—and know that I love you all.

–Lauren

Read This First

Just to say thanks for buying and reading my book, I would like to connect with you by giving you FREE tickets to our next virtual event!

Scan the QR Code Here:

SCAN ME

(Or follow the link to functionalmedicineunlocked.com)

Foreword

There are certain people God places in your life at pivotal moments, people whose presence quietly changes the direction of your future. For me, Dr. Lauren Duroy has been one of those people.

Before finding this community, I remember praying for a life that felt different from the one I was living. I prayed that one day I would be able to do work I truly loved while still being present with my family. I prayed for the freedom to homeschool my children, to build a peaceful home, to make bread in my kitchen in the middle of the day, and to create a life rooted in purpose instead of constant survival.

And now, somehow, that is the life I get to live.

Today I wake up doing meaningful work that changes lives. I get to support families, help children heal, and build something deeply aligned with my faith and calling. While I give all glory to God for where I am today, I also know that He uses people to guide us, sharpen us, and encourage us along the way, and Lauren has undeniably been one of those people in my story.

What makes Lauren so remarkable is not simply her intelligence or expertise, though both are extraordinary. It is the atmosphere she creates around her. She calls people higher. She makes you believe that the vision inside of you may actually be possible.

Attending her masterclass in Dallas impacted me in ways I never expected. I thought I was attending for education and business mentorship, but what I experienced there became so much more. What began as a room full of professionals became genuine connection, deep encouragement, and relationships that still remain in my life today. Many of the people I met there are still people I speak with regularly.

But even deeper than that, the Lord used that experience personally in my life.

There was an unintentional deliverance that took place while I was there, something I was not seeking or expecting, yet something I deeply needed. Through the environment Lauren cultivated, through the vulnerability, truth, encouragement, and connection surrounding that experience, God met me there in a profound way. I left lighter, freer, clearer, and changed not only professionally, but personally and spiritually as well.

That is the kind of impact Lauren has on people.

She has created far more than a mentorship space. She has created a place where people feel seen, challenged, supported, and inspired to step fully into the work they were created to do. The resources, relationships, wisdom, and encouragement that have come from being part of her community have genuinely changed my life.

Lauren has an incredible ability to combine wisdom with humility, excellence with compassion, and leadership with genuine care for people.

This book is a reflection of that same spirit.

If these pages encourage you even a fraction of the way Lauren's mentorship and presence have encouraged me, then they will leave a lasting mark on your life as well.

Forever grateful,

Kelsea Hutchings, APRN, CPNP-PC, BC-FMP

Little Lanterns Pediatrics

FUNCTIONAL MEDICINE UNLOCKED

Root-Cause Protocols + Profit Strategies
for Purpose-Driven Practitioners

LAUREN DUROY
DNP, APRN, FNP-C, FIM-P

Contents

Disclaimer

This material is intended **for educational purposes only.**

Clinical caution should always be exercised when applying any information contained in this text. The content assumes that the provider reading it is already trained, licensed, and fully aware of the potential risks, contraindications, and side effects associated with patient care, diagnostic testing, supplementation, and clinical interventions.

Nothing in this book is meant to replace the clinical judgment of a qualified healthcare professional, nor does it constitute medical advice for any specific patient or situation. The author explicitly disclaims any liability arising from the improper application or interpretation of the material presented.

Providers should always rely on their own training, scope of practice, and state/national regulations when making clinical decisions and should also be aware and diligent that supplements and herbs are not extensively studied to know all potential interactions and side effects, and therefore they simply cannot all be covered or mentioned.

Introduction

"The newness of life is not brought forth by the passage of time, but rather, the passage of the biases in our minds."
– Lauren Duroy

My name is Lauren Duroy. I hold a Doctor of Nursing Practice (DNP) degree, and I am an advanced practice registered nurse (APRN). I am dual board-certified in family and functional medicine. Most importantly, I am a daughter of the Most High, once broken and overwhelmed, having been both a patient lost in a system that didn't know what to do with me and a member of a profession that ruled me.

I am the owner of the Academy of Functional Medicine and the Academy of Functional Medicine, which offers certification for a variety of professionals, including coaches, nurses, physical therapists, medical doctors (MDs), doctors of osteopathic medicine (DOs), chiropractors, nurse practitioners, physician assistants (PAs), and more. If you are reading this book and unsure whether it's meant for you, I assure you that it is. We have a pathway and business plan that works for anyone, regardless of their background. Our programs are designed to accommodate busy and even overworked professionals, those with advanced medical backgrounds or those just getting started. Those from rural America and those in busy metropolises. Those who want to scale 7 figure empires, and those just looking to start a meaningful passion project. No matter your background, you are welcome to reach out to me and meet many of these students in our private Skool group: https://www.skool.com/functionalmedicine/about.

Initially, I didn't envision our programs reaching such a broad audience, but I recognized that diverse perspectives are essential in the field of functional medicine. Traditional methods of healing often conflict with the principles of healing that functional medicine promotes. Incorporating various practitioners has proven to be immensely beneficial, and our programs now reflect that inclusivity.

I hold a Bachelor of Science from the University of Oklahoma and a Bachelor of Science in Nursing from Oklahoma City University, along with my Doctor of Nursing Practice. In addition, I am a certified business coach, and I assist practitioners and coaches from various fields (not just functional clinics) in building their profitable passions. I am also the published author of *Living Between the Lines*, a Christ-centered, self-led cognitive behavioral therapy book to help patients overcome anxiety and depression.

I have been featured on various media platforms and have spoken to a diverse group of medical professionals, including nurse practitioners, MDs, podiatrists, and surgeons. I've appeared on Fox News, the CW, and PESI, as well as at several speaking events across the country.

My journey into functional medicine began as a quest for personal healing. I had what I describe as an "invisible disease." If you are reading this, you may relate to that experience or feel called to advocate for those who are suffering in the grey area of pain and a lack of definitive diagnosis or effective treatments. This "unheard pain" often falls into a ten-minute appointment with providers who don't know what to do and, therefore, either exhaust their resources trying to diagnose the problem or resort to gaslighting clients, telling them that the labs are normal, so there must be nothing wrong.

This book is for providers and caregivers who, even when lab results come back normal and the scans are negative, still know that something is terribly wrong with their patients because they believe their testimony and can see that there are questions that conventional medicine is not prepared to answer.

One of those questions is “Why is this happening to me?” As a provider, you know there must be an answer, a better way, and it's not just a coincidence that you’re reading this today. You likely have a natural intuition that holistic treatment can enable the body to heal itself. You understand and believe that if the body is given the right conditions, it can recover. Merely pushing a pill or adjusting a number on a chart does not address the root cause of the suffering people experience.

You aspire to be the kind of person who is genuinely called to help others heal. I don’t just want to teach you through this book; I also want to reach you on a deeper level. I want you to know that you can make a significant difference in your clients' lives. I speak from personal experience—I didn’t begin teaching functional medicine because it was trendy; it became my passion after it helped me heal.

I suffered from severe and debilitating IBS, and despite numerous tests, labs, and scans, everything came back normal, and no answers were revealed. No path to healing lay before me. During my last conversation with a colleague about my results, they looked at me and said, "Nothing's wrong," and it felt like they were suggesting that I should just give up the act. On the one hand, I felt utterly defeated because it was clear they didn’t know how to help me. I feared my IBS, anxiety, and chronic pain would control my life indefinitely. On the other hand, I felt liberated. That moment gave me the permission I needed to step out of the box I didn't know I had been put in when I started my educational journey over a decade before.

I could hardly eat without it being a battle. Whenever I went out, I was anxious that others might think I was making it up if the food triggered severe pain or that I was high-maintenance, having to choose only certain restaurants. I was anxious about being judged for avoiding certain foods. I feared others might think I was anorexic or bulimic because, at one point or another, I was verbally accused of each concern. I tried to avoid the bathroom after meals because I was thin and didn't want to give anyone more reason to believe my relationship with food was anything besides avoiding physical pain. At times, these fears consumed my thoughts.

I was additionally dealing with anxiety and depression, and I noticed that as my intestinal symptoms worsened, so did my mental health struggles. The foods that triggered my IBS would undoubtedly leave me feeling depressed, irritable, and unmotivated. I never believed it was a coincidence, though other providers suggested that my symptoms were simply a result of my anxiety, instead of the gastrointestinal symptoms also impacting my mental health.

The experience even impacted my spiritual health. I felt ashamed that God was not miraculously lifting my depression and anxiety. Matthew 6:24 transformed my cognitive beliefs. When I read *"Therefore I tell you, do not worry about your life, what you will eat or drink, or about your body, what you will wear… Look at the birds of the air; they do not sow or reap or store away in barns, and yet your heavenly Father feeds them. Are you not much more valuable than they?"* for the first time, it was as if God was speaking directly to me. Those words transformed my mind. Yet, I would still fall into bouts of negative thinking and feel deeply ashamed that I could not take my thoughts captive and not worry. I feared I had only shallow belief, and subconsciously, I was in disbelief of His healing power.

However, once it hit me that conventional medicine didn't have the answers I needed, I also realized that my struggles weren't my disobedience or lack of being a good enough Christian but a mess He was going to turn into a message. He was guiding me through the ordeal so that I could help future patients heal His temple because we are His temple here on Earth (1 Corinthians 3:16).

I knew that God had bigger plans for me than allowing me to deteriorate in my twenties. This realization empowered me to explore alternative options, which led me to discover functional medicine. Initially, I was very skeptical. I fully believed that if it was actually effective, I would have learned about it in my conventional medical training.

However, when conventional medicine failed me, I approached alternative options with humility, and it completely transformed my life. I spent hundreds of hours pouring myself over peer-reviewed journals that had been pushed out of the mainstream narrative, and slowly started implementing. Within the first month, my symptoms of IBS had dramatically improved, and over the next three to six months, I stopped experiencing flare-ups altogether. I also noticed a significant reduction in my pain, anxiety, and depression. Having struggled with severe depression since childhood, this shift was monumental for me. I didn't know at the time that what I was practicing was already classified as "Functional" medicine. I was just overjoyed to find relief.

When I began helping clients, my hesitation at offering such treatments was somewhat amusing. My first client seemed like a great fit, but I was hesitant to even suggest it. I was still struggling with believing that what I experienced was real and not coincidence. I felt like a pseudoscience provider suggesting things that conventional medicine proclaimed were impossible. But yet, I told them, "I haven't helped anyone else with this before, only myself. Are you sure you want to try this for you?" They responded enthusiastically, saying they would do anything to find help.

What I want to share with you today is that the transition to a new life isn't brought forth by the passage of time; it's brought forth by the passage of the biases in our minds. We must relinquish some of our traditional views on healing and transform our mindsets to benefit both our patients and the future of healthcare. We must also recognize that we are engaged in a spiritual battle for our patients just as much as a mental and physical one.

I believe we are called to reclaim health from the enemy. This struggle began in the Garden of Eden with Adam and Eve, and this sneaky attack from the enemy continues today in several ways, including hiding root causes of disease in modern-day food. The forbidden fruit symbolizes our modern "food," including high-fructose corn syrup, preservatives that extend shelf life, and artificial additives that enable food to last for years on a shelf or become addictive due to their highly palatable tastes, which God never intended. These substances are subsequently highly devoid of nutrients and can directly contribute to issues like ADHD and anxiety in our children, yet they are consumed regularly.

This is additionally comparable with the results we see in other aspects of life when we search for things by our own understanding and not the Lord's, which leads to death of the soul and the body. It is all a perfect example of how we think we can do things better and smarter than God, hence the correlation with the Tree of Knowledge.

These foods were developed through the human understanding (knowledge) of what is a good idea, not God's. We eat from the Tree of Knowledge every day in this nation instead of leaning on the Tree of Life and trusting God's plan for how we should be nourishing our bodies. You can be certain the enemy is there every step of the way to steal, kill, and destroy not only our lives and health but also the lives of our children and their children's children.

Same trick of the enemy, different day. The serpent told Eve before she ate from the Tree of Knowledge, *"You will not surely die."* However, that was the moment in time when humans, made in the image of God, lost their immortality and inherited an expiration date and suffering. And what was their next "transformation"? They became ashamed and hid themselves from the glory of God, the same way that food today makes us feel depressed, anxious, and even ashamed when it takes over our choices. Same trick, different day.

Trust that we will get into how food and the gut-brain connection have physiologically influenced our minds, further exposing the enemy's plan to destroy us. You cannot convince me that this is not an attack from the enemy. We need to change our perspective on prevention because the truth is that our society is on a path to extinction.

In increasing areas of the United States, the life expectancy of children is now lower than that of their parents. We are arguably on the path toward extinction, and if we want to be a nation of redemption, we must change how we approach prevention.

One of the first things I want to do is help you eliminate biases in your thinking and empower you to be an agent for change. One way I like to illustrate this is by comparing an eagle to a kiwi. You can search for pictures of these birds; you probably know what an eagle looks like, but a kiwi is a flightless bird native to New Zealand that lacks good vision. The kiwi wanders the ground and, due to its inability to fly, is very vulnerable to predators. This vulnerability has led to the kiwi being placed on the endangered list.

On the other hand, eagles were almost completely extinct at one point, dwindling to around only a couple hundred mating pairs. We had to change our perspective and expand our ability to identify the root cause of disease to discover the cause. It was found that the eagles were consuming water contaminated with pesticides that washed off food meant for humans, which was diluted in their water supply. The mother eagles were drinking this very diluted (though tainted) water, which contained DDT (a harmful pesticide), causing them to be unable to lay viable eggs.

Once we recognized the cause of the problem, we could take steps to save the eagles, and they are now rebounding and are no longer endangered. We must adopt the same approach when it comes to looking at how what we ingest is leading to our demise.

We can't just accept the gaslighting that tells us these issues are all in our heads or that food and chemicals don't have real effects on our health. If such contaminants can wipe out an entire species, who are we to claim they won't negatively affect us in areas such as fertility or gut health?

Another reason I like to use the eagle and the kiwi as examples is that they are both birds. They may even occupy the same earthly location, yet their experiences of life are vastly different. While the kiwi scuttles around in the grass, the eagle soars thousands of feet in the air. As John C. Maxwell puts it, "We eat at the level of our vision." My goal is to elevate your vision.

You are reading this book because you are called to a higher vision for the future and already have a greater awareness of what's happening in our world. I want you to understand that the vision you hold is significant and you have been called to it.

When you're like an eagle facing the murmured criticism of kiwis, remember that they are merely expressing views from their own limited perspective. While they may have their own truths based on personal experience, they cannot see where you are coming from or where you are headed.

When I first heard about the concept of root causes, I thought it was naïve. As a provider of conventional medicine, I believed I was addressing root causes when I prescribed steroids to reduce inflammation. However, I failed to realize that although the steroid alleviated the inflammation, it did not address the underlying cause of the inflammation. I had been looking at things from the perspective of a kiwi. The steroid was not adding life to a person, but merely allowing their body to keep going while the underlying cause of the inflammation stayed seething in the body. The medication also causes compounding side effects, like weight gain, insulin resistance, etc.

I share this to emphasize the importance of having a different perspective. Once you adopt this viewpoint, you won't be shaken when you hear from naysayers. When you understand that the kiwis simply cannot fly up, you realize that they simply cannot understand your perspective. If you're looking to start your own business, for instance, you will encounter people who say, "That's impossible," or "You don't have the knowledge."

You will likely encounter your own negative thoughts, such as: *I'm not made for this* or *I'm not smart enough.* This is when you have to remember that while some kiwis peck you from behind, the most influential ones set up nests in your mind. The naysayer is oftentimes your own quiet voice. I want you to know that holding on to a higher vision isn't necessarily easy, but when you're called to it, your life will never function as it should until you answer that calling.

While eagles soar at great heights, one might mistakenly believe that it's more challenging for them to maintain that high altitude. The kiwi certainly would. The truth is that they use less energy soaring at higher altitudes than they do trying to stay at the same level as others. This is why when you are built to soar, and you lower your perspective, you will annihilate the rate at which you are effective.

Don't try to fit into the view of the world or conform to the beliefs you may have been taught, especially if you've been criticized or told that your ideas are invalid or based on pseudoscience. I understand this struggle; I've been there.

You will often face criticism for trying to rise above, but I urge you to maintain your perspective. Don't let the limited vision of others diminish your purpose. If you allow their thoughts and perceptions to dictate your actions, you allow them to incarcerate you in a lower version of yourself. This will prevent you from fulfilling your passion and calling to help others.

I've lost opportunities and years of my life by listening to the naysayers. Some of the concepts we're going to discuss might seem counterintuitive to what you've been taught, especially if you're a conventional medicine provider. I encourage you to conduct your own research, review the studies, and discover that everything in this book is backed by peer-reviewed science. Just because something is different, it doesn't mean it's not viable or effective. The testimonies and stories you will encounter may challenge your beliefs, but I encourage you to investigate further and adopt a new perspective. This shift is essential for making a meaningful impact in the world.

You are called to this mission at a significant time. There is a growing demand for functional medicine. It's referred to as the "opportunity switch" of the century in the healthcare industry. Providers certified in it are in great demand. Currently, functional medicine is a multi-billion-dollar industry and is projected to grow more than eightfold in less than a decade.[1] While earning predictions should never overshadow the importance of saving lives, I want you to recognize that this is an opportunity for you to grow your passion for healing while supporting your family. You're being called to something that can benefit you and your patients in multiple ways.

Many people falsely assume that functional medicine is too competitive and saturated with practitioners, but that is a misconception. Consider the statistics: there are over one million conventional providers, but only about 60,000 functional practitioners. Even with this number of conventional providers, there is still a shortage of healthcare professionals to meet the demand, and that is not yet considering those who additionally require functional intervention.

The need for functional medicine is increasing. In addition, people are growing weary of the conventional healthcare model, including the experience of being processed like cattle in and out of appointments. They are ready to address root causes rather than to continuously depend on large pharmaceutical companies to feel better. The dissatisfaction with side effects and risks associated with traditional medications is prompting a movement toward more educated decision-making about their health.

As trust in conventional providers diminishes, the call increases for you to meet these unmet needs. Remember, we are at a pivotal moment where everything is evolving.

For example, the statistics surrounding mental health are alarming, with one in four adults affected by mental illness. Alzheimer's disease (AD) impacts up to one in five adults and one in ten men by the age of forty-five. Additionally, depression affects around 10% of the population.[2] From 2000 to 2021, deaths from stroke, heart disease, and HIV decreased, whereas deaths from AD increased more than 140%.[3] This is despite our increased ability to keep people living longer, even with advanced diseases. Treating the symptoms of this terrible disease is not enough.

Child health statistics are even more concerning, as 5% to 18% of children suffer from conditions like fatty liver disease, and the prevalence of diabetes and obesity among children continues to rise.[4] Nearly 50% of the U.S. population now relies on some form of prescription medication, highlighting the urgent need for effective interventions.

Autism rates have also skyrocketed; it was once considered to affect one in two thousand children, but as of 2025, the CDC reports that it now affects one in 31.[5] This underscores the necessity for a new perspective on treatment, and functional medicine offers promising solutions.

Mark Hyman, a leader in this field, states, "We need to start thinking in terms of systems, not symptoms." This approach is crucial as we work on treatment protocols that consider the affected systems rather than merely treating symptoms or categorizing diseases based on them. This requires changing and altering how we look at treatment. But, change can be a good thing. Winston Churchill once said, "To improve is to change; to be perfect is to change often."

If we want to be a nation of redemption, we have to change the way we look at prevention and intervention. This perspective not only echoes my beliefs about healing, but it also echoes my beliefs about business.

One evening, around 7 p.m., when I was still in full-time conventional family practice, I remember sitting at my desk, overwhelmed by my workload, feeling burnt out from going through countless patient charts, and depressed that I knew my family had probably already finished dinner without me... again. I felt crushed by the pressure and crushed by my failure as a mother and wife.

Feeling defeated and unable to chart any longer, I picked up my phone and started mindlessly scrolling. I came across a message from Wayne Dyer that resonated deeply with me: "If you change the way you look at things, the things you look at change." I felt a sense of conviction—it struck me that I should be grateful for what I had, yet my reality felt so painful. I was struggling to see my child and often putting in sixty-hour weeks on a forty-hour salary, leaving me miserable.

I even dreaded returning from vacations because I knew I would face an overwhelming backlog of patients. My feelings shifted when Romans 12:2 (NIV) came to mind: *"Do not be conformed to the patterns of this world, but transformed by the renewing of your mind."* In that moment of reflection, I received a profound message from God: "If you lead with your human perception, you will fall to deception. But if you lead with divine connection, you will rise to perfection." I realized I needed to change my perspective in every aspect of my life and allow God to show me the way to a purpose-filled life, one where career and family could feel aligned. I knew at that moment I already had everything I needed to make it happen. I just had to let go of biases on how it "has to be" and keep an open mind of how I could find my path to balance.

Having already undergone my own healing journey with IBS, I had been helping some patients along the way, but balancing this with a full-time job was challenging. It was then that I decided to go all in, and I hired my first real business coach. She charged me $18,000, or $1,500/month. The price was steep, and I could only make the first payment after the Discover card said I could. That $1,500 was my last bit of access to monetary funds, as I was already living paycheck to paycheck. The plan to pay the second payment would depend on my ability to implement what she was going to teach me. However, I knew I had to get out, and I realized her plan would be faster than me burning myself out trying to figure it out on my own. That is when I built the Passive Clinics System™. This business model transformed my life, enabling me to match and surpass my Nurse Practitioner (NP) income in less than a year with minimal overhead and using only pockets of available time.

Before implementing this system, I often felt weighed down by student loan debt and the heart-wrenching sound of my little boy crying, "Mommy, don't go," as I prepared to leave for work. I had to pull away from him each morning, telling him, "Mommy has patients waiting." It was grueling, and I still cannot share those moments in my life without tearing up, despite that being just a little over three years ago now. The shift in perspective not only changed my professional life but also improved my overall well-being.

I wouldn't see him until that evening, and I felt like a complete failure. I had tried so hard to do well at life, but I was nowhere near where I expected myself to be after years of hard work and advanced degrees. I had checked all the boxes, taken out the loans, put in the time—only to realize I'd been fed a line. I was searching for my purpose, yet I found myself running someone else's circus.

However, I had decided that things were going to change, and they did. In less than three months, I was making $10,000 a month. In six months, I achieved my first $20,000 month, followed by my first $20,000 day just a couple of months later. It was then that I knew I could break free. This was great because I was just about four weeks away from delivering my second baby boy. Yes, that is right: I did all of this while pregnant, but I was determined that my second baby boy would not go through the first few years of his life with only fleeting moments with his mother.

My two sons became my reason, not my excuse, to double down and take some risks in life.

But then, a really incredible thing happened. I started to have colleagues and friends across the nation who reached out to me to find out what I was doing and who wanted me to teach them. I was happy to. But, at first I didn't honestly know if it would work for others with different locations, schedules, backgrounds, etc., like it did for me. But we were all continuously blown away and exceedingly excited when it worked for them as well. That was the beginning of the business education branch of the Academy of Functional Medicine.

If it feels like you're chasing diseases, pills, and numbers, yet you still want to be elevated to a higher level, it's no coincidence you're here. Friends, if you are reading this book now, it is because you are called to something better, and the encouraging truth is this: if you've done "all the things" and you still feel like you are in a setback, it's because you've been set up. You are not a failure. Now that you are awakened to a better way, all you have to do is transition the power from others to yourself in small, powerful, focused efforts.

And here is the big thing: I am not some kind of "unicorn." You can do all of that, too. As I have shared, since that time, just a few years ago, I have not been the only one to use this system and start earning an incredible income working fewer hours than I would in a full-time position. I have now had the honor and privilege of coaching hundreds of other "Kingdompreneurs" to build their dreams using the same system, and I want to help you reach that success, too.

The information in this book aims to help you both understand how to heal at the root cause and break free from the system that constrains you. You can live your purpose and escape the circus of daily life. You can find balance because, just as an eagle soars to great heights with efficiency, you, too, can achieve your goals and be more effective in what you do.

All it takes is a shift in how you approach your practice and the way you help people. This includes the business tips I'll introduce throughout this book, as well as guidance on identifying root causes of illnesses so you can assist others at a higher level.

As a thank you for purchasing this book, we invite you to join us for our next Passive Clients Business challenge. It will give you the exact blueprint you need to break free from the system like I did, without feeling like you're going back to school or taking on a second job!

SCAN ME

SCAN THE QR CODE

or visit functionalmedicineunlocked.com

Chapter 1

Root Cause Investigation

Functional medicine operates on the principle that symptoms are reflections of underlying imbalances. In contrast, conventional medicine tends to focus simply on alleviating the symptoms themselves.

In functional medicine, we aim to identify the root causes that disrupt optimal function across body systems. To illustrate this, I'd like to present a case study.

CASE STUDY: CHRONIC FATIGUE & THE IMPACT OF ENVIRONMENTAL EXPOSURE

Patient was a forty-four-year-old woman who was suffering from chronic fatigue. She reported feeling inadequate as a mother and wife because she barely had the energy to go to work and slept all evening as soon as she got home from work. She additionally contracted cold-like viruses on a regular basis, sometimes every couple of weeks. In a humorous moment, she joked that she "just goes around licking doorknobs" because she wanted to see me, emphasizing her ongoing health challenges.

Lab Workup

Her thyroid panel, inflammatory markers, and basic labs were normal, except her eosinophils were elevated. There were no risk factors to suspect sleep apnea, and she was negative for chronic viral infections, such as the Epstein-Barr virus (EBV). From a functional standpoint, elevated eosinophils can be a sign of parasitic infection, but that was not the case for her, as that was also negative.

History

Through further investigation, I discovered she had been exposed to severe mold in her workplace. After learning this, I highly suspected that the mold was responsible for her array of symptoms.

Interventions

I implemented a liver cleanse, voiding all the toxins we could, along with a microbiome rebalancing for her gut. I also provided support for her mitochondria with CoQ10 and helped boost her immune system by restoring vital nutrients, such as vitamin D. As a result, she began to feel significantly better, though not perfect.

However, once she removed herself from the exposure by finding a new job, she experienced full remission, and her remaining symptoms completely resolved. Her energy returned, and her immune system function improved. This outcome demonstrates the effectiveness of our twofold approach: we not only focused on detoxifying her body, but we also removed her from the harmful environment.

Discussion

When investigating and identifying root causes, multiple contributing factors need to be considered, based upon intake assessment and patient risk factors or past exposures. The treatment protocol selected should be guided by the root cause as revealed by testing or assessment. This differs from the conventional medicine approach where treatment protocol is often initiated based primarily on diagnosis or symptoms. This distinction can be challenging for practitioners transitioning into functional medicine because two patients with the same diagnosis may require very different treatment approaches depending on the underlying factors contributing to their condition. It is important to keep this understanding in mind throughout the functional medicine process.

Instead of asking "What is the treatment for this disease?" the functional practitioner also asks, "What factors may be contributing to this disease development?". The following list incorporates many of the areas commonly investigated without a functional medicine model. However, it is intended as a starting point. Not every test or assessment will be appropriate or necessary for every patient. Testing should be individualized based on the patient's history, symptoms, risk factors, clinical finding, and the likelihood that results will meaningfully influence management:

1. Systemic inflammation and oxidative stress
2. Genetics and epigenetics
3. Nutritional imbalances
4. Gut dysfunction
5. Toxic exposures
6. Impaired detoxification
7. Chronic stress and dysfunction of the hypothalamic-pituitary-adrenal (HPA) axis

8. Immune dysregulation and chronic infections
9. Mitochondrial dysfunction
10. Hormonal imbalances
11. Psychosocial and spiritual factors
12. Insulin resistance and sarcopenia

Also, please note that these are not listed in order of importance. It is imperative that you change your mindset from relying on set protocols based on symptoms to protocols that are tailored to the affected *systems*. It's essential to note that functional medicine differs significantly from conventional medicine in that there isn't a one-size-fits-all protocol. We don't just substitute supplements for medications. While we do use supplements, herbs, and natural remedies, our approach prioritizes eliminating root causes first and foremost.

For example, in conventional medicine, hypertension has a set protocol with first-, second-, and third-line medications, depending on confounding metrics like age, medication interactions, or comorbidities. In the Functional Model, we search for the root cause, which could be any number of the ailments listed above. Based on patient risk factors, we will first test the most likely cause, then treat based on that imbalance, allowing the illness to self-correct. The body has the power to heal itself when provided with the right environment. That is our overall goal.

That first case study was a forty-four-year-old patient whose root cause of chronic fatigue was mold exposure. In another case, a patient's chronic fatigue may have been related to issues such as genetics or epigenetics, or possibly nutritional deficiencies, specifically those related to B12 methylation. Most often the cause is a mix; for example, they may have nutritional deficiency and gut dysbiosis, which is an imbalance in the microbiome.

From my experience, it is more common to have multiple root causes than just one. Patients can present with a single issue or a combination of factors. Our primary goal is to identify the root cause (or causes) and then tailor our treatment protocols accordingly. We aim to get very specific regarding the nutritional, psychological, spiritual, and supplemental needs of each patient.

Systemic Inflammation and Oxidative Stress

A very important, possibly the most important, root cause worth examining is systemic inflammation and oxidative stress. Inflammation is attributed to the development of the majority of chronic diseases.[6] When not resolved within the body, this inflammation leads to a decreased ability to detox, autoimmune diseases, higher susceptibility to acute illnesses, decreased immunity, and several other issues within the body.[6] One could almost say that chronic inflammation is not just a root cause of disease but possibly the root cause of disease, and in functional medicine, we are looking to overturn what caused it to happen.

Oxidative stress damages DNA, mitochondria, and proteins, leading to aging and disease progression. These processes are commonly triggered by poor diet, chronic infections, and environmental stressors, chemicals, or toxins. This will be a very common theme throughout our review of the literature. It's helpful to explain the importance of screening to find more than one root cause of inflammation.

One way to conceptualize this is through the idea of allostatic load—how various stresses (physical, mental, or spiritual) affect our bodies. Genetics plays a role in how we manage allostatic stress load. I like to describe this as each person having a different-sized "cup" to handle these stressors. The way our genetics influence our capacity for physiological, spiritual, and mental stress is crucial in understanding our overall health. While the cup is “filling up,” we may have small hints that something is wrong, such as increased pain, vague symptoms like fatigue, or brain fog. Once a disease is present, we can diagnose it, but by then, the body is no longer compensating, and water is already spilling over.

Some people are born with a significantly larger capacity for handling inflammation and allostatic stress, which we can think of as having a "larger cup." Others, however, have a genetically smaller capacity, or "smaller cup." This difference explains why some people can smoke, eat unhealthy foods, and neglect their health while still living into their nineties or even over a hundred without apparent health issues like cancer. These individuals often have a larger genetic cup that allows them to manage more physiological, emotional, and spiritual stress. Conversely, someone with a smaller genetic cup might experience autoimmune diseases, difficulty losing weight, or other health problems more easily since their smaller capacity can overflow more easily when faced with damaging properties.

This overflow typically manifests as symptoms, indicating that the body can no longer handle the demands placed upon it. To address and improve these issues, a core strategy in functional medicine is the "5R approach," which helps identify and resolve gut and gastrointestinal dysfunction. This approach is also applicable for overall well-being, including detoxification from environmental toxins, and is discussed in the gastrointestinal (GI) chapter in fuller depth.

This is not exclusively applicable to treating "gut issues" because gut dysbiosis is also often a root cause for several issues, like joint pain, neurological decline, mood disorders, and autoimmunity. The treatment for the dysbiosis will be based on gastrointestinal testing results. However, inclusion of this treatment may be based upon interventions for other diseases and is not exclusive to having GI issues.

Genetics and Epigenetics

Let's start by discussing genetics and epigenetics. Certain genetic predispositions may increase susceptibility to specific conditions, meaning some individuals may be at higher risk than others. In functional medicine, we often look at genetic polymorphism variants, which can influence detoxification processes and lead to hormonal and neurotransmitter imbalances.[7]

Testing for methylenetrahydrofolate (MTHFR) polymorphism reveals information on how well B vitamins and folate are being methylated. Poor methylation means these vitamins cannot be utilized. This not only leads to deficiency but also to increased inflammation related to elevated homocysteine and methionine deficiency. If our bodies struggle to methylate the proper amount of vitamin B12 and folate, they cannot break down homocysteine into methionine, as both are necessary for that process.

Excess homocysteine in the body is inflammatory and results in less methionine, which is anti-inflammatory. Consequently, individuals may experience symptoms such as brain fog, fatigue, irritability, mood disorders, and even more severe neurological issues like tics and ADHD.[7] We go into more depth on this in Chapter 5.

Catechol-O-methyltransferase (COMT) plays a significant role in how our body responds to stress (which can be a root cause of disease in and of itself) and pain perception. It can also cause more significant complications for sleep, mood disorders, and hormonal changes, which we will explore in more depth going forward.

The ADRB3 rs4994 polymorphism is a variant that increases a person's risk for obesity and is predominantly strong in East Asian cultures. This kind of information can empower a patient to at least understand the root cause of their struggles, which can empower insights into the types of workout plans or nutrition plans they can be on that would best fit them.[8] There are also several other genetic tests that you can order to reveal risk for issues such as inflammation, the best diet for individuals, and food intolerances. I will often order the 3x4 genetics profile, but there are several out there.

Nutritional Imbalances

The second area we will investigate is nutritional imbalances, particularly micronutrient deficiencies. Deficiencies in nutrients, such as zinc, magnesium, and various B vitamins, can disrupt cellular function as much as genetic polymorphisms. It's essential to inform patients that if a vitamin or supplement hasn't worked for them in the past, it may be due to a lack of necessary cofactors for absorption rather than a lack of its effectiveness. We don't guess; we test. To delve deeper, we can order a NutrEval or a similar test to assess nutritional status and the availability of absorption cofactors.

Epigenetics refers to how environmental factors like nutrition, age, stress, and toxins can affect gene expression over time. While our genetic makeup doesn't change, the expression of our genes can be altered.[9] Environmental chemicals and lifestyle choices alter these genes and increase the risk for disease through alterations in our DNA methylation and expression, known as epigenetics.[10] Food is one such thing that can alter our epigenetics.

Diets high in processed foods and low in nutrient-dense sources can contribute to these deficiencies and systemic inflammation,[10] preventing cells from functioning properly. Additionally, food sensitivities and intolerances can provoke immune responses and increase gut permeability, resulting in a condition known as "increased intestinal permeability" (formerly known as leaky gut). This occurs when the tight junctions in the gut start to separate, allowing inflammation to enter the body.[11] This can lead to even more disease and imbalances, such as autoimmune disease, mood disorders, or neurological diseases (which we will delve into more later).

As we discussed in the introduction, this all began in the Garden of Eden. It started with food not intended for consumption and grew into so much more. It grew into death. I see this as the devil sitting right there in church with us when we "celebrate" with foods that don't honor the temple. I must stress that I do not mean to shame anyone for this. We have been conditioned to believe that these foods are safe for consumption. We've been tricked, but once our eyes are opened, we must have the heart to strive to correct these things, even if it's just one step at a time.

Sugar, especially processed sugars and high-fructose corn syrup (HFCS), is a great example of this, and this is not even considering the impact of foods mixed with high-fat and chemically processed ingredients. Sugar alone is proven to be neurotoxic, cardiotoxic, hepatotoxic, and a leading cause of obesity, diabetes, inflammation, and other diseases, like yeast overgrowth.[12] Even just 25 grams/day for women and 38 grams/day for men is associated with increased risk for disease, which is roughly half of one 20-ounce soda.[13]

Processed sugars are a leading cause of insulin resistance and metabolic dyslipidemia, independent of the presence of obesity. This means that a person can be a healthy weight and still experience insulin resistance and increased risk for neurodegenerative diseases like Alzheimer's and endocrine disorders like diabetes.[14] It's sneaky, no doubt. I have been there before, thinking it was okay to eat as much sugar as I wanted as long as I stayed a healthy weight—until a diagnosis of insulin resistance (pre-diabetes) hit me in my mid-twenties. I spent a year on metformin before I decided this was not going to be my destiny.

Yeast overgrowth is another common illness, often stemming from sugar and carbohydrate overindulgence. Symptoms may include gas, bloating, constipation, and abdominal pain.[15] They can even become more systemic, such as brain fog, irritability, sugar and carb cravings, achy joints, itching of the ears or skin, low libido, persistent canker sores, or fatigue. While many of these are vague and can encompass several other diagnoses, like hormonal imbalances, the one that stands out the most to me as a practitioner is carb or sugar cravings. I will almost always run a comprehensive stool analysis on someone who proclaims they "can't get enough" sugar or carbs.

Gut Dysfunction

Gut dysbiosis and gastrointestinal pathogens are other root causes of disease and inflammation addressed in functional medicine. This imbalance can further increase intestinal permeability and is often associated with chronic infections that disrupt digestion and immune function. Causes can include a history of antibiotic or proton pump inhibitor (PPI) use, a lack of being breastfed as a child, viral or bacterial gastroenteritis, or eating the standard American diet (SAD)—highly processed foods that are high in fat, sugar, and processed carbs and low in fiber and natural prebiotics and probiotics.[16] This is not an exhaustive list of causes, as there are several root causes for dysbiosis. I hope you're now catching on to the notion that food is more than just calories or macros (fats, carbs, or protein). It's even more than vitamins and minerals. It is literally the core of our health.

For example, gram-negative bacteria that are overgrown in the gut and shouldn't be there can cause various issues, including inflammation. Their presence can disrupt the balance of other microbiome populations in the gut. Additionally, poor stomach acid production or insufficient enzyme and bile flow can lead to nutrient malabsorption and gastrointestinal symptoms.[11] These factors directly affect our gut-brain and gut-immune axes, which are central to systemic health, mental health, and disease prevention. This is why we say that our immune system is largely located in the gut and the enteric system, or the nervous system in the gut, is the second brain.

Toxic Exposures

A fourth factor to consider when identifying the root causes of disease is toxic exposure.[17] In today's world, exposure to chemicals and pesticides is very common. In fact, hundreds of these substances are found in umbilical cords when a child is born. This means we are exposed to toxins even before we are born. Chronic exposure to environmental toxins can include pesticides, mold, heavy metals, and plastics. Plastics can break down into harmful components, such as BPA or phthalates.[18] We will discuss this further in the chapter on chemicals.

It's important to note that when a company claims to have a BPA-free or phthalate-free product, they might be substituting the BPA with a chemical that hasn't been studied yet. While we may lack evidence that these substitutes are harmful, it doesn't necessarily mean they are safe; it's a case of being innocent until proven guilty. These new chemicals could still be detrimental to our health.

Air pollutants also pose a risk, especially for those living in urban areas, where exposure levels are typically higher. All these pollutants can impair cellular function and lead to hormonal imbalances, including mitochondrial dysfunction. Even low-level, chronic exposure over time can trigger dysfunction, neuroinflammation, or hormonal disruption.[18]

When a patient says, "I've used this product for years, and it never bothered me before," it can simply be that they have now been exposed long enough for their body to no longer be able to cope. Functional medicine emphasizes both reducing this exposure and supporting natural defense systems. As systems are healed and rebalanced, the body can start to heal.

Impaired Detoxification

The fifth root cause of illness we will explore is impaired detoxification. The body's ability to process and eliminate toxins may be compromised due to genetic variations, nutritional deficiencies, or chronic stress. Nutritional deficiencies can create an overload of the chemicals we are exposed to.

Typically, our detox pathways in the liver operate in two pathways. However, if these pathways are not functioning efficiently, it can lead to a buildup of reactive metabolites and ineffective elimination through the bowel, kidneys, lymphatics, and skin. The first pathway is known as Phase I (or Functionalization). In this first phase, toxins are modified using oxidation, reduction, and hydrolysis to form reactive sites. The second pathway is Phase II (or Conjugation), which binds these activated compounds with water-soluble groups so they are able to be eliminated from the body by urination, bile production, and feces.[7] Hepatic Detox Profile testing can be ordered for a more comprehensive assessment.

Chronic Stress HPA Axis Dysfunction

The sixth root cause is chronic stress and its relation to hypothalamic-pituitary-adrenal (HPA) axis dysfunction. This dysregulation leads to cortisol imbalance, sleep disruption, and immune suppression. Each of these symptoms can increase the risk of illness. Chronic stress can elevate cortisol levels, which can also contribute to insulin resistance, subsequently leading to hormonal imbalances. Patients are often surprised to find that their anxiety and depression may stem from insomnia caused by chronic stress. This stress can be both physiological and psychological. Chronic stress diminishes resilience and impairs digestion.[19]

When we are under severe stress—such as during a physical threat—our bodies shunt blood flow from the intestines to more vital areas, like the brain or heart. This response, while natural, becomes problematic when people remain in a chronic state of stress. Similarly, prolonged exposure to cortisol, our body's natural steroid, can also lead to dysfunction.[19] This can result in imbalances in gut health, constipation, inflammation in the body, and weight gain, leading to further complications.

Stress is both a direct root cause of disease and an amplifier of other dysfunctions. Therefore, we must address stress in nearly all patients. In fact, some treatment failures occur because this aspect is not implemented. In the programs I teach to both my patients and students, we follow a comprehensive protocol that focuses on mindset and stress reduction at multiple levels. This means we aim to optimize the body so that individuals feel less stressed, while also improving mental and spiritual well-being, since all these factors are interconnected.

Immune Dysregulation and Chronic Infections

Immune dysregulation and chronic infections are significant factors to consider. Chronic or reactivated infections often go overlooked. I've diagnosed numerous clients with the Epstein-Barr virus who were completely unaware of it. Many were in their fifties, sixties, and seventies, and some were even nearing the end of their lives without ever understanding why they had relapses of illness throughout their lives.

Reactivation of the Epstein-Barr virus and subsequent flares can be prevented by supporting immune function. A lack of documented initial infection can make correctly diagnosing later relapses even more elusive, which is common. The virus begins as a mononucleosis (mono) infection and can even be misdiagnosed as a strep infection, as the clinical presentation of mono is very similar to strep. Interestingly, if a patient has an active mono infection and is given amoxicillin, it will cause a body-wide rash. It is not uncommon for this to become a misdiagnosis of antibiotic allergy when the clinician treats for strep, but the patient does not have strep and instead has active mononucleosis. Therefore, a history of taking amoxicillin for the treatment of "strep" and a subsequent rash should alert the provider to screen for Epstein-Barr.

Once contracted, the virus stays dormant and can reactivate when the immune system is compromised, sometimes triggered by another virus, bacterial infection, or stress. It has even been identified as a leading root cause of many chronic diseases, such as multiple sclerosis.[20]

Lyme disease is another example of a chronic infection that can become problematic if not treated correctly from the beginning. Additionally, Candida, or yeast overgrowth, is highly prevalent, especially in populations consuming high amounts of sugar and carbohydrates. Low-grade parasitic infections, often dismissed in conventional medicine, can also be a root cause of chronic diseases, contributing to infections or illnesses. There have been several cases of autoimmune diseases being reversed that were initially caused by parasitic infections in the gut.[21,22]

All of these factors contribute to ongoing immune activation. Autoimmunity often occurs when the body loses immune tolerance and begins to attack its own tissues. Conditions like inflammatory cytokines, mast cell activation, and histamine overload may also be present and exacerbate the situation.

Mitochondrial Dysfunction

Mitochondrial dysfunction is also a critical issue to consider when identifying the root cause of disease, especially for the more vague diagnoses. Mitochondria are the cell's energy factories, and when they are impaired, symptoms like fatigue, brain fog, and muscle weakness can arise. Mitochondrial damage can result from nutrient depletion, toxic exposure, or chronic oxidative stress. When we support mitochondrial health and reduce inflammation, the body can function more effectively. Unfortunately, conventional medicine often overlooks this vital aspect.[23]

Professional experience contributed to my understanding of mitochondrial health. During my time in conventional medicine, I encountered many patients who started taking statins and then reported feeling extremely fatigued and experiencing muscle cramps and various issues. When I consulted a more experienced colleague, they dismissed the complaints as being "all in their heads," but I had difficulty accepting this explanation. I noticed a consistent pattern in my clients—after starting the medication, they felt significantly worse. This prompted me to conduct my own research, which revealed that mitochondria require CoQ10 to function properly, which statins admittedly deplete the body of.

I began supplementing CoQ10 for my patients who are on statins after discovering peer-reviewed studies that confirm statins can deplete the body's supply of CoQ10. When CoQ10 levels drop, patients often experience symptoms such as muscular cramps, brain fog, and fatigue.

I have consistently observed that adding CoQ10 for patients on statins can prevent these symptoms from occurring when they first start the medication or even reverse them in those who are already experiencing them.[23,24] This highlights the importance of mitochondrial function, which we must address as a root cause of health issues.

Hormonal Imbalances

Hormonal imbalances are another significant root cause we investigate. These imbalances can stem from many of the factors we've discussed previously. For example, gut dysbiosis can lead to hormone dysregulation because certain neurotransmitters in the gut play a role in breaking down excess estrogen and in the production of hormones such as progesterone. If these processes are disrupted, patients may experience estrogen sensitivity or dominance. "Estrogen dominance" is a term accepted under the Functional Model as a relative excess of estrogen in relation to progesterone levels and is associated with several increased risks, including autoimmune disease.[25]

Thyroid imbalances are particularly important, even in cases where thyroid-stimulating hormone (TSH) levels are within normal limits. It's essential to check not only TSH but also T3, T4, and rT3 (reverse T3) levels to get a complete picture of thyroid health. We will go deeper into the significance of these values in our hormone discussion. Other hormonal issues we need to address involve the adrenal glands and sex hormones, as they can lead to fatigue, mood disturbances, menstrual irregularities, and weight gain. As noted, these conditions often relate to deeper underlying issues.[25]

Psychosocial and Spiritual Dysfunction

At the Academy of Functional Medicine and the Academy of Functional Medicine, we also focus on psychosocial and spiritual factors. We believe that true healing involves the mind, body, and spirit. If we ignore these aspects, we may not achieve lasting healing, and patients can face continual setbacks.

Emotional trauma, unresolved grief, lack of community, and disconnection from one's purpose can all have physical manifestations, such as headaches, insomnia, upset stomach, anxiety, irritability, decreased libido, elevated blood pressure, and even cognitive impairment.[26] So, it very much makes sense that if this stress stays in the body, we are more likely to develop chronic disease, as the damage continues, causing inflammation.[26]

Studies show that the happiest people often feel a sense of purpose in their lives, while those more prone to anxiety and depression frequently lack this sense of purpose, regardless of past traumas. Interestingly, individuals who transform their trauma into a meaningful message and serve a higher purpose can recover more significantly compared to those who feel aimless.

The concept of spiritual purpose aligns with the idea that serving others often contributes to our own healing. A lack of purpose and spiritual imbalance can lead to both mental and physical health issues. We also recognize that mental health can positively or negatively affect physical outcomes based on our mindset. For instance, simply thinking about stressful situations can increase cortisol and increase the risk for insulin resistance, potentially stemming from spiritual imbalance.[27]

Insulin Resistance and Decreased Muscular Mass

This is likely one of the most overlooked causes of dysfunction out there. There is a horrible misconception that you can replace healthy exercise and activity with a good diet. While a healthy diet is undoubtedly key, it does not negate how necessary exercise is in building muscle and decreasing insulin resistance.[28] Having a good amount of muscle mass is one of the leading indicators of longevity and health.

In the current health environment, this is especially important, as the trend with GLP-1 medications is taking the nation by storm. These medications are great at decreasing weight, but their use often results in sarcopenia, which is a loss of muscle mass. This negatively impacts overall health and leads to the deterioration of metabolic health, further increasing the person's long-term risk for chronic obesity. Without that muscle, the person's metabolism is wrecked. They gain weight back quickly and become hooked on the medication for life.[29,30]

This strongly demonstrates our bodies' need for lean, healthy muscle and how much we are harming ourselves by ignoring it. A noticeable decrease in muscle leads to an increased risk of falls, lower self-esteem, and various health complications, including a decrease in longevity.[28] Insufficient muscle mass can disrupt hormonal balance, metabolism, and cellular function. Therefore, physical activity is crucial for every health program. If someone is not physically active in their daily life, they should aim to include an average of at least eleven minutes of exercise each day, as their body allows.[28]

Chapter Conclusion

Our ultimate goal is to create sustainable, long-term health by aligning daily habits with healing. In the programs I teach in our board certification course for the Academy of Functional Medicine, we discuss "steps for life." It's important to help clients recognize that small, consistent changes over time can lead to significant improvements—this is what we refer to as the "slight edge."

If you're just a bit healthier than you were yesterday, you have more energy and feel better overall. This slight improvement in well-being can empower you to pursue greater health goals with even more strength and determination. This may come down to small, frequent exercises daily until the client can do a full workout.

Diet is also an undeniably important part in reducing insulin resistance. At times, when starting with someone who is on a completely processed diet, I might suggest a simple change: eat whole, healthy foods for one meal a day while allowing the other two meals to follow their usual choices. After a few weeks of this approach, I then recommend increasing it to two meals of whole foods. This method is one example of how I help people take gradual steps toward better health for long-term longevity, making it less likely that they ever feel like they've "fallen off the wagon."

Business Practice Pearl

Success leaves clues. There are patterns that all successful people have followed since the beginning of time; honestly, we would be naïve not to follow them as well. I have spent years studying the most well-known and successful self-made millionaires and billionaires, and from that, I discovered three pillars that all of them tapped into: fortitude, passive income, and leverage.

Let us start with fortitude. This pillar is essential to every business that I help others design for themselves. Fortitude includes knowing when to reach out to others who are steps ahead of you. At every step of the way, I help transform my students into the next-level entrepreneurs that they already know in their souls that they are. Throughout the book, I will share some of the mindset pearls I gave them with you, as you are currently a valued student of mine as well.

This mindset of fortitude is critical because if you are not investing in your mental stamina as a business owner, your odds of making it are nonexistent. The best way to cultivate this is to surround yourself with mentors who already have a strong sense of fortitude and business knowledge and are self-actualized. I say that with confidence because even the richest man in the world, King Solomon, had mentors. His first mentor was the Lord, and I advise you to keep God as your first mentor (above me or anyone else)—and as your first business partner as well.

The next was his father, David. In 1 Kings 3, we learn that Solomon learned from his father's guidance and would even gather together the elders in times of need. Having a business coach is essential. Even with my success, I still invest in coaches who are levels ahead of me to help me transform, growing in a few months more than some do in an entire lifetime. The higher I want to go, the more I spend, but I don't wait until I can afford it before going there.

I spent $18,000 on my first year of coaching. Then, months later, I spent $10,000 for a two-day conference just to get the knowledge I needed to go to the next level and be in the room with people who can afford such an event. But this was *not* a cost. Both were an *investment*. We are the average of the people we spend the most time with, so I paid to spend time with those ahead of me so that my future self would come sooner.

The more you learn, the more you know that time lost not earning money (the cost of inaction) is the most expensive cost you'll ever have. For example, right after that last investment, I had my first $20,000 day. If I hadn't gotten hold of that knowledge sooner, I wouldn't have had that day as quickly as I did, and that alone would have been my greatest loss, not to mention the ability to run that play over and over. I was initially nervous about those kinds of investments. But what I have learned is that the more you value time over money, the more your bank account grows.

You can do the same. I don't share to brag; I share to show you what is possible and the real shifts I had to make internally to get to my first seven-figure year. When you know that a four-minute mile has been run, you know it's possible, so you can do it, too. And this isn't just me; I have students like Jen or Dr. Charles, who both made their first $4,500 within weeks of learning and implementing this system.

Or take Aleiah, a health coach who earns two to three times what a medical doctor makes a month because her clients achieve incredible results without prescription medications. She implemented the full system without hesitation in spite of the fear of failure. Or consider Courtney, who, after investing in other systems that took her nowhere, made her first $2,000 within weeks with mine. Then there's Delisa, who made $17,500 in her opening week of clinic.

Those are just a few examples from the hundreds that I have taught this method to. However, for all of them and their clients, the cost of inaction would have been much greater had they not invested in their health and wealth. I am going to give you the same blueprint we all use here in these chapters.

All of my successful clients had a special attribute: they were coachable and action-based. Be coachable and *implement* what you are taught. Do not just spend time learning. Let me repeat that last part in case anyone missed it: Be coachable and implement. I have seen many people learn a system and then either partially implement it or do it in their own way, thinking it's the best approach. How many of those plans do you think have actually worked out for people? None. Not one.

You don't get to tweak a plan until you have mastered it. Once you have, you can tweak and trial different versions of the system for your niche or offer. Otherwise, you are guessing, which leads to stress and wasted time. Even when my coaches assigned me tasks that I didn't feel I had the time or skill to do, I completed them. I did this not only because it grew my capacity, but also because the other part of building a business is this: it's not what you think it is.

My coaches knew what I didn't yet know because I hadn't done it. It wasn't that I hadn't learned it; I hadn't done it yet. There is a huge difference. The real learning occurs in taking action, which is why I say to start before you're ready. You won't understand what you're doing until you have the *muscle memory* of doing it. Most of us have to spend some time figuring it out through trial and error, even when we have the blueprint. This means that there will be a time frame where the fruit from the labor takes time to grow (albeit a smaller time frame if you invest in a business coach).

If you wait until you are ready, you will get frustrated with the waiting and the small speed bumps that you could have already overcome if you had started sooner, so focus on action and impact rather than the details of getting started. That's why they say the best day to start was yesterday, but today is the next best option.

The other advantage to starting before you are ready is that you never know when a big break might happen, like a person reaching out to you for help or a podcast wanting to put you on their show. If you don't have a way to monetize that moment, you've lost a possibly once-in-a-lifetime opportunity.

Furthermore, business building is like swimming. It is a skill that you cannot master by reading a book. So, on top of that, find a coach who will inspire you and even push you to take action.

You can be the best provider out there, but if you don't know how to market yourself or get in front of people, you will never be able to help the masses. Business growth is a completely separate skill from practicing medicine or health coaching. And remember, even the richest man in the world had a business mentor. Don't make the mistake of assuming you are any different.

With our next Practice Pearl, we will dive into the next pillar. First, though, let's discuss functional medicine labs and optimal levels.

BONUS TRAINING:

"Finding your calling and implementing principles that took me from launching my business at $0/month to $100K months...

SCAN ME

...in just over three years."

SCAN THE QR CODE

or visit functionalmedicineunlocked.com

Chapter 2

Functional Labs Overview

In the functional medicine model, we do not simply evaluate lab results based on whether they are within the normal range; instead, we look for optimal levels. These optimal levels represent how the body should ideally operate and are often more stringent than conventional benchmarks.

When I first began exploring this approach, I found it challenging to accept because I had been conditioned to think in terms of different established ranges. In the diagram that follows, you will see a comparison between some of the most common conventional and functional medicine lab ranges.

Functional Versus Conventional Medicine Lab Values

Functional Versus Conventional Medicine Lab Values

Lab Marker	Conventional Range	Functional (Optimal) Range	Why It Matters
TSH	0.4 - 4.5 µIU/mL	0.5 - 2.0 µIU/mL	High-normal TSH often indicates early thyroid dysfunction (especially in fatigue, weight gain).
Free T3	2.0 - 4.4 pg/mL	3.2 - 4.2 pg/mL	T3 is the active thyroid hormone; low-normal = low metabolism and poor energy.
Free T4	0.8 - 1.8 ng/dL	1.2 - 1.4 ng/dL	Even with "normal" TSH, low free T4 can indicate subclinical hypothyroidism.
Reverse T3	8 - 25 ng/dL	< 15 ng/dL	High levels block active T3—often an indication of stress, illness, or inflammation.
Ferritin (Women)	12 - 150 ng/mL	50 - 100 ng/mL	Iron stores below 50 often cause fatigue, hair loss, and cold intolerance—even if "normal."
Vitamin D (25-OH)	30 - 100 nmol/L	50 - 150 nmol/L	Below 50 is suboptimal for immune, thyroid, and mental health function.
B12	200 - 900 pg/mL	600 - 1000 pg/mL	Low-normal levels can cause fatigue, brain fog, and neuropathy.
Fasting Insulin	2.6 - 24.9 µIU/mL	2 - 5 µIU/mL	Higher levels indicate insulin resistance—even if glucose looks okay.
Fasting Glucose	65 - 99 mg/dL	65 - 85 mg/dL	Higher-normal glucose often precedes metabolic dysfunction.
Hemoglobin A1C	< 5.7%	4.8 - 5.2%	Optimal range prevents glycation and long-term inflammation.
CRP (hs-CRP)	0 - 3.0 mg/L	< 1.0 mg/L	Low-grade inflammation is a silent driver of chronic illness.
Homocysteine	0 - 15 µmol/L	6 - 8 µmol/L	Elevated levels increase cardiovascular and neurodegenerative risk.
DHEA-S (Women, age 30-50)	35 - 430 µg/dL	150 - 250 µg/dL	Supports mood, hormone balance, and stress resilience.
Estradiol (Women)	15 - 350 pg/mL (varies)	50 - 150 pg/mL (depending on cycle phase)	Functional range supports hormone balance without excess.
Testosterone (Total, Women)	15 - 70 ng/dL	35 - 55 ng/dL	Low-normal levels = fatigue, low libido, muscle loss. Some providers will keep levels higher than this. I do recommend advanced HRT training if supplementing testosterone in women.
Cortisol (AM Serum)	5 - 25 µg/dL	13 - 17 µg/dL	Optimal morning cortisol is critical for energy, mood, and inflammation control.

***These levels may vary from lab to lab or provider to provider.*

Vitamin D

Another important optimal level for obtaining health is maintaining vitamin D levels above 50 ng/mL. Vitamin D levels even impact seemingly unrelated disease processes. For example, normal levels have been associated with a reduced risk of breast cancer in women. Furthermore, a healthy level of vitamin D during infancy can decrease the lifelong risk of developing type 1 diabetes. Vitamin D receptors in the gut also play a significant role in inflammatory bowel disease and chronic disease in general.[31,32]

By focusing on these optimal levels and guiding patients toward them, I noticed significant improvements in their well-being. Many patients would express feeling unwell even when their lab results were within normal range. Once I adopted a functional perspective and considered optimal ranges, they experienced dramatic improvements.

The key distinction in this approach is that conventional lab ranges are based on a sick population and statistical averages; they do not reflect the health of people who feel great. In contrast, functional ranges are derived from what is optimal for health, energy, and prevention—essentially enabling not just survival, but genuine thriving.

Labs Specific to Functional Medicine

When I started ordering functional medicine labs, I felt uncertain about whether it was evidence-based to do so, as I had never been taught that this was an option for my patients in my conventional training (I wonder why not). However, after years of application and thousands of hours of reading peer-reviewed journals and other clinicians' patient outcomes, in addition to my own patients' results, I have come to realize that these tests provide valuable and empowering information, allowing patients to achieve healing at levels that exceed the possibilities within conventional medicine.

Functional medicine labs are specifically designed to uncover underlying imbalances and root causes of symptoms, rather than simply ruling out diseases. They assess how the body functions across interconnected systems, such as digestion, detoxification, hormones, metabolism, immune response, and environmental exposure. This approach facilitates a truly personalized system of healing.

Examples of functional labs that are not even found in conventional labs include comprehensive stool analysis (different from a regular stool analysis, with attention focused on identification of dysbiosis in the microbiome), organic acids test (urine sample to determine underlying imbalances), zonulin (for determining increased intestinal permeability), DUTCH test (for in-depth hormonal insights), and nutritional evaluation or food sensitivity.

While we will go into the use of each of these tests in this text, it must be noted that our full board certification spends hours discussing them, providing in-depth training that is best done with visuals and didactics. However, I mention them here so you can get a broad understanding of how we ascertain the information we do and the science that backs up the protocols.[33]

One important lesson I share with my clients and students is that in the conventional medical model, we often analyze health by breaking it down into specific systems. For instance, an endocrinologist may focus solely on TSH levels or A1c and insulin, while a rheumatologist looks primarily at CRP or RH factor, and a cardiologist assesses LDL cholesterol levels.

However, we must remember something fundamental that we were all taught as kiddos: "The foot bone's connected to the leg bone, and the leg bone's connected to the hip bone..." So on and so forth. The point is that our bodies are not made of isolated systems; they form an intricate network of interconnected systems. The same blood that nourishes the foot also supplies the gut, and the same nervous system serving the gut also innervates the brain. These systems are intertwined, so they influence one another.

Therefore, it makes sense to investigate labs that reveal root causes and how these interconnected systems interact. One of the first such tests was the comprehensive stool analysis.

Comprehensive Stool Analysis

One of the most common brands of these is the GI MAP, or the GI Effects test. This is a stool sample test. My choice between brands or options depends on the specific needs of the client, the cost of the tests, and what I aim to target for them specifically. You can compare them and see the intricate differences.

In general, we conduct these tests to assess for gastrointestinal disruptions, such as gas, bloating, indigestion, irritable bowel syndrome (IBS), constipation, or diarrhea. However, as you will learn going forward, gut dysbiosis is also a root cause for many diseases, such as autoimmune disease, neurological diseases, as well as hormonal imbalances and mood disorders, so this test tends to be a significant part of those treatment plans as well.

We are assessing for pathogens, such as parasites, *H. pylori*, and yeast, as well as commensal bacterial overgrowth. Commensal bacteria is healthy in the right amount, but it can cause illness in the presence of overgrowth or depletion. I also want to note that some of my patients have had normal stool analyses from conventional testing sites, despite showing an overgrowth of pathogens on the GI map. These patients benefited greatly from functional intervention despite "normal" conventional stool testing. Therefore, I know from experience that there is a need for more in-depth analysis than what conventional medicine has incorporated.

For instance, a patient may not have overt diarrhea when suffering from a chronic infection of *Clostridium difficile*. When I test for *H. pylori* or *C. diff* under conventional labs, the results will come back negative, while a GI map may reveal underlying overgrowth. That being said, if the client has a severe onset of abdominal pain or blood or mucus in the stool, signaling an acute infection, you need to refer to conventional intervention with antibiotics and possibly even emergency intervention.

The GI map has a much higher sensitivity for detecting the organisms we are trying to find by using quantitative PCR analysis and not simply culture.[34] In this regard, a low-grade, chronic infection can disrupt the body even if it doesn't show up in standard lab tests or present as a severe, acute infection.

We're also examining microbiome diversity. While we need certain beneficial bacteria, like lactobacilli, an overgrowth of these can be detrimental. Therefore, we're not just looking for their presence, but also their quantity. These are the commensal bacteria. I like to describe them as the Goldilocks bacteria because you don't want too much or not enough. You want their levels to be "just right."

We assess inflammation in the gut as well, focusing on zonulin, which helps us determine if a person has an increased intestinal permeability. When you order your test, you can choose whether to include zonulin; it is optional, but it is always beneficial to add it for clarity in understanding the level of intestinal healing that needs to be taken on and if it may be contributing to symptoms.

Another important marker in the analysis is secretory IgA (sIgA), which helps us monitor overall immune response, or the lack thereof. This assessment is crucial for understanding gut integrity, immune function, and microbiome health, as well as how well the gut protects the rest of the body. These factors are significant for conditions such as autoimmunity, IBS, skin issues, fatigue, food sensitivities, and mood disorders.

Low sIgA can indicate a weakened mucosal immunity, possibly due to an immune system that has been overwhelmed for an extended period of time. Other potential causes for low sIgA can be zinc or vitamin A deficiency, chronic stress, or genetic factors.[35] Low sIgA increases a person's risk for other infections and worsens the body's ability to cope with what is going on.

Elevated levels indicate an elevation in the immune response from the mucosal immunity of the digestive tract that could be from autoimmune disease, gut dysbiosis or infection, inflammatory conditions such as celiac disease and Crohn's disease, or chronic infections, whether viral or bacterial. This testing is most often done via stool analysis, but salivary analysis is another option.[35] The root cause must be evaluated based on thorough patient analysis and root cause intervention.

Organic Acid Test

Another commonly ordered Functional test is the organic acids test, which gives a comprehensive evaluation of metabolic functioning, gut health, cellular health, neurotransmitter balance, and detoxification pathways, as well as a secondary check for yeast and fungal overgrowth. It is a urine sample. While some results from the GI map and the organic acids test overlap, I often order both tests. This approach provides confirmation when both tests yield similar results and strengthens our understanding of the findings.

The organic acids test (OATs) goes deeper, exploring neurotransmitter metabolites, mitochondrial function, oxalate metabolites, glycolytic cycle function in the Krebs cycle, intestinal microbial overgrowth, amino acid metabolites, detoxification functioning, and metabolism.[36] For example, we can understand at a deeper level how and why bacterial overgrowth may be leading to imbalances in neurotransmitters that affect the body and mind. If you have advanced training in it, like in our course, you can also leverage it to see windows into possible genetic polymorphisms.

DUTCH Test

Next is the DUTCH hormone test. This is also a urine test, and it assesses levels of estrogens, progesterone, testosterone, DHEA, cortisol rhythms, and other hormone metabolites. It helps identify not only hormone levels but also how your body metabolizes those hormones.

It's important for those who may be suffering from PMS, perimenopause, PCOS, fatigue, low libido, or stress-related symptoms to recognize that stress can significantly impact our hormones. While we will delve into some of this information in the hormone chapter, there is always more to consider.

Nutrition Testing

Another commonly ordered test is nutrient testing, such as NutrEval or SpectraCell. These tests provide deeper insights, particularly if there are concerns about vitamin deficiencies. They evaluate and analyze over 125 biomarkers for an in-depth analysis of the body's nutritional status.[33]

PRO TIP:

I recommend that if someone has gut dysbiosis, IBS, or any gut symptoms, it's not always advisable to jump straight into nutrient or hormonal testing. Correcting gut health often improves the body's ability to regulate hormonal imbalances and absorb nutrients, which will alter both statuses. While nutrient testing is useful, it may not always be the first step to take, especially when the root causes of conditions like hair loss, immune dysfunction, anxiety, depression, or chronic illness have not been identified—factors all of which can be significantly influenced by nutrient status.

Mycotoxin and Home Toxin Testing

Environmental toxins and mycotoxin panels can be a key tool in discovering the root cause of a disease, though they are, at times, scrutinized because we are all exposed to mold at various points in our lives, whether from buildings or foods such as dried cranberries or nuts. The debate continues over the level of exposure necessary to cause stress in the body, and people differ in their ability to naturally detoxify once exposure is removed. It's essential to approach this from the perspective of allostatic stress load, as some people may have a smaller genetic tolerance than others [37]

For instance, I previously shared a case about a patient who had a smaller genetic capacity compared to her colleagues, who did not display any symptoms. In her case, a clinical evaluation was necessary rather than solely relying on test results. There have also been cases where patients were convinced mold was the problem, only for their tests to come back entirely negative for exposure. At any rate, we can test for mold exposure to the body in blood work, as well as environmental testing in the air.

Heavy Metal Testing

When testing for heavy metals, the literature can sometimes be confusing. However, hair testing is generally more specific for those with suspected chronic exposure, like tobacco users, those who vape, or those with a profession that increases exposure, such as car mechanics or manufacturing workers. Blood work tends to be better suited for discovering a recent acute exposure.[38]

Additionally, volatile organic compounds (VOCs) can be found in items such as paint or candles, and children may be exposed to them from a young age. Testing for these compounds in the home air is crucial because they can contribute to environmental overload that disrupts hormones, immunity, and mitochondrial functions.[39]

These types of tests are particularly important for those experiencing recurrent unexplained illnesses, cognitive decline, fatigue, or autoimmune flares. The advanced thyroid panel test is commonly used in functional medicine, although it is also available in conventional practices.

Full Thyroid Panel

As previously mentioned, this panel includes TSH, free and total T3 (free triiodothyronine), free and total T4 (free thyroxine), reverse T3, and TPO Ab (thyroid peroxidase antibodies). It plays a crucial role in identifying both overt and subclinical thyroid dysfunction, as well as autoimmune thyroid diseases. An almost non-negotiable lab test that should be part of the thyroid panel is vitamin D, given the strong association between low levels and the development of autoimmune Hashimoto's.[40]

Specifically, TPO antibody levels may indicate autoimmune thyroid conditions. Thyroid dysfunction can manifest in various symptoms, with the most common being fatigue, hair loss, unexplained weight changes (both loss and gain), constipation, and brain fog. These are often the symptoms that lead people to suspect an imbalance in their thyroid function.

When conducting a full thyroid panel, you might discover that a person is producing sufficient T4 but not converting it into T3, or they may not be producing enough T4 in the first place. Another condition may be that the cells of the body are too inflamed to utilize the T3, in which case thyroid disease can be reversed or improved just by getting rid of the root causes of inflammation, such as toxic exposure or gut dysbiosis.[41]

Food Sensitivity Testing

Another set of tests to consider is food sensitivity testing, which includes IgG, IgA, and even IgE panels for acute reaction risk. The IgG panels specifically assess delayed immune responses to foods, chemicals, and food additives. IgE (or Type I) is more widely done in conventional models and is an immediate response, which can include severe reactions. These reactions include mast cell activation and are histamine-driven. They are immediate, within 2 hours, and range from hives to swelling of the throat, wheezing, or even anaphylaxis.

IgG is delayed and may include symptoms of bloating, fatigue, headaches, joint pain, brain fog, skin issues, and upset stomach.[42] Despite some controversy, most practitioners find this type of testing to be valuable because it can reveal triggers that standard IgE tests cannot identify. IgA is also delayed and includes gastrointestinal symptoms such as gas, bloating, diarrhea, but also sinus congestion. A chronic runny nose in children is very often a reaction to milk. Testing for IgA can be done with stool or blood.

However, it's important to note that food sensitivity tests can have low specificity and sensitivity; that is, there can be false positives and false negatives, respectively. Therefore, always relate and correlate these tests to the individual's unique situation, especially if there is significant uncertainty regarding food-related triggers. For instance, if someone is experiencing eczema and suspects it may be linked to food, the testing can offer a starting point for identifying potential culprits. From there, you can proceed by gradually reintroducing foods that show a lower reaction rate and monitor how the patient responds.

Remember, food sensitivity testing is not an absolute diagnosis; rather, it serves as a helpful indicator. I also often check for gluten sensitivity (different from celiac disease) as well, especially in people with autoimmune diseases or chronic digestive issues like diarrhea or constipation. Gluten sensitivity testing is more accurate.

Foods high in histamine, such as asparagus, avocado, and wine, may trigger symptoms of itching and flushing in those who are sensitive. DAO (diamine oxidase) genetic testing can help determine if patients effectively break down histamine.[43] In susceptible individuals, the DAO enzyme that helps break down histamine in the body is deficient. This deficiency leads to a buildup of histamine to trigger symptoms that are associated with histamine intolerance, such as flushing of the skin or easily breaking out into hives. If gut issues are not addressed, some individuals can react that would not react otherwise if clearance is an issue of digestion instead of genetics.

When considering the root cause, it is also important to note that when a disease has been able to progress for a long time, the state of inflammation and dysregulation associated with the root cause may pave the way for further issues. Someone who is autoimmune, for example, might not get instantaneously better just by removing gluten from their diet; that does not mean it was not a piece of or even the root cause from the beginning. After years of exposure, mitochondrial stores become depleted, and dysbiosis ensues, and you may have more than one thing to correct by the time the patient gets to you.[44] Sometimes, you have to correct all aspects before the patient starts seeing real results. Not always, but occasionally. It is also important for your patients to understand that healing the root cause is not as instantaneous as symptomatic treatment, but it will often result in more powerful results.

Homocysteine

Homocysteine testing is especially significant, as it's a crucial marker for methylation status and the presence of long-term inflammation. In conventional medicine, practitioners are taught that high homocysteine levels correlate with increased cardiovascular risk and cognitive decline. However, they are not often taught how to correct it or that elevated homocysteine can result from a lack of vitamin B and folate methylation, which impairs the body's ability to use the nutrients properly. Addressing the MTHFR polymorphism that causes this is vital for preventing heart disease, chronic inflammation, dementia risk, blood sugar instability, and metabolic syndrome.[45]

Autoimmune and Inflammatory Testing

Another group of tests to consider includes autoimmune and immune system assessments, many of which are also used in conventional medicine. Tests like ANA assess chronic inflammation, while rheumatoid factor, HLA-B27, and anti-CCP help evaluate autoimmune conditions. Cytokine panels and secretory IgA tests, conducted via stool or saliva, are also useful for assessing gut health.[46] Low or high levels of sIgA can indicate chronic infections, stress, or immune dysfunction, making this data crucial for individuals suspected of having autoimmune diseases or chronic conditions, such as increased intestinal permeability.

One practical tip from my experience is that many clients appear to have autoimmune issues despite negative results on tests like rheumatoid factor, ANA, or CRP. Often, these markers can be nonspecific, showing no reactivity until the disease has progressed significantly, so it's essential to pay attention to the patient's concerns. If they feel something is still off, it's worth investigating further.

Insulin and Glucose Testing

Lastly, important testing for blood sugar and insulin panels should not be overlooked. These tests typically evaluate fasting glucose, fasting insulin, and hemoglobin A1c, which provides an average of glucose levels over the past ninety days.

Another great indicator for early disease may be using a fasting insulin level (with a goal of < 6) and an insulin-to-glucose ratio < 0.3. Both of these are more specific indicators for early disease and allow for a wider window of opportunity for intervention for insulin resistance and chronic illness.[47]

C-peptide is a valuable marker for identifying insulin resistance or metabolic stress even before a diabetes diagnosis. It is released from the pancreas at the same time as insulin and is therefore a great indicator of resistance with elevated levels.[48] This is particularly important in cases of polycystic ovarian syndrome (PCOS), weight gain, energy crashes, sugar cravings, and hormone imbalances.

If a patient reports consistent hunger that seems insatiable, it's important to consider the possibility of insulin resistance. Checking the insulin-to-glucose ratio is crucial.

I have a personal experience that relates to this. While in my twenties, I experienced hirsutism, which is excessive hair growth, particularly on my arms. Despite being in a healthy weight range, I consumed a lot of sugar from a young age and developed insulin resistance early on, even though I wasn't overweight. The point I am trying to make in sharing this is that one cannot always determine insulin resistance just by looking at a client's weight. This issue was uncovered through the ratio of my insulin to glucose levels.

Genetic Testing

There are several genetic tests you can implement, but we will briefly review the two most common, just to increase your awareness, and then dive deeper into them as they apply to patient care.

MTHFR stands for methylenetetrahydrofolate reductase. It screens for polymorphisms that alter the patient's ability to convert B12 into its active methylated form. This deficiency hinders the regulation of B12 and can result in a lack of other cofactors needed for producing serotonin, dopamine, and methionine, which serve as anti-inflammatory markers in the body. Typically, homocysteine should be converted into methionine, but this process can be disrupted. We will delve further into this in Chapter 5.

COMT, which stands for catechol-O-methyltransferase, is another common genetic test. When there is a deformity in this gene, the enzyme that is essential for the breakdown of catecholamines, like dopamine, norepinephrine, and epinephrine, does not work as it should. This causes issues in mental health, pain perception, and impaired cognitive functioning, such as seen in autism. We will discuss this further at a later time, but just know that it is another polymorphism that can greatly benefit from nutritional replacement.

Chapter Conclusion

Hundreds of tests can be performed. The purpose of this chapter is not to go over every possible test, but to explain some of the more vital testing under the Functional Model. Please also remember that not all tests are necessary and are often an expense for clients. A good patient history determines the root cause being searched for. Also, if you are not a prescriber, there are options for you to partner with labs that allow testing to be ordered under an attending physician. We give guidance for this in our board certification course, as well as how to avoid practicing outside the scope of practice for those who are not prescribers.

Business Practice Pearl

The next pillar of a successful functional business is having a passive element. This is how to design a business so that it works for you, rather than you working for it. Every practitioner should have a level of passive income in their practice. One of the biggest mistakes I see clinicians make is starting their own practice with a ton of overhead (mortgage or rent, employees, lab equipment, etc.) but no income coming in yet, thinking this is freedom. Talk about stress. It's not less stressful just because you are working for yourself. It's actually the opposite when you have a ton of overhead. So, before you take on a mortgage or even buy a practice with a current clientele, have a way to generate passive income to cover when (or if) things don't go as planned. If you don't, you'll likely find yourself back on the job hunt.

The reason this is true is that none of us (even the richest people in the world) have more than twenty-four hours a day. We do not have enough hours in the day to keep trading time for money and get ahead without hitting burnout.

Also, I want you to know that whether you have a formal education or not, passive income in functional medicine is not above you. Consider this: even millionaires who are formally educated don't often use their degree to build their real wealth. They don't use their degree as a source of income, at least not in terms of getting a JOB (just over broke) or becoming wealthy. They use their drive, background, and experience to go to the next level, which is being a communicator, where they earn one-to-many.

Communicators teach, inspire, lead, and change lives, going one-to-many. They are highly paid for their skills because their work has a significant impact. Your impact is no less. These are the top 3–4% of the most successful people in our society. Even a neurosurgeon cannot beat this outcome because they can only perform surgery on one brain at a time. Communicators have one product or message that they build once and sell repeatedly to many at the same time. If you are only selling your time as a provider, you cannot go one-to-many because you can only book so many appointments in a day.

If you have a degree, that is a great start; you just are not done with your journey if you want to reach financial freedom, which is actually just time freedom, not being tied to trading dollars for days. You only need to take one more step: turn that medical mind into a gold mine, start helping the masses, and become a communicator. I consider this to be essential for every practitioner with a calling for large impact.

Many of my students become "communicators" in functional medicine by implementing passive clinics. This can come in the form of speaking opportunities, subscriptions, communities, or courses being sold passively, and it doesn't only benefit them. Some charge for supplements and get paid when a patient purchases the supplements, which is largely passive. I personally do not do this because I do not want to be incentivized, or accused of being incentivized, to keep anyone on a supplement for income and not what is in the patient's best interest.

My goal is to heal and not keep them on a supplement for life. However, many clinicians do implement this strategy with great success, and one could argue that it allows them to pull down their overall charges to clients, benefiting the patients. So, I am not saying you should remove that from your plan as I have; just be cautious and stay true to healing, not dealing.

This plan of one-to-many does not only benefit the provider. As a matter of fact, research shows that patients only retain about 10–20% of what they hear during appointments. By offering them recorded videos or course materials, they can revisit the information at their convenience, reducing the need for them to repeatedly say, "I'm so sorry, I forgot that!" It's not their fault; it's just human nature. They gain more, and you don't waste your time repeating the same things you have for years.

You also get to sell one thing, sometimes with great value, for the cost of less than one appointment or a month of health insurance (that doesn't pay out when you need it), but when it is passive (like with paid traffic or using search bars on the internet), you earn a large income without having to charge each person a lot.

For example, you can build a course once and sell it over and over for years, saving lives every year you provide it. Let's say this course is a "mid ticket," meaning the cost is $500 to $2,500. You may only need to sell a few a month to make a great income, with each one taking only a few minutes or hours of your time a month (after it is built), versus working forty hours a week for a salary. In the next chapter, I will show you how you can make thousands on even small tickets with my favorite tool: leverage, which is the third and final pillar of every successful business.

BONUS TRAINING:

The Power of Passive Income & Leverage.

SCAN ME

SCAN THE QR CODE

or visit functionalmedicineunlocked.com

Chapter 3

Food and Environmental Toxicity

CASE STUDY: ADHD and Children

Twelve-year-old boy with failing grades and a history of multiple notes from school on his hyperactivity. Parents report he seems wound up as if he is being driven by a motor most of the time when he is not medicated with Adderall. Parents recently learned of the potential cardiac side effects and that his weight being in the 60th percentile may be correlated and became concerned. They would like to try stopping medication while on summer break and treat more naturally. Patient denies abdominal pain, bloating, heart palpitations, or aversion to eating, though appetite was not great. Intervention included stopping all food dyes and high fructose corn syrup, cognitive behavioral intervention, reading and focus training, Patient returned to school 2 months later, was off medications, and performed well in school without teacher concerns for hyperactivity. Parents reported the patient felt like a new child.

Discussion

There are numerous cases of children alleviating their ADHD symptoms, resulting in dramatic improvements in both school performance and family functioning, simply by removing red dyes from their diets. While intervention tends to be much more complicated, there are scenarios such as the above case study that highlight the toxic effects of "edible" chemicals. Such experiences serves as an incredible demonstration of how badly the "generally recognized as safe" (GRAS) initiative is severely lacking. Thankfully, legislation is now being put in place to remove these harmful dyes and other chemicals from our food. However, let us not forget the past so that we do not allow it to repeat. Understanding where we came from is crucial as we look toward the future, especially when it comes to the need to be critical thinkers moving forward in a world corrupt with big industry ruling large sectors of our economy.

When I refer to food dyes, I'm talking about all artificially made dyes in food. Their effects on children were often overlooked or pushed aside for decades, leading to an epidemic of childhood diseases, including hyperactivity, impulsivity, and oppositional defiance.[49] The dyes include Blue 1 and 2, Green 3, Red 40, and a slew of others. The dosage correlates with symptom severity, but the amount is not reported in foods, which are often advertised directly to children.

Lastly, removing some of these chemicals from our diet doesn't mean they'll be replaced with something healthier. To my knowledge, there has not been a significant change in how chemicals can be initially used, and I would remain cautious of how loopholes might be exploited.

Edible Toxins

Let's discuss what I refer to as "edible toxins." It's important to note that from the very beginning, babies are already exposed to a plethora of chemicals. As you may recall, more than 90% of maternal and cord blood samples from deliveries contain what we call "forever toxins," meaning that our bodies can't easily detoxify from them.[50] This highlights the importance of eliminating current toxic overloads that we can control and explains why people are getting sicker and sicker at a younger age, as we are being exposed at an alarmingly increased rate to these toxins, even before birth.

The modern food supply contains over ten thousand chemicals, including preservatives, artificial colors, endocrine disruptors, plastics, phthalates, and synthetic sweeteners. The Environmental Working Group (EWG) is an excellent resource that identifies several top offenders found in our food and water supply, such as BHA, BHT, propyl gallate, and titanium dioxide, the latter of which has been linked to an increased risk of cancer and is often found in candies marketed to children.[51]

While federal regulations are removing some of these chemicals from the food supply, it's important to remember that when one is removed, manufacturers often find another chemical to take its place. We need to remain cautious because they don't always need to list additives as ingredients if they're sprayed onto packaging. For instance, BHT, a preservative, can be sprayed on cereal bags. Since it isn't directly added to the food, it may not be listed as an ingredient, which means you might not even know it's there.

It's essential to use critical thinking when evaluating whether products contain harmful chemicals. Take, for example, pre-popped bags of popcorn. They tend to stay fresh longer than popcorn popped on the stove (which typically goes stale within a day) despite not always having preservatives listed in the ingredients. This difference could indicate the presence of preservatives that have been added in covert ways.

We will discuss functional medicine protocols for environmental detoxification and focus on proper dietary choices, supplementation, and lifestyle adjustments to reduce toxic burden and assist clients in detoxifying.

Sodium Benzoate

One of the next chemicals to discuss is sodium benzoate, a preservative commonly used in foods and pharmaceuticals to prevent the growth of bacteria, yeast, and fungi. Sodium benzoate is prevalent in a majority of chemically processed foods.[52] Toxicity in excessive doses is known to cause abdominal pain, CNS depression, nausea, and vomiting.[52] When mixed with ascorbic acid (vitamin C), it forms benzene, which is a carcinogen. While commercial drinks claim not to contain levels known to induce disease, caution is still advisable. People with liver disease or those who eat a diet high in preserved foods may reach toxicity more quickly, and long-term data is not yet available to evaluate the safety of microdosing over extended periods of time.

This substance also significantly decreases levels of brain-derived neurotrophic factor (BDNF) and alters levels of protein kinase A (PKA) in the prefrontal cortex of mice, which suggests potential effects on humans as well.

Brominated Vegetable Oil (BVO)

BVO has been used in lemon-lime, citrus, and fruit-flavored drinks to stabilize the flavor for years. This chemical was recently removed from drinks in September of 2025. However, it's important to note its history and the resistance from organizations meant to protect us. Furthermore, current patients may still have a significant history of exposure, and therefore screening for past exposure is still significant to practice.

BVO was first used in the 1920s, and it was classified as a "generally recognized as safe" (GRAS) food additive in the late 1950s. It was revoked from the GRAS list in 1970, but its use continued by arguing there was not sufficient data to declare it unsafe. On July 3, 2024, the FDA banned its use in commercial food, and companies had about one year to change their formulary.

Recent studies found an increase in TSH in mice after just ninety days of consumption. This was dose-responsive, indicating significant thyroid toxicity,[54] which may explain why hypothyroidism is one of the most common diseases in our time. This is especially concerning now that BVO is not easily removed from the body and can cause other symptoms, such as chronic headaches, fatigue, and even loss of muscle coordination and memory.[55]

This is particularly concerning when we recognize that many children have been encouraged to drink sodas like Sprite or 7-Up because they are perceived to be a healthier alternative, as they are caffeine-free. People think they are making smarter choices, but in fact, they are ingesting chemicals now known to be toxic, such as brominated vegetable oil. This serves as another example of how we cannot simply assume that because something is allowed, it is healthy or even safe. The goal of big companies like this is sales over service, and we must not let our guard down or become complacent.

Nitrates and Nitrites

Research has shown that certain additives can increase cancer risk. Consequently, they have not been approved for use in several countries for years. For example, nitrates and nitrites, commonly found in American processed meats, like sandwich meats and hot dogs, are known to increase cancer risk. Consuming just two servings a week can raise the risk of colon cancer in adults and leukemia in children, making it comparable to the risk of lung cancer for smokers.[56] Other studies have found a decrease in sperm count and testicular toxicity.[55]

Xenoestrogens

Xenoestrogens, which include substances like BPA, propylparaben, phthalates, plastics, and pesticides, bind to estrogen and testosterone receptors in the body. They are found in lotions, plastics, cosmetics, and other personal care products. Their name is derived from their ability to mimic true estrogen in the body. Xenoestrogens have been linked to increased risk of breast cancer, leiomyomas, endometriosis, and reproductive tumors in women.[57] They are also linked to higher rates of testicular cancer and decreased sperm mobility in men.[58]

This interference can block normal hormone function. For instance, exposure to xenoestrogens can lead to gynecomastia in men, characterized by an increase in breast tissue, and hormonal imbalances in women. Additionally, xenoestrogens are linked to stubborn weight loss issues and elevated levels of sex hormone binding globulin (SHBG).[59]

They do this by binding to endogenous sex hormones (both estrogen and testosterone), driving up the SHBG and decreasing its ability to bind and transport actual hormones in the body. When someone has high SHBG, their testosterone levels may drop, resulting in mood swings, decreased libido, and low energy levels because of the increased levels of unbound (labeled "free" in labs) hormones in the body. Both progesterone and estrogen also play crucial roles in supporting dopamine and serotonin, which are vital for overall mental health.

Propylparaben, a preservative often found in foods such as store-bought corn tortillas, is another xenoestrogen. This substance is an endocrine disruptor linked to early puberty in girls, weight gain, and difficulty losing weight. It is associated with an increased risk of breast cancer and estrogen-dominant cancers due to its xenoestrogen properties, which disrupt hormonal balance similar to excess estrogen.[59]

Xenoestrogens are able to act as if they are estrogens in the body, modulating the direct effects of estrogen and androgen (testosterone) receptors. Propylparaben may also cause developmental issues in children and reproductive health complications, as well as potential allergic reactions.[60]

Bisphenols (BPAs) and phthalates are used in food packaging, but they can also be present in topical applications, like lotions and creams. These chemicals may not always be listed as ingredients, as they are part of epoxy and plastic resins. Nevertheless, they are associated with serious health conditions, including pregnancy-induced hypertension (known as preeclampsia), liver damage, elevated levels of lipids, such as total cholesterol and LDL, and an increased risk of thyroid disease due to endocrine disruption.[61]

Moreover, exposure to these substances can lead to decreased antibiotic resistance and a lower response to vaccines.[62] In several other studies, maternal exposure during pregnancy was found to lower the lung capacity of infants.[63,64]

Perfluoroalkyl and Polyfluoroalkyl Substances (PFASs)

These are some of the "forever chemicals" that the body is not able to break down or detoxify easily, if ever. They are included in several cosmetic and cookware products and are often found in water sources, which is one reason why a double-osmosis water filtration device is essential to almost all detox strategies.

The contamination in our soil raises concern for the human consumption of root and leafy vegetables, as well as our meat and egg supply. While some of this is avoidable and some is not, it is important to be aware and avoid exposure as best as we can and realize that it is the overall toxic load of all chemicals that makes a big difference in our health.

PFASs are found in drinking water, foods, non-stick cookware, clothing, stain-resistant carpet and upholstery, food packages, and even cosmetics. They can harm the immune system and fetal development, potentially increasing cancer risk and the potential for causing gender-based physiological differences, as they are easily accumulated in fetal tissues and suspected of having developmental impacts.

These substances may also be sprayed onto packaging, affecting the food without being added as ingredients, thereby impacting our health.[65] Other risks include the development of NAFLD, or non-alcoholic fatty liver disease,[66] elevated cholesterol levels, and increased risk for thyroid disease.[67]

PFASs are a risk to our health because they alter our ability to produce antibodies, making it harder to fight infections. The decrease in immune regulation also increases the risk for cancer, which is why they are identified as potential carcinogens. PFASs are also associated with hormonal disruption, including the reproductive system and thyroid gland. Children are especially at risk, particularly those still in the womb, as it has been associated with increased risk for birth defects and learning and behavioral issues.[68]

Teflon is a very common, though easy to avoid, PFAS found in microwave popcorn to prevent the popcorn from sticking to the bag, cookware, cosmetics, hairstyling tools, couches, and cookware. The chemical is known to cause "Teflon flu," which presents as flu-like symptoms of body aches, coughing, sore throat, and even dyspnea, typically within a few hours of exposure and lasting one to two days with high exposure or in those with significant sensitivity.[69]

BHA, BHT, and TBHQ

BHA (butylated hydroxyl anisole), BHT (butylated hydroxytoluene), and TBHQ (tertiary butylhydroquinone) are preservatives widely used in the food industry that can increase cancer risk and alter immune function. While they are marketed as "antioxidant preservatives," their negative health impacts are well-documented. TBHQ is particularly common in processed meats and is also found in cereals to prolong shelf life.

These chemicals inhibit the oxidation of fats and oils, preserving the color, fragrance, and taste of baked foods. These effects alter cell signaling in the body and put us at increased risk for chronic inflammation, organ damage, and neurodegenerative diseases.[70] They are hepatotoxic (liver toxicity), nephrotoxic (kidney toxicity), and neurotoxic (toxic to our nervous system) in humans, and they can enhance the development of NAFLD.

Food Dyes

Food dyes and colors have been linked to an increase in ADHD symptoms in both children and adults. They are neurotoxic and can cause behavioral problems beyond ADHD, such as defiant behavior. Commonly studied dyes, like Red 3, Red 40, Yellow 5, Yellow 6, Blue 1, Blue 2, and Green 3, are often used in candies marketed to children. These products are strategically placed at checkout counters, where children are likely to ask for them while the parent is under stress from an hour or more of shopping, are more likely to give in, and they themselves may want a quick sugary "dopamine hit." They can also be found in baked goods, snacks, cereals, and sodas.

While these products have been advertised to children for decades, Red 3 has been proven to cause cancer in animals, and Red 40, Yellow 5, and Yellow 6 are known to be contaminated by the carcinogen benzidine and/or other carcinogens. Yellow 3, specifically, has been found to be genotoxic, causing damage to DNA.[71] On a personal level, I believe it should be a federal crime to knowingly advertise products with these substances to children. Thankfully, attention has recently been raised on their danger, and many companies are switching out the use of these dyes, although we cannot be certain if the alternative they choose will be any safer.

Titanium Dioxide

Titanium dioxide, used as a colorant in candies, ready-to-eat baked goods, and ice creams, has been part of our food supply for decades, and while some states have recently tried to outlaw it, it is still allowed in foods that are frequently consumed. It is linked to changes in the gastrointestinal tract and immune system and is also associated with an increased cancer risk due to its ability to stimulate tumor formation in the gastrointestinal tract.[72] It was banned from use in the food supply by the European Union in 2021 for concerns about potential genotoxicity but continues to be used in commonly sold candies and foods in the US.

Sweeteners

Sweeteners, such as aspartame, neotame, saccharin, and sucralose, are known to contribute to weight gain and metabolic changes. These sweeteners disrupt gut flora, leading to an imbalance in the microbiome that can alter the breakdown of carbohydrates and fats, ultimately promoting weight gain.[73] Additionally, they can cause our bodies to release insulin in response to the perceived sweetness, leading to insulin resistance over time, as the body feels "tricked" with each consumption. More specifically, the chemical is found to induce insulin signal transduction of liver tissue.[74]

Saccharin has been found to cause urothelial bladder tumors in rats. While this does demonstrate the significant impact that the chemical can have on health and opens the question of what we may be missing on other impacts it may have, it is important to note that this does not directly correlate to humans because of differences in our urine composition.[55]

Aspartame is another chemically derived sweetener. Short-term side effects can include dizziness, headaches, blurred vision, and gastrointestinal issues. The link between aspartame and cancer continues to be examined.[55] One 2021 study found that aspartame has a potential increased risk for cancer and provides no benefit in the prevention of diabetes. It was found that long-term aspartame exposure increases tumor cell aggressiveness, indicating that it may advance an existing tumor in humans.[75]

A 2023 study found an increased risk for stomach cancer in diabetics with prolonged use of saccharin and sucralose, which is a subset of the diabetic population.[76] This review of studies highlights the diversity of subsets of populations that may be at risk but are often difficult to control for or study. Therefore, caution is advised, as we cannot be certain what is being missed in the literature.

Stevia has been thoroughly tested and has not been found to cause the same reactions in the body as other sweeteners and has conversely been found to be antioxidant, anti-inflammatory, anti-hyperglycemic, anti-hyperlipidemic, and hepatorenal protective.[77] However, it is important to note that substances can be thought safe for decades before adverse effects are discovered. While, at this time, it is a smarter choice than other sweeteners, keeping up to date on non-biased studies (which are hard to find) is recommended.

Pesticides

Pesticides are another significant source of chemical exposure. Numerous studies have shown that people living near areas where pesticides are heavily used, such as farms or golf courses, have a higher risk of developing Parkinson's disease.[78] Also, women living near agricultural fields have exhibited an increased cancer and Parkinson's risk, as have families residing close to golf courses, due to the pesticides applied for maintaining the lawns.[79]

Pesticides can produce immediate health effects, including skin irritation, respiratory issues, nausea, vomiting, dizziness, and exacerbation of asthma, as well as neurological symptoms like irritability, headaches, and muscle twitching. Long-term effects associated with pesticides include depression, ADHD, reproductive problems, and an increased risk of Parkinson's disease, non-Hodgkin lymphoma, leukemia, and other cancers.[80,81]

The bald eagle serves as a powerful example of the harm pesticides can cause. At one point, the eagle was on the brink of extinction, reduced to only about four hundred mating pairs. Many might assume that hunting was the primary cause, but in fact, the eagles had not been hunted for twenty years before their most rapid period of decline. Researchers had to shift their perspective to understand what was truly endangering these birds.

They discovered that pesticide runoff from agricultural crops was contaminating the eagles' water supply. This water, diluted from pesticides meant for human consumption, was being ingested by mother eagles. Specifically, the pesticide DDT (dichlorodiphenyltrichloroethane) was found to disrupt the calcification of the eggs, which ultimately resulted in their non-viability. The inability to reproduce effectively led to the drastic population decline.

Following the identification of this issue, reversals in pesticide usage allowed for recovery, highlighting the importance of the effects of pesticides not only on wildlife but also on human health, as it was found to be.[82] In 1972 it was banned after decades of use. However, its impact on increasing the risk of cancer, endocrine disruption, and long-term intergenerational effects had already taken hold, as it was found to be a toxin that accumulates easily and does not readily clear from human adipose tissue or the environment. Yet another strike on the guesswork of approving chemicals for our consumption and environmental exposure prior to sufficient testing.[83]

Pesticide exposure in general has been linked to various developmental and behavioral problems in children, lower IQ levels, and disruptions in gut flora.[84] A study by the European Environmental Agency found that at least two types of pesticides are present in the bodies of 84% of people, indicating that our bodies do not easily eliminate these toxins. What is worse is that the toxic levels were considerably higher in children than adults.[85] To mitigate exposure, it's advisable to choose organic fruits and vegetables whenever possible.

Many people are rightfully concerned about pesticides on fresh produce. However, when organic is not an option, organic sprays are available that can effectively reduce the ingestion of pesticide residues without leaving harmful residues. Encouraging clients to invest in their health through organic options is important, but for those on a tighter budget, using these sprays can still allow for the inclusion of fresh fruits and vegetables in their diets while decreasing risk. The goal should be to promote healthy eating without inducing fear regarding food safety.

Heavy Metals

Now let's move on to heavy metals, which can also be found in our water and food supply. These metals can increase the risk of neurological symptoms, such as tinnitus, Parkinson's, and Alzheimer's, as well as tingling or numbness in the extremities, headaches, memory loss, and tremors.

Heavy metals are commonly present not only in toxic substances like tobacco but also in our general environment and food. Symptoms tied to heavy metal exposure can include skeletal pain and reduced bone mineral density.[86] For instance, a potential root cause for eczema may be heavy metal exposure. Some studies have even linked vaccines to an increased risk of eczema in children, potentially due to the heavy metals contained in them.

Please refer to Chapter 5 for more information on detoxifying from heavy metals.

MSG

Monosodium glutamate (MSG) is one of the most commonly used additives in our food supply, particularly in fast food and buffet cuisine, and is associated with an array of symptoms and illnesses. It can cause gastrointestinal (GI) upset as well as headaches, nausea, depression, and anxiety. It is also known to be hepatotoxic, neurotoxic, genotoxic, and an endocrine disruptor.[87,88]

Consuming MSG can increase the risk for diabetes.[89] Some people may experience immediate reactions, such as flushing, sweating, facial pressure or tightness, and even numbness and tingling sensations. Others might not notice any symptoms until they have ingested a significant amount of MSG, at which point they may report feelings of nausea or headache.[90] MSG can also trigger increased intestinal permeability syndrome, which increases the risk for chronic inflammatory diseases due to its effects on the gut.

The Milk Controversy

Staying on the topic of dairy, casein is a compound found in milk that has been found to have undesirable effects on certain individuals. Some individuals are genetically unable to break down casein efficiently, which can result in neurological effects that are comparable to those of morphine. Those with food addiction tendencies may be at a higher risk because they experience an instant high from consuming casein, followed by long-term side effects.[91]

This doesn't necessarily mean that everyone needs to eliminate dairy from their diet. Choosing responsibly sourced dairy, such as A2 milk, which is produced by cows that only produce the A2 beta-casein protein, is thought to have fewer side effects and better digestibility.[92] Cow's milk contains great nutrients and proteins, and it has been shown to be anti-inflammatory in those who are not reactive to whey or casein proteins.[93]

However, it is undeniable that a large population of people, some studies estimate around 70% in some populations, are intolerant to milk proteins. Therefore, it is a product that needs to be assessed very thoroughly. It is often a cause of skin reactions, like eczema, gastrointestinal discomfort, and respiratory reactions, like a chronic runny nose, wheezing, coughing, and even shortness of breath.[94]

Limiting dairy in healthy diets and fully eliminating it when potential for interaction is present is a good goal; just be careful not to eliminate the nutrition it provides when possible. For example, yogurt's live active cultures and excellent source of butyrate should not be eliminated when tolerated, as real yogurt tends not to have the amount of casein that cow's milk does. Goat's milk is also an alternative that may be better tolerated by some individuals. There is also great data and clinical results on raw milk being tolerated well, even when dairy intolerance with commercialized milk is present.

If someone is not ready or willing to reduce their dairy intake, or if dairy has benefits for them, trying organic dairy products can be a helpful option. However, people with a genetic predisposition to struggle with casein digestion should consider eliminating it entirely. The strongest indicator for testing is a person's reported addiction to casein.

For those with dairy or casein intolerance, avoidance is the best strategy. However, enzyme supplements like DPP-4 can help break down casein, as it does gluten, in case of accidental exposure. It's also worth noting that studies with opiate blockers in mice showed no behavioral changes when exposed to casein, indicating that casein morphin chemically resembles morphine and can similarly affect the neurological system.[95]

While milk can be a part of a balanced diet, it does come with potential risks, and it's important to work with people to determine the best approach for them. If a person isn't ready for a complete overhaul of their diet, meeting them where they are can be beneficial. Many might be open to reducing certain foods while keeping other elements of their diet intact. Dairy may be one of those trade-offs for a better choice, even if not perfect.

Detoxification

Once exposure to toxins has been proven, the first step is to identify where the patient is being exposed and eliminate the exposure. The next important step is preparation for detoxification. This includes getting adequate sleep and hydration, ensuring regular bowel movements, and a healthy, functioning liver. Milk thistle, alpha-lipoic acid, glutathione, or N-acetylcysteine (NAC) can aid in liver detoxification.[96]

Organic acids testing is a fantastic tool that can help identify nutritional deficiencies, metabolic disruptions, or mitochondrial dysfunction that may be getting in the way of full body functioning and detox. It also gives a window of assessment into gut health, including bacterial or yeast overgrowth. It resembles an emissions test for a car. Just as a car's emissions depend on the proper mixture of gas and oil, the presence of organic acids in the body can indicate levels of various nutrients.

For example, if we do not see the expected emissions from vitamin C, it suggests a deficiency in that vitamin or the processing of it.

Conversely, if we notice an excess of certain emissions, it can indicate an overgrowth of yeast or other microorganisms, which can be detected in urine samples.

This testing also includes a section on neurotransmitters, helping us understand whether the body is producing the right balance of neurotransmitters. When evaluating heavy metals and magnesium levels, I prefer hair testing, as it is more accurate for long-term exposure. If there are concerns about short-term exposure, urine testing may be appropriate. However, in functional medicine, we typically look for long-term accumulation.

In addition to testing, exercise and lifestyle choices are crucial components of any detox process. Binders like charcoal for chemical detox and zeolite for heavy metal detox can be great benefits, as are natural foods that help to detox, like oregano, parsley, or basil.[97] Exercise boosts serotonin and dopamine levels, reduces inflammation, enhances blood circulation to the liver, and improves oxygen and nutrient delivery to the brain. It also significantly aids in detoxification and supports the lymphatic system. One reason a sedentary lifestyle can inhibit effective detoxification is due to the lack of muscle movement that stimulates the lymphatic system.

Lymphatic drainage processes can aid in toxin elimination, but exercise serves as a natural alternative through the natural contraction of muscles that move the lymphatic system as well as the sweating process. Maintaining a whole food diet, such as a low-FODMAP, Mediterranean, or anti-inflammatory diet, can also make a significant difference in liver toxicity, with special attention being made to avoid processed foods and sugar. As a matter of fact, one of the primary toxins to address is sugar, which is prevalent in our society and acts as a neurotoxin.[98]

Sugar can lead to increased agitation and hyperactivity, and it can severely impact health, including causing yeast overgrowth. We often focus heavily on calorie intake and weight management, but in doing so, we may be neglecting our overall health. Sugar is inflammatory and has been linked to heart disease, tooth decay, reduced memory, hormonal disruptions, sleep problems, and potentially even acne.[99,100]

The inflammation caused by sugar is a significant issue, and it's also associated with fatty liver disease. While many people might monitor cholesterol levels, it is essential to recognize that carbohydrates—especially sugars—are often responsible for fat accumulation in the liver. The liver struggles to process and eliminate toxins, resulting in fatty deposits.[98]

Ultimately, there is no one-size-fits-all approach to health protocols. It's essential to ensure that testing, observation, and treatment plans are sustainable for life. Some people may come to us already having made significant health changes that they can maintain over the long term, but if you have a patient who seems unmotivated, I highly recommend having regular check-ins to ensure they are staying engaged. The moment someone feels uncertain about their ability to continue, it's crucial to intervene, focusing on shifting their mindset and helping them view their journey from a different perspective.

Consider introducing milestones that acknowledge how far clients have come and also focus on health improvements beyond their initial goal. For example, do not focus solely on weight loss but also on decreased risk for heart disease, improved neurological health, energy levels, mood changes, etc., and how small efforts add up to a big impact.

If the client feels the need for a controlled break from their new habits, that is perfectly okay in moderation. Just avoid calling these breaks "cheats." Instead, refer to them as "treats." You never want to cheat on your own health because doing so signals to the mind a sense of failure, guilt, and shame. But it is fair to use the word "treat," as the occasional treat is not inherently bad. Focusing on mindset and avoiding the incorporation of shame is imperative for a holistic approach to care. There are several more mindset shifts we help our clients make at the Academy. This one in particular is imperative, as shame is, after all, the root of disease, as evidenced in the Garden of Eden and discussed earlier in our opening conversation.

When addressing issues like yeast overgrowth, even a small amount of sugar or bread (which tends to be the most tempting treats) can hinder progress. Additionally, the longer the client is off carbs and bread, the fewer cravings are felt, and even a small amount can refuel cravings that may have diminished. However, it's essential to look at the bigger picture. If a patient requires a mental break, it's more important for them to take one so they do not give up overall. While results may take longer, getting there later is better than never.

PRO TIP:

When enrolling patients into your programs, it is important to understand why they might decline beforehand. One common fear that creeps into a patient's mind is the fear of "starving" or battling intense cravings. This fear often stops people before they even start. However, functional medicine interventions have an incredible built-in solution for this. Yeast overgrowth and gut dysbiosis are often major sources of these cravings, and they are fixable with proper treatment. Explain to patients ahead of time that they will not have to rely on brute "willpower," because cravings will naturally be reduced with most treatment interventions.

This sets them up for success and helps remove the fear of failure and shame that can subconsciously prevent clients from initiating change. As a result, it becomes easier for them to achieve results and easier for you to grow your impact-driven clinic.

Example Detox Strategy:

Phase 1: Prep + Drainage Support for the first 1–2 weeks.

- Begin avoiding toxins, chemicals, and alcohol.
- Maintain adequate hydration (typically 80–100 oz. of purified water a day or half the client's body weight in ounces, adjusting accordingly in obesity).
- Supplements to consider:
  - Initiate Binders BID-TID that can help remove toxins such as:
    - Activated charcoal
    - Bentonite clay
    - Spirulina, chlorella, blue algae
- This is a great supplement for immunosupport and detox when sourced right; however, caution that quality matters, and this must be third-party tested, as contamination is common and can cause serious rashes, as well as neurotoxic and nephrotoxic side effects if not properly sourced.
  - N-acetyl cysteine or dandelion root extract for antioxidant effects
    - NAC is the precursor to glutathione, which can also be supplemented orally, but glutathione bioavailability is much greater via IV (intravenous) or IM (intramuscular).
- Lymphatic massage or dry brushing daily
  - Combine with a sauna or warm Epsom salt bath to further open the ducts.
- Diet:
  - anti-inflammatory, whole foods, high fiber (if tolerated and no SIBO, which is described in our gastroenterology chapter)
  - Cruciferous veggies are important for detox.

    - Adding basil, thyme, cilantro, or parsley to foods is helpful.

Phase 2: Replenish (next 14–21 days, longer as needed)

- Consider one or a mix of the following supplements for gut repair.
    - Marshmallow root or zinc carnosine: both are most beneficial in initial phases as they form a protective, gelatinous barrier around the mucosal lining
    - Aloe vera: tends to be best in constipation-dominant and can exacerbate diarrhea
    - L-glutamine: most commonly used longer term and after the initial phases. It helps to seal the tight junctures of the GI tract.
    - Proper probiotics and prebiotics (follow the 5R method in the gastroenterology chapter).
- Supplements to consider for mitochondria repair if testing indicates mitochondria dysfunction may be hindering detoxification process:
    - CoQ10, magnesium, or carnitine
- As a final note, testing for genetic variants like MTHFR and replacing methylated B12 and folate, or other vitamins, may be necessary. A lack of methionine can lead to significantly inhibited detoxification pathways.

Chapter Conclusion

Globally, over ten thousand chemicals are used in food processing and packaging. This includes dyes, flavors, preservatives, and chemicals involved in the processing and packaging stages. Many of these chemicals can migrate into food during these processes, exposing us to substances that often aren't listed on ingredient labels because they aren't directly added to the food. For those interested in researching this topic further, a good resource is bcpp.com and peer-reviewed articles.

When examining the root causes of illness, one phenomenon to consider is bioaccumulation, which is the process by which the rate of chemical intake exceeds the rate of excretion. Since children are exposed to these chemicals even before birth and their livers are not fully developed until age one or two, bioaccumulation can occur rapidly. These chemicals are not only present in food; they can also be ingested through contaminated water or inhaled from air pollutants.

While it's challenging to completely avoid exposure to these substances, as we need to breathe and drink water, we can take steps to minimize our exposure. Using water and air filters and opting for whole, organic foods as much as possible can help in this regard. This process can be quite individualized, so you will need to work with your clients on a case-by-case basis.

Finally, let's discuss a key principle: progress over perfection. One of the main obstacles that even well-informed people face in adopting a root-cause approach rather than a symptom-based model is the fear of not being perfect at it. I want to encourage you: you will never feel perfect while implementing these changes. Don't let that stop you from helping others and possibly starting your own health journey simultaneously.

In Philippians 3:12–14 (KJV), Paul encourages us that even he was not perfect prior to taking action, but he emphasizes the need for progress over perfection. He tells us, *"Not as though I had already attained, either were already perfect: but I follow after... forgetting those things which are behind, and reaching forth unto those things which are before, I press toward the mark for the prize of the high calling of God in Christ Jesus."*

Forget past failures. Forget past inhibitions. You are new again in your excitement, and that is the secret: to never give up and to keep pressing forward. This truth also applies to those of you who want to start your own business. Zig Ziglar, the famous motivational speaker and successful businessman, once said, "You do not have to be great to start, but you have to start to become great."

I encourage you today to take this as your sign to get started. Focus on the impact you were meant to make, rather than fearing you will not do it "perfectly." None of us ever do. More importantly, it is not about you. It is about your calling and the fact that others need you to step forward. Simply put, other people's fate is waiting on the other side of you saying, "It can wait."

Business Practice Pearl

Leverage is the second pillar of a successful functional practice or business, and it can be applied in many ways. One way is by purchasing the experiences of others so you can learn from their mistakes. This allows you to stop wasting time and reach a return on investment more quickly. You will always spend one of two currencies: time or money, and you will spend the one you value least. Successful people value time more because they know it is a truly irreplaceable resource. You can always make more money. You can never remake time. You can only save it for the future.

I have invested six figures into learning from business coaches, and it got me to where I wanted to be faster than I would have gotten there on my own. To be honest, more than I ever would have gotten on my own. Despite my quick adoption of the strategies, I have a firm belief that I would have never figured it out on my own. The cost of inaction would have been in the millions if I had waited until I felt "ready" or until the investment felt "comfortable." As the saying goes, stand on the shoulders of giants.

I applaud you today because you are already practicing this form of leverage by purchasing this book. This is one reason I believe my students often get financial results even faster than I did. They invested in me and did not have to spend the extra time or money I did trying to figure out what works for our exact niche. That is leverage, shortening the distance from point A to B by exerting less energy than if you did it on your own.

For example, I spent hundreds of hours reading peer-reviewed journals and courses, gleaning the information from those resources that are backed by good evidence. Then I implemented what I learned and found what worked and what didn't (because, trust me, there is some woo-woo in the functional medicine arena). Finally, I placed only the information that is helpful in this book, which you can read in a few hours. Even going all in, by going through our fully accredited board certification and CEU course, can be done in a fraction of the time I spent learning viable protocols, as the course is a literal forty-eight hours of real time.

As I mentioned, I have invested well over six figures in learning from different business coaches. About half of that money spent helped, while the rest did not move the needle much. With that said, I never complained or asked for a refund from my coaches, even when I didn't feel they delivered what I expected. Why? Because I am responsible for my outcome. If I believe for a moment that others hold that power, I lose the momentum I set forth and have control over.

If it's meant to be, it won't just be. If it's meant to be… it is up to *me*. As the owner of my businesses and practice, I am the only one who can take responsibility to learn what I need in the moment and figure out how to apply it. I am not looking for a million ideas to each make me a dollar; I am looking for that one idea that gets me my next million dollars. Quality over quantity.

If I learn one thing that helps me move the needle, I can figure out how to make back my investment. This gives me motivation and builds my innovation to be better, and I can apply that new skill to other aspects of my business. There is always a way to leverage the knowledge you gain in bigger and better ways.

Trust me, you'll either watch someone else do it or you will figure it out. Winners know that *they* are the common denominator. The rest expect the common denominator to be someone outside of themselves. However, if you expect someone else to carry you further than you can carry yourself, you'll never make it. That's one reason why there is only 1% at the top. That is the fortitude of a successful business owner leveraging the experience of others—standing on the shoulders of giants.

I also teach my students to leverage other people's audiences. If you don't have anyone in front of you to purchase your offer, it doesn't matter how good you are; you do not have a business. There are a ton of people out there, like YouTubers, social media influencers, or group owners, who know how to build an audience but are not monetizing that traffic. If you go to someone for a collaboration and provide a way for them to monetize, they will happily share their audience with you. That is when things get fun and very passive.

For example, you build your offer and course, then collaborate with someone who has an audience of ten thousand on one of the many platforms out there. In our live conferences (which are free to you by scanning the QR codes at the beginning or end of this book), we go into the details on how to properly do this. But, for reference, let's say 10% of their audience sees your offer, so one thousand people. Let's assume, since you are starting out, your offer converts (lands sales) at 15% (the market average goal is 30%). That means that 15% of a thousand people, or 150 people, bought your offer. Even if it was only $47, you earned $7,050 and added a sizable audience of buyers to your email list.

This brings me to my next point: start building an email list! I see so many business owners who are not leveraging this. Do not be like them. An email list is the best thing you can leverage because one email send can possibly earn multiple sales. Plus, it's the only thing you actually own. Instagram, Facebook, YouTube, all of those platforms can shut you down in a moment without even a notice. It happens all the time, and people earning a great income lose it overnight. There are ways to safeguard against that, and an email list is one such way.

One-to-many, friends; that is leverage. That is the impact. That is freedom from working hour to hour, chart to chart, and missed moments with family. What price could you put on that? If you are like me, you can easily see how learning this skill was worth the over six figures I invested in several different experts to hone this. However, I am happy to share with you the blueprint so you don't have to go to all of those different experts. Again, that is leverage.

Now that you have an email list and a front-end offer converting, you can build higher-level programs or courses. But here is one more piece of knowledge: never spend any time building anything before you have sold it. There is a strategy that I implement called beta launching. That means that people purchase the course or product before I spend a moment of my time building it. I cannot count the number of practitioners who come to me with 101 really great courses and not one sale. Why? They spent time building something they assumed people wanted because they knew it was what they needed. You have to sell them what they want (because they won't buy it unless they want it) and give them what they need. There are several advantages to beta group launching. One advantage is that the clients typically get a good discount for being the "test pilots" and can give feedback on what they want to learn next. That is how you know you are building what your clients and potential clients will want. Do not underestimate the power of this.

The other reason I say not to build it first is simply that you won't have many (if any) issues building the program, but selling it might be a challenge, especially if you do not have a proven model to work off of. You don't want to waste time and energy building a course that doesn't sell. It's the fast path to burnout. Honestly, do you want to be a course builder or a business owner? No sales, no business. That's as simple as the math gets.

Chapter 4

Functional Gastroenterology

Functional gastroenterology focuses on the treatment of diseases specifically involving the GI tract, such as Crohn's, IBS, ulcerative colitis, etc. However, the gut has also been found to be the root cause of a lot of diseases once never thought to be associated with the gastrointestinal system. As we look at specific charts, you'll see that certain strains of bacteria can increase the risk of autoimmunity, while a lack of others can be linked to anxiety, depression, Parkinson's disease, and various neuroinflammatory disorders.

While we go into a deep dive within our full program, there are a few simple principles you should know that are of great importance. For example, several deficiencies in the microbiome have been associated with increased risk for diabetes, and overgrowth of gram-negative bacteria is associated with several neurological diseases, such as autism, Alzheimer's, and autoimmune disease.[101] Causes for dysbiosis can be related to diet, alcohol consumption, acute gastroenteritis (common with traveling), or even less obvious causes, such as past viral infections and vaccinations.

After vaccination, some people may experience gastrointestinal disturbances, such as diarrhea, indicating a change in gut flora. While this alteration is typically temporary, it may persist in some cases. Additionally, those with conditions like IBD (Inflammatory Bowel Disease) or other gut issues may not respond well to vaccinations and may have a heightened risk of adverse reactions or inflammatory responses afterward.[102]

It is also fair to note that a lack of diversity initially in the gut microbiome prior to vaccination will also decrease the efficacy of vaccinations.[102] That is not to form an opinion on a very controversial space, but to identify good science and potential root causes for the root causes, if you will.

CASE STUDY: THE POWERFUL INTERVENTION OF SIMPLE DIETARY SCREENING

To illustrate these concepts, I want to share a case study of a young female who experienced anxiety and chronic diarrhea, with a family history of ulcerative colitis. She was on biologics for hair loss, which was suspected to be autoimmune in nature, although she had no positive markers at the time. As I mentioned earlier, it's common for patients not to present with autoimmune markers. Despite her treatment, the root cause of her symptoms remained unidentified, and symptoms only mildly improved at best until she came to see me.

Labs

Upon evaluation, I discovered she had chronic diarrhea and tested her for gluten intolerance. While she tested negative for celiac disease, the results showed she was positive for gluten intolerance. I also ordered a full thyroid panel, complete stool analysis, and GI map. When her labs came back showing severe hyperthyroidism, I ordered a selenium level and iodine level.

Intervention

After we rebalanced her gut health and removed gluten from her diet, she experienced a rapid improvement in her symptoms. However, this quick response also led her to experience some constipation due to a loss of muscle strength in her digestive system, which made normal bowel movements challenging. She required time to rebuild that muscle strength to restore balanced digestive function. She worked with her rheumatologist, as she decided to stop the autoimmune medication she was on.

I rebalanced her GI microbiome by using specific probiotics that addressed her unique needs. Eventually, her immune system re-regulated, and she began to enjoy a more normal life—all from identifying that one root cause. She had endured years of undiagnosed gluten sensitivity (not celiac) that contributed to her compounding issues. As we will learn moving forward, Graves' and Hashimoto's are very similar to gluten sensitivity based on the phenomenon of molecular mimicry.[103] Molecular mimicry is a phenomenon that occurs when a molecule is identified as a threat by the body and attacked, such as with gluten molecules, but then the body identifies similar cells in the body (like the thyroid cells that are molecularly similar to the offending antigen) and begins to attack them as well.[103] I use this case study to highlight that we cannot isolate the body into individual systems; rather, we must consider the body as a whole and how the gastrointestinal system influences overall health.

The Enteric Nervous System: The Second Brain

A significant aspect of the relationship between the body and the gut involves the enteric nervous system, often referred to as the "second brain." This system contains millions of neurons—the second most abundant collection of nervous tissue in the body. The enteric nervous system communicates back and forth (bi-directionally) with the central nervous system, which comprises the brain and spinal cord.[104]

Many people think that the brain mainly influences the gut; however, in reality, about 90% of signaling is afferent, meaning it travels from the gut to the brain via the vagus nerve, rather than efferent (from the brain to the gut). This demonstrates that the gut has a significant impact on brain function and the brain is more of a receiver of information in the gut-brain connection.[104]

The Microbiome

The entire gastrointestinal tract is involved in this process, starting with the mouth. We like to summarize this with the phrase "from the gum to the bum," indicating the full length of the digestive system. A key clinical insight to consider is that dysbiosis can begin in the mouth. For example, the overuse or regular use of mouthwashes can disrupt the balance of oral bacteria. While mouthwashes can kill harmful germs, they can also eliminate beneficial bacteria, which are essential for maintaining a healthy microbiome.[105] This disruption can lead to an overgrowth of harmful microbes, which increases the risk of conditions such as cardiovascular disease, autoimmune disorders, and IBS.

PRO TIP:

It is important to point out to your clients that letting a dysbiosis go without treatment can cause subsequent damage. It is not just about the immediate symptoms but the long-term impact. Since dysbiosis is a source of inflammation that can lead to secondary disease, your clients' knowledge of this can help with compliance. I always say I am an information broker for my clients. Once they are informed and aware, they then take the power to transform their lives.

The gut microbiome is incredibly complex, consisting of more than thirty million microbial genes, which is actually more than the total amount of human DNA.[106] To put this into perspective, there are approximately 39 trillion microbes in the human gut, compared to just 30 trillion human cells.[107] This means that we are arguably more microbiome than we are our own cells.

An essential aspect of the gut microbiome is that it has a form of memory. If the gut flora has been dysregulated for an extended period, it becomes more challenging to restore it to a healthy state, as it tends to revert to its previous imbalance.[108] Consequently, younger people who seek help often experience better results than those who have struggled with dysbiosis for a long time. This emphasizes the importance of urgency in implementing treatment programs as soon as possible and that healing may take longer based on a person's history of dysbiosis.

The gut microbiome consists of trillions of microbes, including bacteria, fungi, and viruses, as well as commensal bacteria. These are the so-called "Goldilocks bacteria," as both an excess and a deficiency of them can be harmful. The gut microbiome plays a crucial role in digestion, nutrient absorption, immune system regulation, hormone metabolism, inflammatory pathways, neurological functions, and mood regulation. In fact, about 90% of serotonin, a key neurotransmitter, is produced in the intestines due to microbial activity, and it interacts with receptors of the brain via the vagus nerve.[109]

Dysbiosis: Causes/Risk Factors

Gut dysbiosis refers to an imbalance among these microbes, and several common causes should be screened during initial patient evaluations. These include:

- Poor diet (standard American diet)

- Medications such as:
  - Antibiotics (arguably the most detrimental influence on the microbiome)
  - Proton pump inhibitors (PPIs)
  - Non-steroidal anti-inflammatory drugs (NSAIDs)
  - Oral contraceptive use (greater than six years)
- Chronic stress
- Environmental toxins
- Infections (bacterial and viral; history of and/or current infection)
- Symptoms such as bloating, constipation, or diarrhea
- Lack of being breastfed as a child
- Cesarean delivery at birth
- Maternal gastrointestinal issues

Symptoms

The consequences of gut dysbiosis can manifest in various forms, including constipation, diarrhea, gas, bloating, brain fog, fatigue, skin conditions, autoimmune reactions, chronic inflammation, and neurologic diseases. There are also significant ties between an imbalanced gut and the development of Parkinson's, autism, and multiple sclerosis.[110]

For instance, I have worked with a client who had severe multiple sclerosis and was told they would be in a wheelchair within a year without medications. It was of their own accord, prior to working with me, that they declined prescription medications. They had found significant improvement after simple dietary interventions and then came to me for additional help. We have since focused on correcting their gut health and eliminating the offending pathogen, and they continue to experience significant improvement several years out without prescriptions.

Basics of the Biome

Two major bacterial phyla in the human gut are Firmicutes and Bacteroidetes. Overgrown levels of Firmicutes are often linked to high-fat, high-sugar diets and are associated with enhanced energy extraction and fat storage, leading to obesity. However, undergrowth is additionally not healthy, as is seen in those on a ketogenic diet. The ketogenic diet, which is high in fat and low in carbohydrates, lends to a decrease in the abundance of key Firmicutes that are butyrate-producing bacteria and essential to decreasing the risk of diseases such as obesity, depression, and diabetes.[111,112]

This is why I often advise against diets that strictly cut out food or macro groups, such as ketogenic or, conversely, extremely low-fat diets, for long periods of time. If used for weight loss, the benefits of a keto diet could outweigh the long-term effects of obesity, but a plan to transition to a balanced diet is advisable. This is not considering more extreme conditions such as epilepsy, where the benefits of a keto diet outweigh the microbiome risk. The ketogenic diet is known to decrease migraine occurrences as well as significantly improve, and at times, achieve complete remission of epilepsy.[113] In such situations, maintenance of severe disease and then subsequent supplementation of deficiencies and proper probiotics is an optimal path. It's vital to maintain a balance between Firmicutes and Bacteroidetes, as both are essential for gut health—the "Goldilocks bacteria" concept reaffirms that both too much and too little can be detrimental.

This additionally serves as an example of how we often "don't know what we don't know" when we go to extremes in diets by focusing on one outcome (typically weight loss) and ignoring that there are likely several reasons why humans have historically eaten from all macro groups. While it may benefit as a weight loss hack to eat a certain way, it may not benefit gut flora, which can cause an array of diseases down the road. I appreciate that this next part is not peer-reviewed for scientific literature. However, I do find it intriguing that even in biblical literature, we are encouraged to eat diversely. Genesis 9:3 (ESV): "*Every moving thing that lives shall be food for you. And as I gave you the green plants, I give you everything.*"

Bacteroidetes are often more abundant in fiber-rich plants, which tend to be lacking in the standard American diet (SAD). This type of bacteria is associated with leanness and a balanced metabolic profile. Again, it comes down to the microbiome. For example, research has shown that transferring gut microbiota from obese mice to lean mice can cause the lean mice to gain weight without changing their caloric intake. Conversely, transferring fecal matter from lean mice to obese mice can result in weight loss, again without altering caloric intake.[114] These findings highlight the clinical significance of gut microbiota in various health conditions, including obesity, insulin resistance, and systemic inflammation. In my personal experience, resolving my insulin resistance was linked to correcting my gut health.

A balanced and slightly Bacteroidetes-dominant microbiome is more metabolically favorable. An unhealthy diet that promotes dysbiosis typically includes high levels of refined carbohydrates, processed foods (especially sugars), and saturated fats. High sugar intake significantly increases the risk of yeast overgrowth, leading to issues such as irritability, neurological dysfunction, and cravings.[115] This creates a self-perpetuating cycle where cravings for more carbohydrates and sugars may be the result of an overgrown Firmicutes microbiome that thrives on those foods. Yes, the gut microbiome can influence cravings, as over 90% of the communication between the gut and brain flows from the gut to the brain, signaling a desire for foods that support its composition.

Impact of Nutrition

Healthy dietary strategies that promote a balanced microbiome include a high intake of diverse plant foods, soluble and insoluble fiber, and prebiotic-rich foods. However, it's important to note that some people may not benefit from these recommendations if they have small intestinal bacterial overgrowth (SIBO), which is a leading cause of IBS and GI symptoms that we will discuss later.

Prebiotics are compounds that feed probiotics; examples include chicory root, garlic, onions, leeks, asparagus, Jerusalem artichokes, green bananas, oats, and apples. This is another reason why we should focus not just on caloric intake, but also on the variety of foods we consume. Prebiotics support the growth of beneficial bacteria like Bifidobacteria and Lactobacilli, which many people tend to lack, thus enhancing microbiome diversity and improving the production of vital short-chain fatty acids (SCFAs), such as butyrate.[116]

Dietary fiber plays a crucial role in maintaining this balance. Soluble fiber can be found in higher quantities in foods like oats, legumes, and fruit, while insoluble fiber comes more from whole grains and leafy greens. The functional benefits of fiber include supporting regular bowel movements, reducing the risk of constipation, and regulating blood sugar and cholesterol levels.[116] Consuming a whole fruit like an apple will result in a more stable blood sugar level compared to drinking apple juice, which can cause a significant spike in blood sugar. The fiber in fruit acts as a buffer against sugar spikes, helping to stabilize blood sugar levels when consumed alongside carbohydrates, regardless of their type.[117]

Fiber also aids in regulating hormones by minimizing the risk of insulin resistance, as it prevents sharp increases in both insulin and glucose levels. Butyrate, a key short-chain fatty acid produced from fiber fermentation, is crucial for fueling colonocytes (the cells of the intestines), reducing gut inflammation, and maintaining the integrity of the gut barrier.[117]

A balanced gut microbiome is essential for overall health, while dysbiosis, an imbalance in the ratio of pharmaceuticals to bacteria, can contribute to chronic diseases. As discussed in our lab section, this ratio can be assessed through stool testing analysis, which provides valuable insights. Diet is one of the most significant factors influencing microbiome health, and incorporating prebiotics and fiber is vital for restoring gut balance. It's crucial to understand the microbiome and its connections, as the metabolic products produced by the microbiome play a significant role in these links.

Inflammation, Lipid Polysaccharide, and Neurological Links

Lipid polysaccharide, or LPS, is a complex molecule produced by gram-negative bacteria that should not necessarily be in the gut. We know there's a direct correlation between the brain and LPS. Researchers have even injected LPS into mice and caused neurologic symptoms similar to those of autism and Parkinson's disease.[118] There is a direct correlation between the gut and the brain, and LPS makes a big difference. Another interesting study tested LPS in people with dementia and found they consistently have higher levels of the molecule, pointing to a probable underlying correlation.[119] Alkaline phosphatase is produced in the liver and the gut to help regulate LPS. However, when the liver is not doing well, it cannot perform this function effectively.[120] LFTs (liver functional tests) are another element in the client's overall health that should be considered when determining the root cause. Clients who have a strong history of ingesting drugs or hepatotoxic diets (such as with alcohol, high-fat carbs, acetaminophen use, or abundant chemicals) may experience improved treatment outcomes if first started on milk thistle for liver detox.

Gluten and Its Effects on Health

Even those without celiac disease may need to remove gluten if they have a history of GI symptoms not otherwise explained. Gluten sensitivity, which can be tested for, can also lead to chronic inflammation and other symptoms, like dysbiosis, joint pain, and/or autoimmune triggers. Gluten, particularly the gliadin components of the protein, can have significant effects on gut health and even mental or neurological health, primarily because it breaks down into gliadorphin, an opiate-like peptide. Some people struggle to break down gliadorphin in their bodies due to a polymorphism related to a lack of the enzyme DPP4, which can lead to its accumulation and potential neurotoxicity.[121]

PRO TIP:

If cost is a concern for extra testing related to gluten sensitivity, patient symptoms may help to narrow down those who are at risk. Real-life experiences illustrate this issue through the phenomenon known as "carb highs." People may feel elated after consuming carbohydrates and crave more, but they often experience a subsequent "carb crash." This crash is frequently observed in people who do not effectively break down gliadorphin.[122] A thorough patient history can reveal if removing gluten may have benefits without having to test. While this is not absolute, it can help give insight.

Interestingly, gliadorphin is chemically similar to morphine—hence the resemblance in their names. Just like morphine, which is given to patients in hospitals, gliadorphin can induce various reactions. When the body successfully breaks it down, the adverse effects are mitigated, but many people do not process it properly.[122]

Historically, celiac disease was the only recognized sensitivity to gluten. However, we now understand that many people can be gluten-sensitive without having celiac disease. Numerous patients have reported feeling emotionally better, experiencing increased energy, and alleviating inflammation simply by removing gluten from their diets. Symptoms such as diarrhea often resolve almost immediately after eliminating gluten.[123] The same issues can also arise with dairy products, as the proteins in dairy, particularly casein, share similarities with those found in gluten.

Research shows a strong association between gluten intake and various mental health conditions, including schizophrenia, depression, and anxiety. Numerous randomized controlled trials and longitudinal studies indicate that gluten-free diets can improve these symptoms across different populations. Furthermore, there is evidence linking gluten intake to symptoms in people with autism spectrum disorder, with significant improvements observed following the withdrawal of gluten.[124] If gluten cannot be eliminated from a diet easily, the enzyme that breaks it down, DPP4, may be added as a supplement for some relief.

A note on wheat/bread/pasta products: The qualitative data overwhelmingly demonstrates that many people who cannot tolerate pasta and bread in the U.S. are able to eat it freely in other countries. One hypothesis for this is attributing it to the U.S. having a much higher percentage of gluten in its products than those sourced overseas. Another potential and probable cause is the use of glyphosate, which is a herbicide used on genetically modified organisms (GMOs). The U.S. does allow GMOs, while European countries are known to be more proactive at regulating and stopping their use; thus, they do not use the herbicide as much. Another possible explanation is genetic variations in the population, but that does not account for those who move overseas and note the dramatic change in their health despite not changing the amount of food they eat.[125]

Short-chain fatty acids (SCFAs)

SCFAs also play a crucial role in our overall health. These are produced by gut bacteria breaking down food, and one of the beneficial SCFAs is butyrate. Butyrate plays a key role in immunoregulation and maintenance of tissue barrier function.[126] Butyrate is beneficial for reducing inflammation, protecting neurons, and fueling colonic cells, which account for nearly 70% of absorbed energy. Consequently, individuals low in butyrate may experience fatigue despite having normal thyroid levels.

Other SCFAs, such as propionate and acetate, are produced by other microbes and have fewer beneficial effects and, in larger amounts, have been associated with autistic-like symptoms and neurodegenerative diseases, including dementia.[115] Interestingly, these microbes tend to be higher in autistic populations. Studies have shown that injecting mice with propionic acid can induce autistic-like behavior in them.[127] While small amounts of this substance are essential for our health, excessive amounts are harmful to our neurological systems, and some scientists perceive this to be a significant window into understanding the development of autism.

Many people choose to be dairy-free, but it's essential to consider individual needs. Some people are intolerant to dairy, and in those cases, it is best to avoid it entirely. However, for those who do not experience inflammation from dairy based on their unique presentations, moderate consumption can actually be beneficial, and A2 milk is recommended.[128]

There are many conflicting studies when it comes to dairy, including raw versus commercial grade, inflammatory versus anti-inflammatory, and cancer-causing versus anti-cancer properties. Therefore, I find that it is important for the practitioner to do their own unbiased assessment of the literature and what is best for the individual. While some may tolerate milk well, others may react with diseases such as eczema.[129] It can be a great source of protein, probiotics, vitamin D, and calcium and has been found to be anti-inflammatory in hundreds of studies.[130]

Other Foods to Consider

Inflammatory foods, particularly ultra-processed and sugar-laden products, should also be considered. For instance, a study by the American

Academy of Neurology involving tens of thousands of people found that even a 10% increase in ultra-processed food consumption was linked to a 16% increase in cognitive decline.[131] While this study is neurologically based, its findings are powerful and do directly relate to gut health. Chemical-laden foods are additionally widely associated with triggering IBS, IBD, upset stomach, and are even connected as a root cause in gastrointestinal disease.

Many people follow the 20–80 rule, aiming to maintain 20% unhealthy habits and 80% healthy ones. However, even this level of unhealthy eating can lead to chronic health issues, necessitating the removal of ultra-processed foods from one's diet.

Food Sensitivities

In addition to gluten or dairy, each person may have their own personal food sensitivities. Other common sensitivities are to soy, nuts, and corn. Testing should be done to identify any underlying triggers. Also, please note that the specificity of these tests for IgG or IgA varies. An elimination diet that does not change more often than every six weeks to three months may be more difficult, but it will more accurately identify actual triggers. Genetic food testing is more reliable, but it does cost more.

Medications That Could Be Contributing to GI Disturbance

Some medications can contribute to gut dysbiosis. For example, nonsteroidal anti-inflammatory drugs (NSAIDs) can exacerbate gut issues and harm the lining in the gut.[132]

Similarly, proton pump inhibitors (PPIs), which reduce stomach acid to alleviate heartburn, can increase the risk of bacterial overgrowth and other gastrointestinal issues, including Clostridium difficile and H. pylori infections.[133] PPIs can additionally lead to various complications with long-term use, including renal disorders, dementia, cardiovascular disease and events, myocardial infarction, and increased risk for fractures. There have been associations with even some cancers, including gastric, pancreatic, colorectal, and hepatic cancer.[134,135]

Lastly, besides the acid in our stomachs protecting us from bacterial overgrowth, it helps break down food so we can absorb nutrients. Therefore, chronically decreasing stomach acid is detrimental to food being broken down and nutrients being fully absorbed. PPIs are also known to increase the risk for micronutrient deficiencies such as hypomagnesemia, anemia, vitamin B12 deficiency, hypocalcemia, and hypokalemia.

Thus, I often recommend discontinuing PPIs as a potential root cause when addressing these concerns in patients. By carefully removing these damaging elements, we can better support gut health and overall well-being.[135] For the functional clinician, long-term use of PPIs in a patient's history should alert you to numerous possible root causes of disease that you can begin to address—most notably gut dysbiosis (as a result of chronically low stomach acid) and micronutrient deficiencies.[134,135]

PRO TIP:

One effective method for helping people discontinue PPIs is to supplement magnesium levels and correct dysbiosis. PPIs diminish magnesium in the body, and low magnesium (hypomagnesemia) can increase the risk of heartburn. Chronically low stomach acid can also contribute to bacterial overgrowth that leads to heartburn symptoms. Some people may find themselves reliant on PPIs because of this cycle, which becomes a self-perpetuating medication dependence.

By increasing magnesium intake and correcting underlying dysbiosis, I have often helped such individuals discontinue PPIs.[136] Be diligent about monitoring magnesium levels during supplementation. Although extremely rare in oral supplementation, hypermagnesemia is associated with the potential to develop cardiac arrhythmias.[137] Always remain within your legal scope of practice, as only licensed medical professionals can recommend discontinuing PPIs or assist with weaning.

GI Intervention: The 5 R protocol

The 5R protocol is a widely accepted method for correcting underlying gastrointestinal issues. The 5 R's stand for remove, replace, reinoculate, repair, and rebalance. A comprehensive stool analysis should be guiding treatment in an individual, case-by-case plan.

1. **REMOVE**

The first step in the 5R approach is to remove any of the harmful factors identified above, as well as the treatment of bacterial overgrowth, yeast, pathogens (like H. pylori), or parasites. The proper supplement will be chosen based on stool analysis. When considering removing harmful microorganisms, these are broken down into four treatment categories:

- Antifungal agents used include caprylic acid, garlic oil, oil of oregano, and olive leaf extract. Typically taken three times a day, prior to each meal, though dosing and frequency may depend upon the supplement brand.
    - It should be noted that garlic oil, especially, has blood-thinning capabilities and should be used with extreme caution, or considered contraindicated, for those on blood thinners or at risk for bleeding.[138]
- Antiviral agents include olive leaf extract, purified silver, cat's claw, monolaurin, osha root (*Ligusticum porteri*), vitamin A, vitamin C, vitamin D, reishi mushrooms, *Echinacea*, and zinc.
- Antimicrobial/broad-spectrum herbs include berberine, caprylic acid, garlic oil, oil of oregano, uva ursi, and olive leaf extract. Typically taken three times a day, prior to each meal.
- Antiparasitic agents include black walnut, garlic oil, oil of oregano, *Artemisia* (wormwood), berberine, goldenseal, gentian root extract, quassia bark extract, and citrus seed extract.

Typically, the client will stay in this phase of treatment for six weeks to three months, depending on their response. Clients will also be removing trigger foods, sugar, and most likely gluten during this phase.

It is also very important to note that during this phase, the client may experience a Herxheimer reaction, where they feel "flu-like" symptoms from the die-off phase. If someone is autoimmune, or the reaction is too much to handle, the dose or frequency may need to be decreased. It is also always a good idea to add a binder in this phase, such as activated charcoal, to decrease the severity of a potential Herxheimer reaction. Glutathione, light exercise, lymphatic drainage, and Epsom salt baths can help alleviate symptoms. While the occurrence can be quite uncomfortable, it tends to be limited to a few days. If symptoms become severe, intolerable, or last more than a few to several days, consider a diagnosis of something more serious or lowering or discontinuing treatment.[139]

2. **REPLACE**

The second step most often involves the replacement of a lacking healthy microbiome, enzymes, pH, or micronutrients, like vitamin D or C. This needs to be a personalized plan based on stool analysis and other testing.

- Enzymes like protease, lipase, and amylase may need to be supplemented to help individuals break down their food and absorb nutrients effectively.[140] These enzymes include betaine hydrochloride, apple cider vinegar, herbal bitters, ox bile, lactase, pancreatic enzymes (amylase, lipase, protease), or pepsin.
    - These are taken prior to meals (and should be started with the "REMOVE" supplements of step 1) to help the body break down biofilm and allow the antimicrobials to take better effect.
- If nutrients need to be replaced, they may not be absorbed well until after the process is complete, so be patient in retesting.
- When stomach acid levels are low (a condition called hypochlorhydria), we can replace it with betaine HCL.[141]

Hypochlorhydria: Low Stomach Acid

Initially, I found it surprising when a patient mentioned using pickle juice for heartburn. My thought was that heartburn typically results from too much stomach acid, so their testimony did not make sense. However, I later learned that heartburn can occur when the lower esophageal sphincter doesn't close properly due to stomach acid levels being too low, leading to acid reflux into the esophagus. Antacids will occasionally help in the short term. As the acid refluxes into the esophagus, it becomes basic enough to no longer cause a burning sensation, but the reflux is quietly occurring.

To determine if a client is in need of betaine HCL replacement, the practitioner can order a Heidelberg pH test. This involves swallowing a capsule that measures pH levels.[141] The proper pH level of the stomach is important for many reasons. Such examples include keeping opportunistic gastric infections at bay and preventing SIBO or dysbiosis, as well as being necessary for the proper absorption of nutrients, such as vitamin B12.[142]

3. REINOCULATE

The third step is reinoculation, which focuses heavily on the gut microbiome. This is a vital part of treatment for conditions like IBS or SIBO. However, reinoculation isn't limited to gut health. For instance, in treating eczema, it may be necessary to reintroduce microbiome elements to the skin using topical products.

Probiotics such as *Lactobacilli, Bifidobacteria,* and spore-based strains are common choices. It's crucial to ensure that any probiotic used can survive gastric acid and reach the small intestine intact, so selecting a reputable brand is important.

Prebiotics are crucial for supporting gut health. These are the fibers and polyphenols that nourish beneficial bacteria. While it's important to reintroduce probiotics into the body, without providing prebiotics for them to thrive, they won't last long.[143]

Another vital aspect to consider is fermented foods, which may not be suitable for everyone. Some people may find that fermented foods cause gas, bloating, or discomfort. In such cases, it's best to avoid these foods until underlying issues, such as small intestinal bacterial overgrowth, are addressed. Excessive gas and bloating following the consumption of foods like beans or fermented products often indicate that there may be an imbalance of bacteria in the small intestine and should alert the clinician to SIBO (which we will discuss later).

Our focus here is to promote a healthy microbiome and support immune function. It's interesting to note that the Bible suggests we were given all the foods of the world to nourish our bodies, yet many of us limit ourselves to just a few options (Genesis 1:29). Eating a diverse diet, often referred to as "eating from the rainbow," is a smart strategy. Aim to include various colors in the nutrition plans—not just for calories, but to ensure a rich variety of probiotics and prebiotics. Studies have shown that diets rich in diverse probiotics and prebiotics correlate with better overall health and lower disease rates.

4. **REPAIR**

The next step is to focus on repair. Our goal is to restore the integrity of the intestinal lining and reduce excessive immune responses. This includes healing the gut lining and the body as a whole, which is essential for reducing inflammation. Several nutrients can support gut health: L-glutamine, zinc carnosine, aloe vera, quercetin (which also assists mitochondrial health), omega-3 fatty acids, as well as slippery elm or licorice. However, caution is necessary with licorice, as it should be DGL (deglycyrrhizinated licorice). This version contains the beneficial properties of licorice without the glycyrrhizin compound that can lead to side effects, such as increased blood pressure. It's still important to monitor patients closely, especially those with existing hypertension.

5. **REBALANCE**

The fifth step is to achieve balance. This step involves looking at various aspects of health to ensure that everything remains regulated.

The focus here is on stress levels, the HPA axis, sleep quality, physical activity, and emotional and spiritual well-being. Many people overlook the importance of avoiding unhealthy levels of stress and incorporating physical activity, but it is a key component of any health plan and a common reason for relapse and treatment failure.

While supplements do not tend to carry high risk, they are not without potential side effects, and drug-herb interactions are a real risk. Do not assume just because an herb or supplement is natural that it cannot do harm, especially when prescription medications are on board. The NIH does have a small database you can access for free.

One of the riskiest medications with any herbs is warfarin. If the client is on warfarin, you must involve the provider managing the medication in the plan of care, and complete contraindications may stop treatment altogether. Other medications with higher risk include several cardiac meds and oral contraceptives. You can start some of your research here by scanning the QR code:

SCAN ME

Specific Disease Processes

The 5R approach is the mainstay for GI treatment. However, there are some caveats to the application of specific disease processes that will now be examined in more depth.

Irritable Bowel Syndrome (IBS)

When dealing with IBS from a functional medicine perspective, we recognize it as primarily a dysbiosis or parasitic infection, and once corrected, it can most often resolve. However, it tends to have rates of relapse, possibly because of the "memory" of the gastrointestinal microbiome, discussed earlier.[144]

IBS is characterized by symptoms such as abdominal pain, bloating, constipation, diarrhea, or alternating constipation and diarrhea, and they are often recognized as nonspecific. Conventionally, IBS is diagnosed as a condition of exclusion, but functional medicine seeks to uncover the underlying causes of these symptoms. It is important to note that it is often due to a mixture of many root causes, possibly even some of the causes we discussed prior to this in the general GI discussion.

Food Sensitivity as a Root Cause

Food sensitivity is a possible underlying cause of IBS that can be identified by testing or elimination diets. Limitations were discussed in Chapter 2 and earlier in this chapter. A low-FODMAP (fermentable oligosaccharides, disaccharides, monosaccharides, and polyols) diet is the most commonly tolerated diet for IBS and eliminates the most common triggers, though it may not be perfect for every client.[145] This diet eliminates most dairy, many fruits, some vegetables, wheat products, beans and legumes, and most sweeteners. Monash is a great app to reference for specifics.

Trigger foods, as well as chemicals like MSG, should be eliminated for at least six months while treatment of the 5R process is underway. Seed oils are another very common trigger for IBS and should be avoided. It is also important to be careful about seasonings, as some can trigger IBS as well. This is where a food diary to identify such details can help, as most individuals differ in their triggers. Oftentimes, clients can reintroduce some of the foods that they once reacted to after healing has taken place, but they should always be cautious about this and aim to never reintroduce chemicals, sugars, or processed foods that are not of benefit, as this can trigger a relapse in both habits and disease state.

Infectious Disease as Root Cause

Post-infectious IBS is known to have an autoimmune etiology and is a common risk factor for IBS. Some bacterial and viral infections will directly inhibit the interstitial cells of Cajal (ICC) in the intestine to stop regulating the migrating motor complex (MMC). ICCs are necessary for regular peristalsis.[146] This is particularly common in SIBO, a later topic. When these are stunted, it leads to constipation dominance. Ginger, effectively chewing food, vagus nerve stimulation, and stress management can help stimulate ICCs.

Post-infectious gut dysbiosis is particularly common among patients who have had COVID-19. Chronic diarrhea from dysbiosis following COVID often goes undiagnosed for years. By addressing the imbalances in gut bacteria, we often find that patients' diarrhea or constipation resolves. It's also important to regulate the immune system, especially in cases related to COVID-19, due to the effects of spike proteins and the immune overreactions they provoke. This imbalance is frequently a primary factor in their symptoms.[147]

Psychosocial Triggers as a Root Cause

Gut-brain axis dysfunction can also contribute to IBS flare-ups, influenced by trauma, stress, and vagal tone issues. However, it's essential to recognize that when the right psychobiotics are not inoculated in the intestine, the gut can also trigger mood disorders or hormonal disruption and exacerbate the entire cycle. This is where a program that identifies and aids in the full treatment is essential.

Prescriptions

Rifaximin (prescription only) is a prescription treatment found to be effective for the treatment of IBS-D (diarrhea-dominant) under the functional medicine model.[148] It is one of the few prescriptions I have utilized as a functional practitioner. When pathogenic bacteria levels are severely elevated, other prescription antibiotics may also be necessary, though most times medicinal levels of herbals are just as effective and better for the overall microbiome. This should be decided on a case-by-case basis.

After the pathogenic or overgrown bacteria are eliminated, retesting is best practice, as it is imperative to start with replacing the good microbiome that was found to be deficient (if found to be deficient) and move on to healing the gut mucosa with supplements such as aloe vera, L-glutamine, and vitamin D (if deficient).[149]

Small Intestinal Bacterial Overgrowth (SIBO)

SIBO is a gastrointestinal disease characterized by the excessive colonization of the small intestine by microorganisms such as anaerobic bacteria and archaea. It accounts for a majority of IBS cases. This overgrowth leads to symptoms such as gas, bloating, constipation (occasionally diarrhea), and gastrointestinal pain.[150] The disease can cause systemic inflammation and neurodegeneration that can lead to symptoms of fatigue and joint pain.[151] The presence of bacteria and archaea that should not be in the small intestine leads to premature food breakdown, resulting in bloating and pain with fibrous food, which is why caution is used to not reintroduce high-fiber foods too soon.

Many clients will have undergone endoscopy but remain undiagnosed, as this disease is found most specifically via breath testing. The SIBO breath test is the gold standard for diagnosis.

Etiology of SIBO

High-carbohydrate diets, antibiotic use, and other factors (similar to those in IBS) can contribute to an increased risk of SIBO. It is common to find that individuals with SIBO have frequently used proton pump inhibitors (PPIs) or antacids for an extended period. The low pH levels of the stomach lead to inadequate food breakdown, further exacerbating intestinal permeability and increasing symptoms. This, in turn, keeps the client reliant on PPIs or antacids. Other risk factors include opiate use, celiac disease, vitamin D deficiency, or pathophysiology that slows gut motility, allowing the overgrowth to commence, such as slow motility seen with diseases like multiple sclerosis.[152]

SIBO Classifications & Specific Treatment Plans

There are three main types of SIBO. The treatment for all three will remain uniform, with the exception of the antimicrobial agents chosen. All treatment plans should start with a biofilm disruptor such as serrapeptase, Lauricidin, garlic, or a combination supplement such as Biofilm Defense or Biocidin. Also, either during or right after antimicrobials are started, it is recommended to start a binder, such as activated charcoal, to help capture toxins in the die-off phase (during the REMOVE phase) of the treatment plan to avoid severe Herxheimer reactions. The three types of SIBO are as follows:

1. Hydrogen-Dominant SIBO: This type shows a rise in hydrogen levels greater than 20 parts per million (ppm) over baseline within 90 to 120 minutes. The most common culprits are hydrogen-producing bacteria, such as E. coli or Klebsiella. Symptoms typically include diarrhea (IBS-D), bloating, abdominal pain, and urgency. Treatment varies by patient but often includes neem, berberine, oregano oil, or a combination of any if resistance is an issue. Bismuth is another option to add as needed, if it is right for the individual patient. These are broad-spectrum and cover most pathogens. In IBS-C, it's important to add prokinetic agents to enhance gut motility and reduce recurrence.[153] The rest

of the 5R protocol should be used to continue effective treatment for all three types of SIBO. In treating the different types of SIBO, the plan stays mostly the same, with the exception that the antimicrobial herbs chosen will change based on the microbes present.

2. Methane-Dominant SIBO: The breath test for this type will show methane levels greater than or equal to 10 ppm at any point, possibly with an early peak. The primary microbial culprits are archaea, specifically *Methanobrevibacter inestini sp*. This type of SIBO tends to result in constipation-dominant IBS, characterized by hard, pellet-like stools, straining, bloating, and slow transit times by paralyzing the interstitial cells of Cajal.

It's important to note that archaea consume hydrogen to produce methane, which may suppress hydrogen levels and lead to false-negative results for bacterial overgrowth if methane isn't measured. Methane gas slows gastrointestinal motility, contributing to constipation and perpetuating the issue.[154]

Treatment may include allicin, derived from garlic, due to its effectiveness against archaea, often in combination with berberine. I say to myself, *Allison does meth,* to remember that methane-dominant is the SIBO most commonly responsive to allicin. In this memory hack, Allison represents allicin (a garlic derivative), and Meth represents methane dominance. Sorry to any Allisons who are reading this. It is nothing personal, of course. A longer treatment duration of up to four to six weeks may be necessary, and prokinetic support is crucial post-treatment, which may involve motility supplements or ginger.

3. Hydrogen Sulfide SIBO: This type typically results in a flat line on traditional hydrogen-methane tests, with sulfate-reducing bacteria being the culprits. Symptoms include a rotten-egg gas smell, diarrhea, gas, bloating, and systemic inflammation.[155] Clinically, this type can sometimes be identified without a breath test due to its noticeable symptoms.

Advanced testing, such as TrioSmart, now includes hydrogen sulfide measurement. It's advisable to avoid sulfur-rich foods like garlic, onions, and cruciferous vegetables. Oregano, bismuth, or neem, alone or in combination with rifaximin, can be effective antimicrobial agents in hydrogen sulfide SIBO.

Increased Intestinal Permeability

Increased intestinal permeability (sometimes known as "leaky gut") occurs when the tight junction of the intestine becomes loose and allows an exchange outside of the intestinal lumen to occur. It's often a consequence of GI dysfunction such as IBS or SIBO, with impaired mucosal immunity typically manifesting as high zonulin and low sIgA revealed on testing. This causes gastrointestinal pain, bloating, and localized and systemic symptoms of illness. Particles of stool-like bacteria, toxins meant for clearance, and undigested food particles are able to escape into the bloodstream, contributing to illnesses such as rashes, chronic fatigue syndrome, asthma, allergies, fibromyalgia, acne, autoimmune disease, and even mental illness.[156]

Etiology

Increased intestinal permeability is often a result of other issues, such as IBS, Crohn's, or other gastrointestinal etiologies, but it can be a direct effect of certain exposures from diet or environment. When evaluating etiology, please also reference the section on dysbiosis earlier in this chapter and remember to rule out or eliminate the root causes identified there. Direct triggers include chemicals, such as MSG, gluten, dairy, and a diet high in omega-6 fatty acids and deficient in omega-3s. The proper ratio of omega-6 to 3 should be 1:1 or 1:4, but most American diets are closer to 10:1 or 20:1.

Omega-6 fatty acids in the American diet tend to be abundant, from the high amount in cooking oils like canola oil, rapeseed oil, and vegetable oils used for cooking and frying foods. Chicken is much higher in omega-6s than omega-3s, as is peanut butter. While omega-6s are not innately bad for us and are actually necessary, it comes back to the need for balance. The SAD tends to be low in omega-3s, which are found in fatty fish, like salmon, flaxseeds, chia seeds, walnuts, and grass-fed red meat.[157,158]

Interestingly, chicken is often viewed as healthy while red meat is demonized, despite the need for more omega-3s in most diets. This lends yet another insight into why a balanced diet should be prioritized over fad dieting. However, please note that moderation is still always key, as a diet very high in red meat also has its detriments, and if the animal is grain-fed, the ratio is no longer omega-3 dominant, but rather omega-6.[159]

Genetic variants, such as NOD2 and ATG16L1, can also be tested as a root cause, as they affect immune function and the body's ability to handle bacterial infections, leading to increased intestinal permeability. Additionally, toxic exposures, such as to mold or glyphosate—which is a pesticide found in non-organic foods—can provoke immune responses and contribute to dysregulation. Unresolved immunologic triggers may also play a role in immune dysregulation.

Lab testing

Key interventions and lab tests include a stool analysis, such as a GI Map. Zonulin testing is the definitive test for identifying hyperpermeability. The complete analysis will help us assess for associated pathogens, inflammation, dysbiosis, and sIgA, which gives insight into the immune response.

Recommended Diet

An anti-inflammatory, whole-food dietary plan is recommended and will often include an elimination diet to avoid triggers, some of which may even be unidentified. Other options include the Paleo diet and various autoimmune diets that are anti-inflammatory, such as the low-FODMAP diet. Our goal is to repair nutrients in the gut and address inflammation. Food sensitivity, whether from experience or testing, can also help guide the proper diet to recommend, keeping in mind the limitations previously discussed.

Treatment Protocol Structure

Phase 1: Remove (first 4-6 weeks)

The same treatment that you see in IBS or other etiologies to remove offending pathogens may be necessary—and please refer to those sections for proper treatment to remove any pathogens or triggers identified. These will be one or a mix of antimicrobials such as neem, oregano, allicin, berberine, bismuth, or rifaximin.

A gluten-free diet is often necessary for these people; in fact, I sometimes recommend it without testing based on the high rate of causation. If they test negative for gluten sensitivity, we can cautiously reintroduce it later, but removing it initially can help reduce body inflammation, possibly due to the decreased exposure to pesticides that are common in bread products.

Step 1 of Phase 1: Dietary Intervention

Beginning dietary modification helps to reduce fermentable substrates and symptom burden.

The most common diet to implement is the low-FODMAP protocol. Keep strictly to the diet for at least 3–8 weeks. The main goal is to avoid fructose, lactose, polyols, fructans, and high-fermentable carbohydrates. Consider a gradual transition in patients who struggle with dietary changes; while this will extend the treatment and delay results, it can improve adherence.

Elemental diets may be bought online and can be considered for refractory or severe cases. But they must be implemented under trained supervision. Another potential intervention is intermittent fasting (16 hours fasting: 8-hour window to eat is a common ratio), which may be used cautiously to support the migrating motor complex if clinically appropriate.

Step 2 of Phase 1: Reduce Bacterial Overgrowth (2–4 weeks)

Herbal antimicrobial protocols can be selected based on symptom severity and tolerance. If tolerated, administering on an empty stomach 10 minutes before meals may improve efficacy.

- Oregano oil (enteric-coated): 150–200 mg twice daily
- berberine: 500 mg twice daily
- and/or allicin (garlic-derived): 450 mg once to twice daily are the most common choices to reduce overgrowth. It is important to avoid whole garlic during the high-FODMAP phase. This may seem contradictory, but it is because the fiber in garlic is not low FODMAP, despite the allicin in garlic being beneficial.

Prescription antibiotics should be used with caution, as they can disrupt the overall flora. However, Rifaximin (550 mg three times daily for 14 days, hydrogen-dominant SIBO)

and Neomycin for methane-dominant SIBO also has good effects.

Yeast or Fungal Overgrowth (Small Intestinal Fungal Overgrowth)

Another common issue is yeast overgrowth. If this is suspected or found on stool analysis, it is crucial to follow a yeast overgrowth protocol and avoid sugars and starchy foods such as potatoes. The low-FODMAP diet is particularly effective for managing yeast overgrowth, especially when organic acid or stool analyses suggest its presence.

Berberine, oregano oil, and caprylic acid are more natural antimicrobials that are effective in yeast overgrowth. Fluconazole is a prescription option that is faster and often covered by insurance.

Parasitic Infection

If comprehensive stool analysis reveals parasitic infection, black walnut hull, wormwood, cloves, garlic, pumpkin seed, papaya seed, neem, goldenseal, barberry, and Oregon grape all demonstrate antiparasitic properties. Many brands carry a blend of a few to several of these ingredients. There are several to choose from. Ensure the one chosen is third-party tested for efficacy, and avoid use in pregnancy.

Phase 2: Replace (next 4-6 weeks)

Replacing bile, digestive enzymes, nutrients, and stomach acid may also be a necessary part of treatment. Most clients will require digestive enzymes, and these are found in biofilm disruptors.

Low Stomach Acid

As discussed earlier, many people have developed dysbiosis as a result of chronically low stomach acid, whether medication-induced or not. In such cases, a pH string test can help identify if hypochlorhydria (low stomach acid) is present. This involves swallowing a capsule attached to a string and then pulling it out after ten minutes. The string is then tested with pH paper.[160]

A less sensitive method of testing is the baking soda test. Have the client mix one-quarter teaspoon of baking soda in a glass of water and drink it. If they burp within two to three minutes, they likely have normal stomach acid. If a burp is delayed by more than 3 minutes, hypochlorhydria should be considered. Betaine HCL with pepsin may also be taken for presumed hypochlorhydria. Have an antacid or baking soda on hand in case it worsens symptoms.

Patient history can also help evaluate whether treatment is necessary. For example, if a patient tells you that acidic foods like pickles help rather than hurt their heartburn and that antacids such as Tums do nothing for them, their symptoms are likely due to low stomach acid. In this scenario, the lower esophageal sphincter does not close sufficiently, and any level of acid in the esophagus will cause symptoms. Coffee drinkers are also prone to betaine deficiency and may benefit from its use, despite fears of increasing stomach acid levels.

Micronutrients

Micronutrient testing can help determine which nutrients need to be replaced. Deficiencies may be revealed through organic acids testing, NutrEval testing, or a thorough patient history.

For evaluating the need for digestive enzymes, start these in anyone with suspected or proven bacterial overgrowth, which can ultimately lead to the development of biofilm within the GI tract. I also recommend digestive enzymes if food particles are seen in stool or on specimens, or if the client belches easily while eating or demonstrates poor nutrient absorption as evidenced by low nutrient levels despite adequate intake. Liposomal glutathione is additionally often a necessary part of treatment.

Phase 3: Reinoculating (3 months to lifelong, depending on response and diet).

Targeted probiotic therapy will be based on the results of the stool analysis and microbial resistance screening. It's crucial to use spore-based probiotics, which can survive the stomach and reach the lower intestines. Additionally, mold and toxin assessment is vital for those for whom it is appropriate. Consider rotating probiotics as the client tolerates, if lifelong use is necessary.

Phase 4: Repairing (4-6 weeks)

L-glutamine is excellent for reducing inflammation and healing hyper-permeability, while zinc carnosine and omega-3 fatty acids also play essential roles in sealing tight junctions in the gut lining. Butyrate levels tend to be low in many people with leaky gut, so supplementing with it can often be beneficial.[161,162] Other options include slippery elm, marshmallow root, or turkey tail for mucosal and immune support.

Phase 5: Rebalancing (final 4-8 weeks)

We also emphasize the importance of nervous system regulation, particularly regarding stress and vagal tone dysfunction. Many providers focus solely on the physical body without considering mental and spiritual health. If nervous system regulation and mindset are overlooked, patients may experience ongoing anxiety, which can affect gut function by diverting the body's focus away from digestion. This ongoing anxiety contributes to gut issues, leading to inflammation that disrupts the immune system.

Mind-body therapies, such as cognitive behavioral therapy and breath-work, are essential for ensuring lasting results in clients. Mental stress triggers the body's fight-or-flight response, which diverts resources away from digestion, spikes cortisol levels, disrupts acid regulation in the stomach, and slows motility in the GI tract. This also increases the risk of intestinal permeability and worsening symptoms, especially those related to IBS.[163] Never forget that the gut-brain axis is a bidirectional highway.

Lastly, note the importance of rebalancing the right mindset for a healthy lifestyle. In my programs, I add and allow my students to resell my Mindset Academy. This is a full program dedicated to rebalancing mental mindset when it comes to lifestyle choices. I have found, from working with clients, that if you can help them to rewire their train of thought, you can help them make changes for life without "falling off the wagon."

Food's Effect on the Gut Lining

Good fats include real butter, cold-pressed olive oil (or olive oil used only at low or no heat), and avocado oil. It can be confusing when discussing the use of these oils, so let me clarify. Healthy fat sources, such as butter, almonds, and cashews, are all rich in monounsaturated fats. Olive oil is an excellent choice, but it's crucial to prioritize cold-pressed varieties and refrain from using it over high heat. Many people mistakenly cook with olive oil, thinking it's healthier; however, it has a low smoke point. This means it can quickly turn into toxic chemicals if overheated. Olive oil is best used in cold dishes, like salad dressings. For cooking at higher temperatures, avocado oil is a better option because it has a higher smoke point and is less likely to break down into harmful substances. Avoid margarine and any overheated oils. Margarine consists of chemical compounds and is not healthier than real butter.[164]

For those struggling to eliminate dairy, goat dairy or A2 milk can be beneficial. Both are easier to digest, providing good options for people who are gradually reducing dairy consumption.[165]

Artificial sweeteners can also disrupt gut health, so stevia is the preferred choice. However, it's important to use sweeteners like stevia in moderation, as we continually discover that many sweeteners, once considered safe, may be linked to health risks, including certain diseases and cancer.[166] When discussing sugar intake, it's essential to adhere to a low-sugar diet for gut health. Sugar is neurotoxic to the brain and a direct cause of inflammation in the gut. Therefore, minimizing sugar consumption is crucial for overall health.

While goals should include a diet completely devoid of processed table sugars, moderation is often implemented and key to getting started or even maintaining. Even then, most recommendations (such as those on labels) suggest a sugar limit that is still excessive even for those starting their health journey. I typically advise my clients to consume no more than 20 to 30 grams of sugar per day, trying to include naturally occurring sugars from fruits and honey and avoiding added sugars whenever possible.

Non-Alcoholic Fatty Liver Disease (NAFLD)

NAFLD is a condition where the liver has accumulated debilitating levels of lipids (steatosis) as a result of high intakes of sugar, trans or saturated fats, and refined carbohydrates.[167] Once a rare disease, its prevalence is increasing rapidly, even among children, with around 10% now affected.[4] Approximately 40% of the entire population is currently affected in America and Southeast Asia.[168] Sadly, this disease can cause cirrhosis, where liver cells die and cease to function. This can lead to symptoms similar to those seen in people with alcoholic cirrhosis, such as spontaneous bleeding, gas, bloating, and swelling in the abdomen, hands, and feet.

Functional Intervention

In interventions for fatty liver disease, the primary focus should be on weight loss (if needed), balancing insulin and glucose levels, and maintaining a high-protein, low-carbohydrate, no-chemical, healthy-fat-balance, fresh-vegetable diet. It is also important to avoid alcohol and limit or eliminate sugars. Supportive supplements may include betaine, NAC, vitamin E, magnesium, and probiotics.

Ulcerative Colitis and Crohn's Disease

Crohn's disease is an inflammatory bowel disease (IBD) that can lead to irreversible damage if not treated early. If someone is diagnosed with Crohn's disease, or it is suspected based on a positive fecal calprotectin level, it is highly recommended that they work with a specialist. The same is true for ulcerative colitis. Even if the client wants to forgo conventional treatment, as a thorough practitioner, you should always make the referral so that the client can get a full set of information and make their own informed decision—and document this discussion. This should be true of any diagnosis that is degenerative in nature. Patients may need to be on anti-autoimmune medication to prevent irreversible damage from IBD; however, the goal is to help re-regulate their immune system so they can eventually wean off or prevent medications altogether, if possible.

Crohn's can affect any part of the gastrointestinal tract, but it most commonly impacts the terminal ileum and colon. Unlike irritable bowel syndrome (IBS), Crohn's involves structured immune-mediated damage with transmural inflammation. This can lead to complications such as strictures, fistulas, and nutrient malabsorption. For instance, people with Crohn's may be unable to absorb vitamin D, even if corrected through supplementation. This resistance to treating low vitamin D levels can be a significant sign warranting screening for Crohn's disease.[167]

Ulcerative colitis is another form of autoimmune IBD, characterized by chronic inflammation and ulceration of the colon lining. It typically starts in the rectum and may extend proximally. Patients often present with symptoms such as bloody stools, urgency, and weight loss. Key areas to address for those with this diagnosis include re-regulating the immune system and examining the balance of commensal bacteria in their gut.

Labs and Diagnostics

Endoscopic findings in Crohn's disease typically reveal skip lesions, a cobblestone appearance, and ulcerations—all of which are absent in IBS. A biopsy is the gold standard for diagnosis in either disease. Occult stool will likely be positive, with gross rectal bleeding, or hematochezia, being common in UC and less common in Crohn's. Additionally, patients may present with anemia, hypoalbuminemia, and elevated white blood cell counts. Autoimmune and IBD panels are recommended, as are C-reactive protein (CRP) and erythrocyte sedimentation rate (ESR), which tend to be elevated. However, a negative result for either CRP or ESR does not rule out chronic inflammation. CBC or H&H is important to screen for anemia.

Functional labs include screening for gluten sensitivity, comprehensive stool analysis (such as a GI-MAP brand), organic acids testing, food sensitivity and allergy panels, and nutrient deficiency panels. Stool should include calcipotectin and lactoferrin. If the client is not yet diagnosed, these tests can provide 80% accuracy and would indicate referral if found to be indicative of IBD.

Root Causes

As both are immune-activated diseases, the root cause should be screened for anything that could be disrupting the immune system. Eliminating gluten is commonly necessary for these individuals since gluten is known to trigger autoimmune disease and be inflammatory in the intestinal lining. At times, this intervention alone may be sufficient for clients to see significant improvement. The next step is to address any imbalances in the gut microbiome, which may include chronic infections from pathogenic organisms, such as *E. coli* or even parasites.

It's worth noting that a negative stool analysis for parasites does not definitively rule them out. The stool sample may not have contained the parasitic infection at the time of testing. So, consider retesting for parasites depending on clinical significance. Biofilms often form with chronic dysbiosis and provide a barrier of protection for the overgrown pathogen.

Interventions

Elimination of all triggers known to induce immune-modulated disease should be initiated. A combination of autoimmune intervention and the 5R protocol should be implemented on a patient-by-patient basis. Treatment with IV immunoglobulin therapy has had some success in treating IBD. That includes an advanced modality not covered here, but it's worth researching or referring to a specialist who performs this. Oral immunoglobulin therapy is an alternative with some positive results. The idea is to decrease the impact of disease by reducing the inflammatory burden on the body, but remission is also a goal.

Mucosal barrier breakdown and increased intestinal permeability syndrome are common among these people and should be addressed accordingly, highlighting the need for agents such as glutamine and/or marshmallow root. They may also have low sIgA levels, indicating the need to remove triggers and repair immune function. Furthermore, sulfur-metabolizing bacterial overgrowth is often a concern, along with an imbalance in the omega-6 to omega-3 ratio, which creates a pro-inflammatory state. Similar to IBS treatment, a low-FODMAP or anti-inflammatory diet could be adopted with benefit, focusing on avoiding foods known to trigger symptoms. Lastly, emotional trauma and chronic stress are often contributing factors in the gut-brain connection and should therefore be adequately addressed.

Business Practice Pearl

One of the things that transformed my life and allowed my business to skyrocket was when I started investing in myself and buying back my time. There are two types of currency, time and money, and you will spend the one you value the least.

If you value your time on this earth (time with family and time doing things that align with your purpose and passion), then don't try to do it alone. King Solomon's journey in the Bible teaches us that he relied on his father and collaborated with elders, even though he was the richest and most successful man to ever live. Everyone needs help if they want to go the furthest they can in life. That is the power of investing to get from point A to point B more quickly, which helps us avoid lost revenue and wasted time. I invested in a coach, but I wish I had done it sooner. Once I did, everything became exponentially easier; I was more inspired and happier with my results. I didn't feel like I was spinning my wheels and burning myself out. So, I encourage you to invest in implementing this principle.

The next tip to save time is making sure you do your market research before you ever build anything out. I shared with you in the last chapter about how beta launches can help you do just that. However, there is a lot more to the research than that. You need to know what people are looking for, not just what they need. We already know you know what they need, but that is where practitioners fail at marketing.

In marketing, we often say, "Sell them what they want and give them what they need." This doesn't mean bait and switch. For example, when I'm potty training my child, I don't try to sell him on the idea of using the potty outright since he isn't initially interested. Instead, I incentivize him with stickers. While he may not want to use the potty, he does want the stickers. I use that desire to guide him toward what he ultimately needs. It's not a trick. He receives both outcomes, but I incentivize based on what I know he wants. We teach various methods for discovering what people want within the program, and we'll cover that in a different practice session.

Let's use a real-time example of this in the thyroid niche. Yes, people want to treat their thyroid and their symptoms to resolve, but that isn't what they really want. They want their hair to stop thinning, but they care about it because they don't want to be embarrassed in public and look more aged than they are. See the difference? Yes, they want to lose weight, but what they really want is to stop having to hide in pictures or fear the random candid picture on social media that "exposes" their struggles.

You can go even further here and talk about how they feel like a failure at trying to stay at a healthy weight when comparing themselves to others. Their deep desire is not to feel like they are failing themselves.

I hope you see the subtle yet powerful difference here. One way to learn this positioning is by learning from clinicians, like myself, who have already worked with hundreds of clients and already know these trends. The other way is putting in the time and speaking with hundreds of people yourself. Both are great, but the former is a shortcut that takes out the guesswork.

In the next chapter, we will discuss how much to charge. I want to preface that by reminding you that your knowledge of health gives your clients the peace of mind that comes from knowing they are taking control of their health. That is priceless, so as you go through the next chapter, really consider: what payment would you accept to be sick, lose your memory or time with family on this earth, or live day to day in pain or suffering?

I have asked myself, *What amount of money would be worth it to me to take back my IBS and anxiety?* The answer is that no number is high enough. If you told me that I would get to trade bank accounts with the richest women on the planet, but I had to go back to a life of IBS and anxiety and could never heal from it, I would not take it. What good are things or money, or even time off, if you are miserable all the time?

The last thought on fortitude that I want to leave you with is this: If you feel bad at the thought of charging for helping to heal, do you *truly* value health? Do you truly value the temple? Is it more important than gold to you? If the answer is honestly yes, keep reading, friend.
Let's go.

BONUS TRAINING:

Gastrointestinal functional medicine.

SCAN ME

SCAN THE QR CODE

or visit functionalmedicineunlocked.com

Chapter 5

Functional Medicine Approach to Mental Health

The first thing we need to understand about mental illness is that it has multiple root causes; it is multifactorial. Traditional models tend to segment mental health conditions, categorizing them separately, such as ADHD, depression, anxiety, and bipolar disorder. However, research indicates significant overlap and shared mechanisms of causation among these conditions. This overlap extends to anxiety, depression, schizophrenia, bipolarism, and even to neurodegenerative diseases, such as Alzheimer's, autism, and Parkinson's disease.

CASE STUDY: WHEN VACATION BACKFIRES, THE CLIENT BECOMES THE LONG-TERM VACATION

A fifty-seven-year-old female presented with severe anxiety and depression for the last ten years. She said, "I didn't use to be this way," and was tearful during every visit. Despite her appreciation for our sessions, she dreaded leaving her home due to severe agoraphobia. In her youth, she described herself as rambunctious, excited, and fun to be around, but now fear had taken over her life, affecting her health and her relationship with her husband. Although he cared deeply for her, the stress of her condition was wearing on him, as she was frequently upset, scared, or anxious.

Prior to seeing me, she had consulted several providers, including psychiatrists, counselors, and therapists, but those traditional approaches had not helped. Remarkably, she did not have a significant family history of mental illness, which left her feeling isolated and unable to relate to others experiencing similar issues. Additionally, she had comorbidities, including hypothyroidism, hypertension, and prediabetes. She also reported symptoms such as "nervous diarrhea" and occasional constipation, and she experienced significant fatigue.

We traced the onset of her symptoms back to a vacation she took in Mexico, during which she experienced traveler's diarrhea. Though she took antibiotics and the diarrhea improved, that seemed to trigger the onset of further symptoms. A stool analysis revealed a parasite and severe dysbiosis in her gut that showed a depletion of healthy microbiome and an overgrowth of pathogens that she may have brought back with her and had been keeping with her this entire time.

To address her immediate symptoms and reduce her dependence on a high dose of benzodiazepines, I prescribed L-theanine. As I worked on correcting her gut health, I was also able to improve her mental health. During our last encounter, she stopped me in public to express gratitude for what I had done. Her husband also signaled his thanks, acknowledging his gratitude for his wife's strong improvement.

This experience illustrates that when we examine mental health, we must look beyond symptoms to consider the systems affecting the brain. In her case, her gastrointestinal health played a significant role in her mental health and nervous system.

Lab Testing

Testing for mental health will depend upon the client's evaluation and intake assessment. Here we will list some of the labs that are always considered to reveal the root cause of mental illness and why each may be considered.

- Functional nutrient testing: consider that with most clients, SAD is not conducive to mental wellness, and most people have deficiencies.
- Comprehensive stool analysis: Consider with most clients, even when GI issues are not consistent. The gut-brain axis plays a part in everyone's mental wellness.
- Organic acids testing: Consider for most. Quinolinic acid is standard and reveals neuroinflammation.
- Genetic testing for MTHFR/COMT: Consider for most, as 50% of the population is estimated to be affected.
- Inflammatory markers, such as CRP and ESR: Helpful, but non-specific
- Insulin resistance can cause irritability and anxious bursts as well and should be considered in the right population.
- Thyroid and sex hormones (DUTCH): difficulties in hormone absorption, production, or utilization can result in significant fatigue and depression.[169] This topic will be covered in Chapter 7. But do not forget the mental assessment for those at risk.
- Heavy Metal Testing: Screen those at high risk for exposure and those in geographical areas known for low lithium.

Now let's get into the different root causes that these tests are searching to uncover.

Root Causes of Mental Illness

This chapter could be a book in and of itself. As a matter of fact, we have a completely different board certification for functional mental health altogether. The root causes of mental health issues extend beyond just the brain. They involve hormonal changes, chronic inflammation, gut health, nutritional deficiencies, and toxicities. We will discuss each of these factors. Note that treatment plans related to each can vary widely based on individual needs.

Every health program, but especially every mental health program, should integrate mind, body, and soul. This holistic approach is vital because we often do not know where health challenges originate, and they can feel like an attack. Part of this struggle is spiritual in nature.

I like to explain this to my patients by comparing it to climbing a mountain. For someone suffering from anxiety and depression, each day can feel like an uphill battle. While some people may be better equipped to handle this journey, for others, it remains a significant challenge.

I used to struggle spiritually because of my anxiety and depression. I often wondered, *Why isn't God healing me?* I believed in Him and had faith, which I felt with a strong conviction. Despite this, I wasn't experiencing instant healing, which made me feel like a bad Christian. Through my journey, I discovered that when I let my physical health take a back seat in my priorities, my anxiety and depression worsened. It felt like I was trying to run up a hill while wearing heavy metal armor. Our bodies can block us from regulating the right neurotransmitters, which means our brains aren't getting what they need.

You can maintain a positive mindset and strive to regulate your spiritual health, but if your body isn't healthy, it's like trying to run uphill in an armored suit while someone else is running in workout clothes.

Both might reach the top eventually, but one will have a much tougher journey.

True healing comes when we consider the whole person and eliminate shame. I work with my clients in mental health to help them remove shame. Brené Brown eloquently explains the difference between guilt and shame: guilt is about feeling bad for something that was done, while shame induces feelings of being innately bad. I assist my patients in transitioning from shame to guilt, ultimately leading them to resolution. This involves helping them realize they are good people through cognitive behavioral therapy (CBT). This is an essential part of the programs I implement, though it's important for each practitioner to find what works best for them and their clients.

Mental health is a significant issue that is growing more and more critical, especially in America. The statistics on mental health disorders are deteriorating rapidly, with more than one in four people experiencing a diagnosable mental disorder each year. For women, the lifetime risk for Alzheimer's by age 55 is one in five, and for men, it's one in ten. If there's a family history, that risk increases dramatically—there's a 50% chance if one parent had Alzheimer's and nearly a 100% chance if both parents had it. Fortunately, we can often identify root causes and even prevent some issues, which makes prevention programs essential for the future. For those called to this work, starting a program focused on prevention would be incredibly valuable. Depression is currently ranked as the third leading global burden by the World Health Organization and is projected to become the number one burden by 2030. The situation is worsening, and it's important to look at societal factors contributing to this trend.

Societal Root Causes of Mental Illness

Mental health issues have societal influences that directly affect self-esteem and self-worth through constant exposure to media such as social media websites that automatically trigger comparison and influence, especially among children and young adults. However, there are additional physiological phenomena that result from this exposure. To begin, blue lights emitted from screens are known to increase anxiety.[169] These lights are not natural to the eye and are focused amounts that are known to suppress melatonin production. This leads to sleep disturbances, hormonal imbalances, and even exacerbation of depressive symptoms and ADHD.[170]

Additionally, when we use phones specifically, the size and distance from our faces when held naturally cause our eyes to converge, triggering our brains to produce more cortisol, which prepares us to focus. Additionally the blue, short-wavelength lights further contribute to suppress melatonin and elevate cortisol further. [171] Extended time frames of elevated cortisol levels lead to increased agitation. This is one reason some report feeling ill after prolonged periods of social media scrolling. It has an impact on our physiological systems, not just our mental health, in the "comparison game." There is a direct correlation between time spent on social media and depression for many reasons.[172]

One unnatural phenomenon of social scrolling is the feeling of "doing" a lot while actually sitting still, giving a perception of being worn out when the body has not been in motion at all. Another is the high rate of comparison to others, which leads to feelings of inadequacy. We are witnessing record spending on mental illness and chronic conditions that are largely preventable. It has been noted that 80% of certain diseases are preventable, including mental illness, yet we continue to see high rates.

Children's mental health has deteriorated significantly over the past decade, with a 63.5% increase in the number of kids requiring psychiatric treatment.[173] Autism diagnoses have increased over 312% since 2000, with studies indicating that 1 in 31 children now falls on the autism spectrum.[174] While it is true that our screening processes have become more precise and we are better at identification, these rates are, nonetheless, alarmingly high. Additionally, 40% of children report experiencing persistent sadness or hopelessness, and 27% have seriously contemplated suicide—this is more than 1 in 4 children.[175]

We also need to look at work-related stress. There is a common misconception that the problem lies solely in the hours worked. However, it's actually the lack of a sense of purpose or impact that many people feel, which is increasing rates of depression and anxiety. Wasting time and lack of purpose are not natural to our creation. In the past, people worked even longer hours but often found greater meaning in their work. Today, many feel stuck in roles that seem ancillary and devoid of purpose, which can lead to depression and anxiety.[176] This is exactly the experience that I see many in the health care field facing when they feel they spend more time doing charts than actually helping people heal. I can say from experience that it is a real challenge and one of the main reasons that I decided I had to leave the conventional model of care and employment.

The movement of people affirming themselves to be whatever or however they want does not appear to be helping the mental health crisis. The simple truth is that self-validation exists in a vacuum, which demonstrates how it eventually collapses upon itself. A lack of purpose beyond self-validation is ultimately detrimental because it narrows our focus to our own desires and disconnects us from contributing meaningfully to society. When life becomes only about "me and my desires," we lose depth, purpose, and meaning. Over time, this inward focus renders us unnecessary to the collective, and the practice slowly fails to validate the very person it set out to affirm.

In Matthew 16:25, it reads, *"For whoever wants to save their life will lose it, but whoever loses their life for me will find it."* In Acts 17:28, it reads, *"For in Him we live and move and have our being."* God is love. Jesus is sacrifice. Therefore, following these scriptures has a much deeper meaning.

However, it is no surprise to me that an argument against Christian theology is that it is centered around a "selfish" God. When in fact, that command is there to serve us, if we look from a strictly scientific, psychological standpoint, because we benefit just as much as anyone else.

Psychological Root Causes

Trauma is another crucial area to explore. Most understand the significance of big "T" trauma, which includes severe forms of abuse, whether sexual, physical, or emotional, as well as the death of a loved one. However, what many practitioners may not realize is that little "T" trauma, subtle psychological wounds, can be equally, if not more, impactful.

When we experience big "T" trauma, we often find ways to process and rationalize it, allowing us to move on. In contrast, little "T" trauma, such as being told as a child that you are "getting a little chunky" or that you are "lazy," can resonate deeply with our self-identity and values and cause lasting harm. It may be essential to focus on these subtle experiences when helping clients, as they can be significant impediments to healing. In my practice, I find CBT to be most helpful in addressing these issues. However, there are other techniques that a practitioner may choose to implement, including referrals to other professionals.

Geography also plays a crucial role in mental health. Geographic location affects school quality, social interactions, and access to resources, all of which contribute to health disparities, as well as nutrients and chemicals in the water supply. For example, locations with low levels of lithium in the environment have been associated with increased rates of suicide. These are all factors to consider when implementing a holistic intervention.

The Role of Inflammation on Mental Health

About 30% of patients do not find relief from standard mental health medications.[177] Inflammation is suspected to be the common denominator for this. Within the conventional medical model, it is recognized that inflammation contributes to this lack of effectiveness. However, the conventional approach often overlooks the root causes of that inflammation. It's important to understand that inflammation itself can heighten the risk of anxiety and depression. Every one-point elevation in CRP (C-reactive protein) over 3, a marker of inflammation, corresponds to a 2.02 times increased risk for these conditions.[178] Keep in mind that CRP may not always be elevated, even when chronic inflammation is present, but either way, it is an interesting piece of data that may very well be opening an underlying connection long overlooked.

SSRIs and related drugs may marginally reduce inflammation; this is not their primary function. However, some studies are exploring whether these mild anti-inflammatory properties of SSRIs may be playing a significant role in alleviating anxiety and depression.[179]

These suggestions make sense, as brain function being aggravated leads to microglial activation in the brain. This leads to inflammation and the release of inflammatory chemicals, such as cytokines, which decrease serotonin by activating indoleamine 2,3-dioxygenase (IDO). This, in turn, breaks down tryptophan—and, therefore, serotonin and melatonin.[180] One way that has been found to effectively decrease this inflammation and have a direct effect on mental health is supplementation with omega-3 fatty acids.[169]

One tool to assess the presence of neuroinflammation is testing for increased quinolinic acid. Elevated quinolinic acid increases glutamate, which is neuroinflammatory and a direct marker of the condition. This test is a part of the organic acids test.[181]

Inflammation from other sources also plays a significant role in anxiety and depression. Cytokines such as IL-6 and tumor necrosis factor (TNF) alpha are known to be elevated in people suffering from anxiety and depression, alluding to an underlying connection.[182] Whether the depressive states cause the inflammatory markers is unclear, but it is clear that inflammatory cascades worsen the situation by reducing serotonin and melatonin levels, which are crucial for sleep and mental health.[180] Neuroinflammation can be screened for by testing for quinolinic acid levels on organic acid tests.

Epigenetics

Epigenetics refers to how our genes are expressed; while our DNA remains unchanged, the way our body responds to environmental factors can vary. Studies show that 80% of health outcomes are influenced by lifestyle and environmental factors, with only 20% being purely genetic.[183] This suggests that one's genetic makeup does not determine one's destiny. While genetics may hold the gun, lifestyle loads it.

Adverse life events can additionally alter gene expression over time and even lead to transgenerational epigenetic inheritance. This concept is interesting from both a scientific perspective and a biblical standpoint, considering the notion of generational curses and blessings discussed in the Bible. It stands to reason that experiences in one person's life can impact future generations, as we often see with cycles of trauma and abuse; thus, epigenetics could play a role in these patterns.

In my approach with patients, I address the mind, body, and spirit. I assist with reframing the mental aspects through cognitive behavioral therapy, then continue by addressing both the physical and spiritual roots of health. Specifically, I focus on gut health and systemic well-being, along with spiritual health through faith and wholeness. This holistic approach is crucial in mental health because research shows that happier people often feel a sense of purpose in their lives. Scientifically, we know that those who are deeply rooted in their purpose have improved outcomes of happiness.[184]

When people prioritize spiritual health, they tend to experience a stronger sense of purpose. I believe this is no coincidence; our bodies are designed in such a way that this interconnection is intentional. I believe that the Lord wants us to co-create with Him and find purpose in our lives. There's a clear link: people who have purpose also tend to be happier, and this reflects God's desire for us to experience joy and abundance.

In my personal journey, I initially focused on treating my IBS without realizing it would help alleviate my anxiety and depression. When I corrected my gut health, I felt a profound sense of freedom. I noticed that whenever my gut became unbalanced, leading to pain, gas, and bloating, I also felt depressed and irritated. This experience felt distinct from other types of pain, like injuring my knee, highlighting the different impacts gut health can have on our mental state.

Functional medicine is amazing because it often resolves multiple issues simultaneously. For example, treating an autoimmune condition can lead to improvements in other areas, including pain. It's what I call the ultimate leverage in health.

I genuinely enjoy helping my patients with all of their health concerns, including those they might not even be aware of. Often, even while we are still working towards a primary goal, I remind them of the improvements they've made—such as increased energy or improved mood—even if the primary issue, like resistant weight loss, is still progressing slowly. By focusing on the overall picture rather than just isolated concerns, we can leverage health improvements more effectively. That's why I believe functional medicine offers profound leverage for health. Patients often seek help for one issue, but as we address it, they experience improvement in other areas they didn't even mention (this is a clinical pearl to help your clients stick with the plan).

The Gut-Brain Connection

Okay, let's dive into a fascinating topic: the gut-brain connection! The basis for the gut-brain connection is the enteric (found in the abdomen) nervous system, the vagus, or tenth, cranial nerve, and the central nervous system (including the brain).

The vagus nerve is a major nerve that originates in the brainstem and extends down through the neck, chest, and abdomen. Everyone has one on each side of their body. It serves as a vital communication link between the brain and various organs in the body, including the heart, lungs, stomach, and intestines. It's involved in regulating numerous bodily functions, such as heart rate, digestion, and respiratory rate, and plays a key role in the parasympathetic nervous system, which is responsible for rest and digest responses. Additionally, the vagus nerve is involved in transmitting sensory information from the organs back to the brain, helping to maintain homeostasis and regulate bodily processes.

A significant number of people with anxiety and depression also experience gut dysbiosis, characterized by conditions such as IBS, Crohn's disease, or ulcerative colitis, which are linked to a history of mental health issues. Notably, around 90% of serotonin, a key neurotransmitter, is synthesized in the gut.[109] When dysbiosis occurs, the microorganisms responsible for producing neurotransmitters like serotonin, GABA, and dopamine can be disrupted, leading to imbalances in these neurotransmitters. Therefore, it's essential to assess gut health, even in patients who report normal digestive function. Stool analyses can often reveal surprising findings.

There is a troubling trend where mental health issues are on the rise, alongside an increase in prescription medications for mental health conditions.[185] This indicates that our current approaches may not be as effective as desired; ideally, we would see a decrease in medication use paired with improved mental health outcomes, but that isn't what we observe.

There's growing research on psychobiotics and probiotics and their effects on mental health, and their impact is becoming more and more evident.

For instance, Lactobacillus species, which are often lacking in the population, are known to produce 5-HT (a serotonin precursor) and help boost norepinephrine levels.[186] They also support gut diversity and lower cholesterol. Lactobacillus species are associated with the secretion of GABA, the body's calming neurotransmitter, and are involved in circadian rhythm regulation, insomnia, and antidepressant effects. This may explain why many individuals with insomnia also experience gut issues, such as IBS.

Sadly, despite this not being mainstream information, this research is nothing new, as studies date back to the 1940s. They discovered then that when scientists altered the microbiome of mice to be devoid of necessary microbiota, the mice developed higher levels of corticosteroids and exhibited fewer social behaviors and more repetitive behaviors, similar to those found in mood disorders, such as autism spectrum disorder (ASD). These mice became known as germ-free mice, and it was found that their symptoms, when induced under the controlled environment, were reversible with fecal transplantation that rebalanced the microbiome.[187]

This discussion becomes really fascinating as continued studies involving fecal transplants in animals have led to significant findings and similar results in humans. Researchers observed dramatic changes in behavior, coining the term "mood transplants." They took gut microbiomes (stool samples) from mice exhibiting autistic symptoms, anxiety, or depressive behaviors, such as social withdrawal and repetitive actions, and transplanted these samples into normally functioning mice. Remarkably, the transplanted mice began to display similar symptoms. The reverse was also found to be true.[187] This has been repeated several times.

As a matter of fact, a meta-analysis of twenty-one fecal microbiota transplant studies showed improvement in anxious and depressive symptoms. These studies all concluded that people with less anxiety tended to have higher levels of Firmicutes and lower levels of Bacteroides, similar to the trends that have been identified in obesity.[188] Other studies have demonstrated that simply starting a probiotic can have beneficial effects on depression.

These results provide strong evidence to support microbiome treatment as a viable option for the treatment of anxiety and depression. However, it must be noted that to maintain the benefits, the root cause of the dysbiosis likely needs to be identified. As a reminder, these causes can include, but are not limited to, the standard American diet (SAD), environmental toxins, pathogenic bacterial or viral infections, sedentary lifestyle, nutritional deficiencies, hypochlorhydria, chronic stress, or medications like antibiotics or PPIs.

Another factor that can result in imbalanced dopamine levels is an overgrowth of gram-negative bacteria that can inhibit dopamine beta hydroxylase, the enzyme responsible for breaking down dopamine, leading to its accumulation.[189] This excess dopamine can cause increased agitation, irritability, and even tremors.[190] This decreases the body's ability to form norepinephrine and epinephrine, as a portion of the dopamine in the body is supposed to be used for this formation, further exacerbating mental illness.[190]

We will dive back into the gut-brain connection in our chapter on neurodegenerative diseases.

The chart below further explains the psychobiotic effects of the microbiome.

Beneficial Psychobiotics (Non-Exhaustive)

Selected microorganisms with documented psychobiotic effects, natural dietary sources, and clinically relevant mechanisms.

Microbe	Natural Sources	Pathophysiological Effects	Psychobiotic Effect
Lactobacillus acidophilus	• Yogurt • Sauerkraut • Kefir	• Anti-inflammatory • Increases opioid and cannabinoid receptors • Significant prevention of *Campylobacter jejuni* pathogen that causes anxiety and gastroenteritis by preventing its adherence to the gut lining	• Reduces host inflammation and lowers levels of GSH and production of LPS (a major driver of immune dysregulation) • Decreases IBS severity and GI, colicky-like pain • Prevention of small intestinal bacterial overgrowth (SIBO)
L. rhamnosus	• 1 × 10^9 CFU	• Secretes GABA [3][5] • Stimulates HPA axis [3][5]	• Reduces depressive-like behaviors in postpartum women and obese individuals across several studies [3][4]
L. casei, L. brevis	• Italian cheeses • 1 × 10^9 CFU × 8 weeks • Fermented foods	• Secretes GABA [3][5] • Decreases cortisol stress response [5]	• Enhancement of sleep [1] • Decreases anxiety scores [5] • Decreases stress in placebo-controlled studies [3]
L. delbrueckii (bulgaricus)	• Yogurt • Kefir		
Bifidobacterium pseudo-catenulatum		• Decreases corticosterone • Increases 5-HT levels and hippocampal expression [5]	• Reverses diet-induced obesity (multiple studies) [3][5] • Alleviates depression-like symptoms in obese mice [5]

CFU = colony-forming units; GABA = gamma-aminobutyric acid; GSH = glutathione; HPA = hypothalamic-pituitary-adrenal; IBS = irritable bowel syndrome; LPS = lipopolysaccharide; SIBO = small intestinal bacterial overgrowth; 5-HT = serotonin. References in brackets correspond to source bibliography.

Beneficial Psychobiotics (Non-Exhaustive)

Selected microorganisms with documented psychobiotic effects, natural dietary sources, and clinically relevant mechanisms.

Microbe	Natural Sources	Pathophysiological Effects	Psychobiotic Effect
L. helveticus	• Yogurt • Kefir • 1×10^9 CFU	• Secretes 5-HT and signals CNS and serotonin receptors [2][3] • Secretion of norepinephrine [3][5]	• Circadian rhythm regulation; anti-depressive and memory-enhancing effects [3] • Many pharmaceuticals act via similar mechanisms • May be inhibitory or excitatory • Affects gastrointestinal transit, blood vessels, and platelets [3][5]
L. reuteri		• Prevention of TNF-α [3] • Decreases pro-inflammatory cytokines [3] • Decreases LPS, IL-6, and corticosterone [3] • Prevents inflammation-induced decrease in hippocampal BDNF *(B. infantis)* [3]	• Enhances mood and memory via BDNF upregulation in the hippocampus, similar in mechanism to ketamine and SSRIs [3] • Reduces risk of inflammation-related diseases • Reduces ASD-like behavior in mice [4]
L. plantarum	• 1×10^7 CFU	• Produces butyrate [3] • Regulates BDNF expression *(L. paracasei)* [3][5] • Reduces brain inflammation [3] • Decreases cytokine levels and corticosterone [3]	• Increases dopamine and serotonin levels [3] - significant decrease of anxiety and depressive behaviors in mice [3][5] • Strengthening of intestinal barrier [3]
L. paracasei	• Cheeses	• Lactic acid bacteria • Produces butyrate • Produces GABA [5]	• Decreases depression and improves cognition [3][5] • Cholesterol-lowering effects [3]
Faecalibacterium prausnitzii ATCC 27766	• 1×10^9 CFU	• Increases SCFA levels [3] • Normalization of CRP, IL-6, and cortisol/HPA axis [3]	• Prevention and therapeutic use in depression and anxiety [3]

ASD = autism spectrum disorder; BDNF = brain-derived neurotrophic factor; CFU = colony-forming units; CRP = C-reactive protein; GABA = gamma-aminobutyric acid; HPA = hypothalamic-pituitary-adrenal; IL-6 = interleukin-6; LPS = lipopolysaccharide; SCFA = short-chain fatty acids; SSRI = selective serotonin reuptake inhibitor; TNF-α = tumor necrosis factor-alpha; 5-HT = serotonin. References in brackets correspond to source bibliography.

Chart Resources:

1. Hoyer D. Targeting the 5-HT system: Potential side effects. Neuropharmacology. 2020 Nov 15;179:108233. doi: 10.1016/j.neuropharm.2020.108233. Epub 2020 Aug 14. PMID: 32805212.

2. Cortes-Altamirano JL, Olmos-Hernandez A, Jaime HB, Carrillo-Mora P, Bandala C, Reyes-Long S, Alfaro-Rodríguez A. Review: 5-HT1, 5-HT2, 5-HT3, and 5-HT7 Receptors and their Role in the Modulation of Pain Response in the Central Nervous System. Curr Neuropharmacol. 2018 Jan 30;16(2):210-221. doi: 10.2174/1570159X15666170911121027. PMID: 28901281; PMCID: PMC5883380.
3. Yong, S.J., Tong, T., Chew, J., Lim, W.L. Antidepressive Mechanisms of Probiotics and Their Therapeutic Potential. Frontiers in Neuroscience. Jan. 2020. Vol. (13) https://doi.org/10.3389/fnins.2019.01361
4. Yu CD, Xu QJ, Chang RB. Vagal sensory neurons and gut-brain signaling. Curr Opin Neurobiol. 2020 Jun;62:133-140. doi: 10.1016/j.conb.2020.03.006. Epub 2020 May 4. PMID: 32380360; PMCID: PMC7560965.
5. Del Toro-Barbosa M, Hurtado-Romero A, Garcia-Amezquita LE, García-Cayuela T. Psychobiotics: Mechanisms of Action, Evaluation Methods, and Effectiveness in Applications with Food Products. Nutrients. 2020 Dec 19;12(12):3896. doi: 10.3390/nu12123896. PMID: 33352789; PMCID: PMC7767237.

Gut-Brain Axis: Lipopolysaccharide (LPS)

Another significant factor in the relationship between gut health and mental or neurological health is LPS. This is particularly relevant for people with increased intestinal permeability, IBS, Crohn's disease, or ulcerative colitis. LPS is a byproduct of gram-negative bacteria that should not be present in our gut, as it can cause neurotoxic effects. Studies have shown that when mice are injected with LPS, they develop symptoms resembling Alzheimer's, Parkinson's, and autism.[191]

It's also worth noting that when these mice are injected with LPS but undergo a vagotomy where the vagus nerve is severed, the symptoms occur less frequently and in a lower percentage of the population. This highlights the significance of the vagus nerve and the bidirectional relationship between the gut and the brain.[192] Inflammation is a byproduct of this process, and it, too, plays a role in the exacerbation of symptoms.

Gut-Brain Axis & Gluten Intolerance

DPPIV is an enzyme in our body that is involved in breaking down certain peptides, including those derived from gluten and casein, which can act like opioid compounds in the brain. In some individuals, when DPPIV activity is low or impaired, these peptides may accumulate and interact with the nervous system, potentially disrupting normal neurotransmitter signaling. Testing can determine if someone is gluten intolerant (not celiac), which can be contributing to symptoms of anxiety, depression, and schizophrenia, such as cognitive fog, emotional instability, and sensory sensitivity.[193] Clinically, patients who crave high-carbohydrate foods and report a carb "high," often followed by a "crash," should be highly considered as having this intolerance.[194]

Additionally, DPPIV plays a role in immune regulation and inflammation—two processes increasingly recognized as critical in the development and persistence of psychiatric disorders.[195] Altered DPPIV activity has been observed in individuals with schizophrenia and mood disorders, suggesting that its dysfunction may create a biochemical environment that amplifies neuroinflammation, disrupts neurotransmitter balance, and heightens vulnerability to mental health symptoms. Therefore, intervention should include the removal of gluten from the client's diet. We will again discuss gluten intolerance in autoimmune disease and neurological disease.[195]

Nutritional Deficiency

Nutrition is often overlooked as simply something to worry about when the scale doesn't produce admirable numbers. However, what we put into our bodies (and leave out) is equally important to our mental health as the thoughts and life experiences we endure. Interestingly, from a functional medicine standpoint, lithium, magnesium, calcium, zinc, and copper deficiencies in the soil and water are all significant risk factors in the development of depression and bipolarism.[196] For example, in regions with lower lithium levels in the water, we see higher rates of suicide. Thus, addressing these deficiencies is a vital component in treating mental health issues.

If you recall, according to the American Neurological Association, a 2024 study found that a mere 10% increase in the consumption of processed foods corresponded to a 16% rise in cognitive decline risk, which is alarming. Even more disturbing is that about 67% of American children's diets consist of ultra-processed foods, which may partially explain the rising rates of anxiety and depression among them.[197]

Vitamin D Deficiency

Vitamin D is crucial for mental health. One study found that people who are deficient in vitamin D are 65% more likely to be depressed.[198] In functional medicine, we aim for optimal levels to be between 50 and 80 ng/mL. Some aim for numbers closer to or past 100 ng/mL. Conventional models often consider a level of 50 ng/mL to be sufficient, but maintaining levels closer to 80 ng/mL is beneficial, based on findings that optimal levels improve depression and other interconnected systems, such as the GI tract, the immune system, and hormonal balance. Vitamin D itself is a secosteroid (pro) hormone, lending to why we see a direct correlation between it and sex hormones and parathyroid hormones specifically.[199] Hormone dysregulation is additionally another root cause for mental illness and instability, discussed further in the hormones chapter.

Additionally, there is a direct correlation between increased susceptibility to IBS and lower-than-optimal levels of vitamin D[169], which affects the gut-brain connection and leads to further disruption of mental status. Numerous studies have linked vitamin D deficiency to depression and anxiety, making it essential to monitor and treat deficiency in the right clients. Kidney disease and hypercalcemia may be contraindications to high-dose replacement.

Magnesium Deficiency

Magnesium also plays a large role in mental health in several ways. It is a vital nutrient, and its deficiency (hypomagnesemia) can lead to anxiety and depression, as well as insomnia and increased constipation—all factors that can affect mental health both directly and indirectly.[201] Magnesium also supports GABA (gamma-aminobutyric acid), which is our main calming neurotransmitter. Therefore, a lack of magnesium can lead to insufficient GABA levels, decreased mood regulation, and insomnia. Additionally, GABA is produced in the gut, so if we don't have a healthy microbiome, we won't make enough of it either, leading to worsened symptoms. Last to note is that magnesium also aids in cortisol regulation, our primary stress hormone. Therefore, without adequate magnesium, we struggle with stress regulation.

Magnesium deficiency is another example of how interconnected our body systems are; we cannot separate them out into compartments that don't affect one another. Deficiency leads to mental ailments and additional symptoms, such as constipation and gastric upset, which exacerbate the original condition and lead to new ones. When we try to break the body up into compartments and ignore its interconnectedness, we see treatment resistance, medication dependence, and the rising incidence of comorbidities as we fail to resolve the root cause of disease. It then manifests into a six-foot trail of polypharmacy and side effects, which often could have been avoided.

Dosing can vary based on the individual. It's essential to monitor the patient while administering magnesium, preferably in glycinate or citrate forms. A typical dosage ranges from 125 to 300 milligrams, taken with meals or at bedtime. Some people may find it calming enough to induce sleepiness, so they might consider taking it an hour before bedtime. Additionally, monitor for any heart-related risks, ensuring that patients do not have underlying heart dysrhythmias.

In the realm of mental health, magnesium deficiency is a nutritional concern that should not be ignored. So, it's crucial to monitor magnesium levels as part of best practices in healthcare. Despite magnesium's amazing benefit profile, it is imperative to note that magnesium supplements do carry risk if used in the wrong population. For example, it can interact with certain antibiotics, diuretics, and bisphosphonates. As a careful practitioner, you need to be monitoring for such medications and educating your patients. Magnesium supplementation may also be an increased risk for patients with heart block, kidney disease, myasthenia gravis, or bleeding disorders.[202] It is also important to note that magnesium can be dangerous in excessive amounts, potentially causing fatal heart arrhythmias. Contraindications can include decreased renal function, pregnancy (class D contraindication), and neuromuscular disease. You must know a patient's renal function is within normal limits before starting magnesium.[203] While it's uncommon for oral magnesium to cause such issues, caution is still warranted.

Magnesium in neuromuscular patients can be detrimental because it can inhibit the release of acetylcholine, leading to muscular deterioration.[204] Another precaution with magnesium is being aware of how it affects calcium and potassium levels. Magnesium is necessary for the production and release of parathyroid hormone (PTH), which regulates our levels of calcium. This means that if magnesium is low, calcium may also be low, and when it is replaced, calcium may naturally increase as well. The same is true about potassium levels because magnesium is involved in the transportation of potassium in and out of the cell, and the kidneys will inadvertently urinate out potassium, leading to hypokalemia. This is why, if you are trying to replace potassium and it is not coming up, you should always check the magnesium level and screen for any hyperkalemia or hypercalcemia before giving magnesium.

Toxicity in hypermagnesemia is considered a magnesium level > 2.6 mg/dL, and electrocardiac changes can occur with levels > 6 mg/dL, including peaked T waves, widening QRS, and PR prolongation, indicating increased risk for cardiac arrest, especially if levels reach above 15 mg/dL. Those with renal failure are at the highest risk for this.[205]

Another important consideration is the quality of the magnesium you use. It's essential to select the right type. Magnesium oxide and citrate are both used for the treatment of constipation because of their osmotic and laxative properties. Magnesium sulfate, on the other hand, is preferred in the treatment and prevention of eclamptic seizures.[203] Magnesium glycinate and magnesium malate are the preferred forms when optimizing joint health or decreasing pain because of the relationship between magnesium and calcium levels and both of their effects on joint and bone health.[206] Magnesium glycinate is often preferred for insomnia, anxiety, and stress-related symptoms because of magnesium's role in regulating the hypothalamic–pituitary–adrenal (HPA) axis. Magnesium L-threonate has the special property that allows it to cross the blood-brain barrier. This further enhances brain magnesium levels to further support brain health and memory.

PRO TIP:

RBC magnesium testing and nutrient testing (instead of serum levels) are the preferred forms of testing for magnesium levels because serum magnesium levels may hide a deficiency, as the body may pull from the RBC to compensate for the serum levels.[201]

B12 Deficiency & Genetic Polymorphism

Vitamin B12 (cobalamin) plays a significant role in mental and neurological health. A deficiency in B12 can lead to feelings of depression and anxiety, and in severe cases, it may even manifest as symptoms similar to schizophrenia. This makes B12 a critical vitamin to focus on, particularly in individuals with genetic polymorphisms such as MTHFR, which impair the body's ability to methylate and process B12. This deficiency can further contribute to severe anxiety, fatigue, and depression.

In people with normal genetic variants, where the MTHFR polymorphism is not present, the MTHFR enzyme (methylenetetrahydrofolate reductase) converts folate into 5-MTHF (methylfolate). Methylfolate is then used in the methionine synthase reaction, where it donates a methyl group to cobalamin (B12), turning it into methylcobalamin (active B12). Methylcobalamin is now bioavailable to assist in converting homocysteine (which is inflammatory) into methionine (which is anti-inflammatory), except in the case of polymorphism or deficiency.

Methylfolate is also essential for the regeneration of tetrahydrobiopterin (BH4), a critical cofactor in neurotransmitter synthesis, as well as for the production of SAMe, the precursor for several vital processes such as DNA repair and the formation of red blood cells.

As demonstrated by the following diagram:

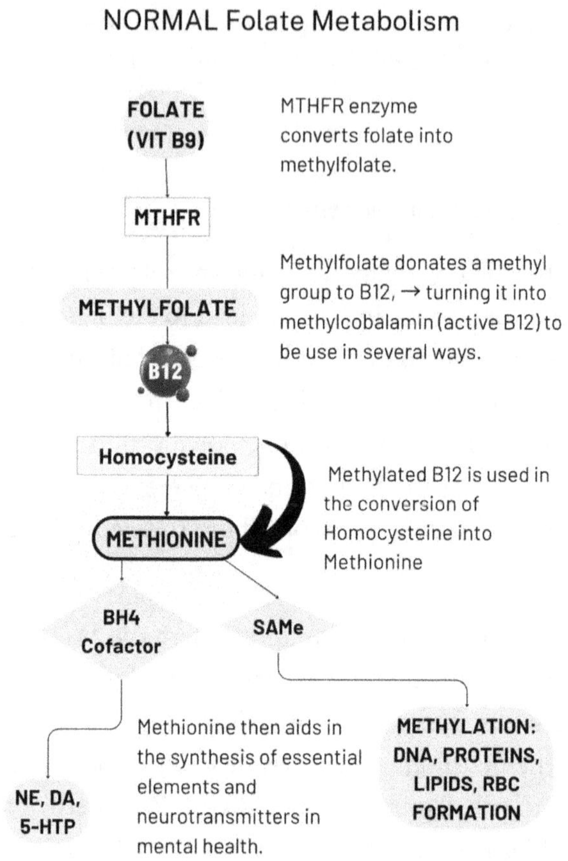

*NE = Norepinephrine; DA = Dopamine, and 5-HTP = the precursor to serotonin
(all important neurotransmitters in mental stability)

However, when a genetic polymorphism is present, the MTHFR enzyme (methylenetetrahydrofolate reductase) cannot efficiently convert folate into 5-MTHF (methylfolate). Depending on the genetic variant, this process is hindered by approximately 30 to 70%. As a result, methylfolate is unable to donate a methyl group to cobalamin (B12) to convert it into methylcobalamin (active B12).

This leads to a significant decrease in the amount of bioavailable B12 needed to convert homocysteine into methionine. Consequently, methionine levels drop and homocysteine levels rise. In addition, less methylfolate is available to support critical processes such as neurotransmitter production, resulting in further imbalance and potential mental health concerns.

This is demonstrated by the following diagram:

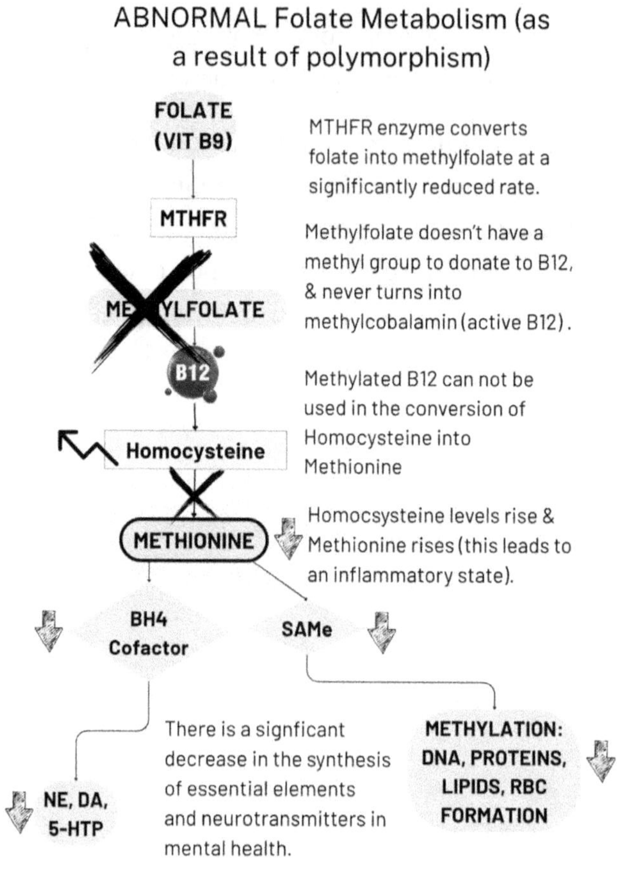

*NT = Neurotransmitter

Since B12 is water-soluble, there are not many studies on the concern for toxicity. To date, there is one case study I am aware of where a woman was given 12 mg daily, and she started to have palpitations and anxiety.[207] At any rate, vitamin B12 and methylation pathways are essential to consider. People with the MTHFR polymorphism struggle to convert B12 into its active methylated form. This deficiency hinders the regulation of B12 and can result in a lack of other cofactors needed for producing serotonin, dopamine, and methionine, which serve as anti-inflammatory markers in the body. Typically, homocysteine should be converted into methionine, but this process can be disrupted.

Whenever we lack methylated B12, it leads to high levels of homocysteine in the body, which can be inflammatory and increase the risk of mental health issues related to inflammation, decreased NT levels, and the effects of a lack of B12 on bodily functioning.

COMT (catechol-O-methyltransferase), another potential genetic polymorphism, plays a crucial role as it affects the body's ability to inactivate catecholamines, such as dopamine and norepinephrine, which stimulate brain activity. Excess dopamine can lead to irritation and agitation.

Niacin/Vitamin B3 Deficiency

Now, let's discuss niacin, or B3. It has historical significance, as its deficiency was discovered to cause pellagra, which posed severe mental and physical health risks resembling schizophrenia, eczema, chronic diarrhea, and even death.[208] It was discovered through dietary changes in prison populations, where symptoms, such as psychosis and eczema, resolved once prisoners were placed on a diet sufficient in the vitamin. This again illustrates how skipping out on a functional approach can lead to an abundance of issues and how the body cannot be broken down by diseases based on symptoms. Overall, this historical data emphasizes a common oversight in conventional medicine of how the focus of prescribing to treat symptoms evades our ability to think in terms of systems.

B3 additionally plays a role in regulating dopamine and helps detoxify metals and other toxins in the body, which can compound neurological disease. Niacinamide is also included in the benzodiazepine weaning protocol. However, it is crucial that only healthcare professionals trained in this area administer high doses of niacinamide, magnesium, and omega-3s to help patients safely reduce their benzodiazepine use.

Omega-3 Fatty Acids

Our functional testing toolbox for both the prevention and treatment of depression and mood disorders includes omega-3 fatty acids, as they are also associated with promoting good mental health. Numerous studies support omega-3's effects on the brain, including promoting neurogenesis and neural repair, preventing neuroinflammation, and improving mood, cognition, and memory. Knowing this, it may not come as a surprise that we will see this supplement come up again in our discussion on Alzheimer's.

The suggested pathophysiology behind omega-3's antidepressant effects starts with the fact that it decreases inflammation, improves antioxidant capacity, and increases membrane fluidity. This promotes cell proliferation, growth, and development, as well as apoptosis for unhealthy cells so that they do not become "zombie cells," taking up energy without giving a positive effect. The regulated activity of the immune system enhances neurotransmitters, such as dopamine and 5-HT (the precursor to serotonin), and enhances neural synaptic plasticity between neurons of the brain.[209]

Heavy Metals

Heavy metals also play a role in inflammation and mental health issues when imbalanced. Exposure to toxic heavy metals has been positively correlated to behavioral changes, including depression, anxiety, irregular heartbeats, stress, lack of confidence, restlessness, and aggression. I recommend hair testing for heavy metals for an accurate assessment.

Since a major form of overexposure to these elements includes tobacco products, I often wonder if this leads to the self-perpetuating need for people to stay addicted. When we treat these issues, our approach must be patient-specific.[210] Lead has also been correlated with the development of mood disorders and, as we will later see, autism.[211]

Some metals are necessary for mental functioning. For example, the treatment of zinc deficiency has come up in the literature as one of the most convincing and effective treatments for anxiety. Zinc is an essential nutrient found in natural whole foods that acts on the GABA-aminobutyric acid, glutamatergic, serotonergic, neurogenic, and immune systems.[212] Several studies have identified a direct correlation between zinc levels and anxiety. One study found that the use of zinc and vitamin E, when used in combination, can ameliorate heavy-metal-induced anxiety disorder.[213]

Nutritional Intervention

Treatment strategies should focus on implementing a low-inflammatory diet, possibly involving an elimination diet and one that indefinitely cuts out processed foods, dyes, and preservatives. Functional Nutritional Testing and OATs can pinpoint where deficiencies may be affecting the individual's mental health, and treatment should follow accordingly.

It is important to note that the elimination of neurotoxic foods is just as important as replacing needed nutrients. For example, ADHD can be triggered by red dyes. Recent legislative changes are removing these from food sources, but we should remain vigilant as consumers since new chemicals may be introduced to replace them that have unknown side effects.

In terms of food, we should prioritize whole, unprocessed options that include plenty of fruits and vegetables. Additionally, for those suspected of having mast cell issues, avoiding high-histamine foods such as wine, avocados, and asparagus is advisable. Genetic testing can reveal if this is an issue for people. A Mediterranean-style diet focusing on whole foods could be beneficial, tailored to the person's specific health needs.

To promote digestive health, we should ensure the diet is rich in fiber, unless the person is dealing with small intestinal bacterial overgrowth (SIBO), where a high-fiber diet could worsen gas, bloating, and discomfort, leading to increased inflammation. Identifying the right probiotic also plays a crucial role—this can be informed by stool analysis, and necessary treatments for parasites or SIBO should be undertaken.

The Most Underused Antidepressant

Exercise has a dramatic effect on our mental health. Movement is quite literally like nature's antidepressant and is the most underused tool we have at our disposal. Exercise directly increases neurotransmitter functioning and endorphin release, reduces anxiety, and improves focus. It is known to decrease the rates of cognitive decline, enhance sleep, and boost testosterone (decreasing cortisol in the long run), all leading to improved mental health.[214]

Mental Health Supplements To Consider

Potential supplements for consideration include omega-3 fatty acids, magnesium (glycinate or threonate), curcumin, resveratrol, and quercetin, which are particularly important for mitochondrial function and overall energy. If a person's diet consists of fewer than daily servings of high omega-3 foods such as fish, walnuts, or chia seeds, then supplementation should be considered. Anti-inflammatory supplements like curcumin, resveratrol, and quercetin are helpful when inflammation is suspected in general and especially if quinolinic acid is elevated.

Additionally, lithium supplementation can be used safely in low doses, either as an over-the-counter supplement or by prescription. B-complex vitamins in their methylated forms are important, especially for those with MTHFR or COMT mutations. Finally, neuroinflammation can be further addressed with supplements like glutathione and NAC.

N-acetylcysteine (NAC) is a precursor for glutathione, which is the most important anti-inflammatory marker in the body. Many people tend to be deficient in glutathione, and this deficiency can be linked to mental health issues. Additionally, B vitamins are essential for mental health.[212] NAD+, whether IV or transdermal, has shown efficacy in memory, Alzheimer's reversal, and anti-aging.[215]

Melatonin may be a viable option to help decrease neuroinflammation, especially if insomnia is of concern. Another option is L-theanine, especially for patients who are anxiety-prone. It has proven to be quite impactful for improving mental health. I've had patients with severe insomnia and panic attacks who have benefited greatly from L-theanine; it's even allowed some to discontinue benzodiazepines. Double blind studies suggest statistical improvement against placebo for the use of L-theanine in stress and depression related symptoms. [216] A typical starting dose is one capsule (100 milligrams) in the morning and two capsules in the evening, which can help re-regulate sleep patterns and promote more restful sleep. The maximum dose is 600 milligrams per day. L-theanine has also shown benefits in treating ADHD and schizophrenia.[217]

Last, but certainly not least, are adaptogens. I commonly use adaptogens like lion's mane, ashwagandha, rhodiola, and holy basil, as they are considerably effective at treating depression and anxiety, PMS symptoms, and mood swings.[218] Clients also report that they help with energy and restful sleep. Some report them being energizing, in which case, I recommend early morning or afternoon dosing. Some report them to be more calming. For them, I recommend evening dosing.

The goal is not to keep patients on these supplements but to alleviate symptoms whilst resolving the underlying cause of their ailment, whether it be gut dysbiosis, heavy metal toxicity, nutritional deficiency, psychological issues, hormonal imbalance, or a mix of these.

Psychological Interventions

Incorporating stress management training, or as I like to say, mental stamina, is also essential. We haven't discussed meditation, music therapy, or yoga much, but incorporating these types of interventions can be very beneficial. Tai chi and other mind-body practices can significantly reduce stress.

One technique I use with my clients is guided imagery. For example, if someone is extremely stressed, I may guide them to enter a meditative state and visualize their stress as a raging fire. They can then mentally decrease that fire, observing the heat lessen until it is just a candle that is flickering gently. If applicable, using non-toxic candles can enhance this visual imagery.

What I find to be most effective in the treatment of dysregulated thoughts or past traumas is cognitive behavioral therapy (CBT). This is simply a restructuring of how a person thinks about negative impacts or occurrences in their lives. It is very powerful, but it can also pull up some fairly deep memories. Therefore, I advise being trained before trying to implement this with your clients. There are many fantastic books on the subject. If you are looking for a more simplified approach, I wrote *Living Between the Lines: Powerful Mind Training for Anxiety and Depression,* which can be found on Amazon.

You can check it out here.

SCAN THE QR CODE

When we get down to the root cause of mental illness, a wonderful benefit is being able to taper off of prescription medications, including some that are particularly dangerous, such as benzodiazepines. These medications, particularly when combined with opioids, are commonly prescribed for chronic pain and anxiety. Unfortunately, there is an ongoing epidemic of overprescription related to these medications, contradicting the principle in conventional medicine of "do no harm." Helping patients transition away from these medications can profoundly impact their lives and longevity.

It's important to emphasize that if you are not trained, experienced, and licensed in titrating antipsychotics, you should never recommend stopping or changing these medications. Furthermore, if a client expresses the desire to stop taking benzodiazepines, make sure they understand that discontinuing them abruptly can be extremely harmful and may even increase the risk of death due to withdrawal symptoms. This process should only be managed by a trained healthcare provider.

However, in the long run, discontinuing benzodiazepines can be very beneficial. It's essential to recognize that there is no such thing as a benzodiazepine or Prozac deficiency. Instead, the focus should be on addressing underlying issues rather than merely masking symptoms.

Summary of the Functional Interventions on Mental Health

One method I like to use is my functional framework for investigating the root cause of mental illness, which I refer to as the "ham and cheese" mnemonic. It can be very useful in the assessment and treatment of neurological disease. When using this framework, be sure to align it with the five R's of functional medicine: remove, replace, reinoculate, rebalance, and restore, but give a mental recall for the other essential aspects of root cause investigation in mental health.

- Functional Mental Health Approach: Remove, Replace, Reinoculate, Rebalance, and Restore
  - H (Hormone rebalancing)
  - A (Amino acids, protein, and antioxidant replacement)
  - M (Microbiome/parasites)
  - M (Metals screening and chelation therapy)
  - M (Medications: PPIs, metformin, other factors to decrease B12)
  - N (Nutrients: essential fatty acids)
  - C (*Clostridium* overgrowth-LPS)
  - C (Chemicals: endocrine disruptors, pesticides, etc.)
  - E (Exercise)
  - E (Exclude food intolerances or chemicals)
  - Z (Zinc and other minerals)
  - S (Sugar)
  - S (Supplements: B vitamins especially)
- And you can't have a ham and cheese sandwich without the bread, so please, consider gluten sensitivity and DPPIV insufficiency.

Please note that we have not discussed all interventions here, as some are better suited to their proper chapter (such as hormones). However, they are very important to mental health, and as a good practitioner, you can ascertain the validity of each intervention for each patient with good history taking and proper screening, as not every possible intervention may be necessary.

Business Practice Pearl

One of the questions I get asked frequently from start-up practitioners is how much they should charge. That is ultimately up to you, but we have already learned that if you stay in the trading-time-for-money model, you can never get ahead. One way to ensure you have a cushion until your passive income grows to replace your living expenses and more is to build cash injections into your business.

Many clients require a higher level of care and want to invest in something they know will change their life, not just cover up symptoms—this is where concierge medicine shines because it gives these people the results they are looking for. They are tired of being run through an office visit like cattle through a chute. They want real results and understand that it takes investing to get there (just like King Solomon). They want out of a system that leaves them feeling unsupported.

It is true that functional medicine is more complex than merely taking medications, so patients sometimes need that higher level of support. But it is worth it, because (as I like to say) functional medicine provides the ultimate leverage. For instance, a client may come to you with IBS issues, and once those are addressed, they might find that their anxiety improves, their depression subsides, or their joint pain disappears. All of these results can arise from fixing just one root cause. This is one reason why diving deep into care and investing in our health is massively worth it.

I've seen this happen countless times, and it can happen for your patients as well. They are not just paying for one issue to be fixed but often several and to potentially get off or decrease several medications. Plus, by focusing on the root cause, we decrease the risk of other health issues arising later in life, as one root cause can lead to multiple illnesses and differing symptoms (just like we saw historically in the pellagra epidemic caused by simple vitamin deficiency). We are not merely applying "Band-Aids," such as prescription medications, to their problems.

For clients interested in high-touch services, you can offer subscription models or courses that allow you to share key information without having to repeat yourself. I have compiled all my core information into courses and provide my clients access to these resources—high value to them and low overhead for me.

When building programs for your patients under the functional medicine model, keep in mind that our approach is not just a quick consultation followed by a prescription. This is a comprehensive, whole-body experience. As discussed earlier, we need to focus on the physical, mental, and spiritual aspects to ensure that the body is in total alignment. This often requires a complete program, meaning that patients are investing in their healing and health. While your expertise is extremely valuable, the real investment is their end goal: a life with less disease and/or fewer prescriptions and a life of empowerment. There is just about no price you can put on this.

In my practice, my goal is not to keep them on supplements for life in exchange for prescriptions. While we cannot ever guarantee that this will be their result, the goal is to fix their underlying issue, not keep them coming back every four months for the rest of their lives. Because of this, my students successfully charge $2,500 to $10,000+ for their programs.

Now, I know you may feel resistance to that, and there are likely a couple of reasons for that resistance: one, you don't know your own worth, and two, your intuition is right. You cannot just raise your prices and expect people to pay that. You have to learn positioning, and I will teach you the blueprint for that in later chapters. First, let's discuss the number one thing that actually stops clinicians from going all in: their internal hesitation and lack of self-worth.

If this is you, no worries. Most of us feel this way at first. But here's the thing: hospitals make tens of thousands of dollars for one visit, while nurses, health workers, and docs make pennies of that, being the ones actually running that show. Your knowledge is expensive. As a matter of fact, many of you spent tens of thousands of dollars, sometimes hundreds of thousands, on your education, and that doesn't include the time you sacrificed learning instead of spending it with family or friends. Even right now, you are sacrificing your time to better help your clients. That is extremely valuable and something most won't do. When you were a student, you put value on that information, enough to invest big time. Why devalue it once you hold the knowledge?

Because of your hard work and through the power of functional medicine, you can alleviate worries about the client's future, such as "What if my diabetes worsens and I end up on insulin injections or I lose a leg?" or "What if my chronic inflammation leads to cancer?" Not to mention the money they can save by not taking off work or paying for health care visits, hospital stays, days lost with family, early death, prescriptions, imaging, and/or new clothing when they are able to stop gaining weight.

Most importantly, you actually decrease the likelihood or severity of an illness or eliminate it altogether. That is more valuable than, say, going on a fleeting vacation or attending a concert to see a famous singer or artist who charges thousands of dollars or even tens of thousands for their appearance or work. I'm not saying those people do not deserve their wealth. I'm simply saying that you do, too.

Does that mean that you have to charge a lot to be successful? No, and actually, in several cases, you can implement what we call "building the business down." This means that some of your services can be lower ticket and part of passive systems that do not take up much of your time but still serve patients at a high level. When you "build the business down," you use the capital from your higher programs to invest in resources to make them more affordable for a wider range of audiences. This is a very successful business plan, especially if you need to replace a job income quickly before you burn out. Once you own a successful business, you can then even move on to offering more charity work. But you can never reach that level if you don't first stop your ship from sinking, being stuck working 40-60 hours in a job that keeps you living paycheck to paycheck.

Knowing the worth of what your system does is not a bad thing. As a matter of fact, even King Solomon, a great man of God (not perfect, but he still made the Lord very happy), charged a high ticket, but he also paid a high ticket. In 1 Kings 3, we see that King Solomon gave the Lord a thousand burnt offerings. While we cannot quantify the cost of that exactly, we can assume it to be a very large amount. It's not about the money; it's about the offer. The willingness to pay means you are willing to pay attention.

The Lord came to King Solomon and gave him the opportunity of a lifetime, telling him that he could have anything he wanted as a result of his dedication. King Solomon did not ask for riches but the wisdom to *serve* his people best. That is your first clue to success: never get tired of being obsessed with how you can serve others the best you can. If you *do* that (not just think about it), riches will follow. God proved that by bestowing riches like no one had ever seen, nor ever will see, on King Solomon in exchange for his desire to serve. Hallelujah!

Does that tell you that riches are evil? Would God be willing to give riches away to his people if they were evil? No, riches are a blessing that we are entrusted with. It is the heart that is either evil or pure. Scripture tells us simply that it is the *love* of money that is the root of all evil (1 Timothy 6:10), not money itself.

Next, Solomon accepted 120 talents of gold, along with precious spices and stones from the Queen of Sheba, in exchange for his teaching her what he knew. His coaching fee was no joke. equating to around 9,000 pounds of gold, which, in today's society, would be approximately $603,092,800 USD as of the writing of this text. Knowledge is valuable.

There are an estimated 62.4 million millionaires in the world today. To earn a million in a year, you must make around $2,740/day (with leverage going one-to-many, that is certainly attainable). I would say your healing knowledge more than qualifies you to be a part of this wealth, and if others can make that in a day, you can make that without worry in a life transformation.

This leads us to another lesson: successful people do not hesitate to pay for the value they want and do not fear that the money will not "come back to them." As a matter of fact, that is something that I believe to be a hidden secret: the more you hoard money, the more you worship it and tell God that there is no way for Him to show up in big ways. I have trained myself to get excited every time I have a large, unexpected expense. Instead of worrying, I get excited to see how God is going to replenish that deficit. Money loses its power over you the more willing you are to both pay and charge. Plus, you attract it more the less you suffocate it by pretending it cannot flow back to you. It is a little like playing "hard to get" in the dating world, at least in terms of energy. It is the exact opposite of what so many people perceive to be reality.

So, if you're a practitioner who aspires to run your own functional practice, I highly encourage you to pursue that goal. It can be incredibly liberating. You gain control over your schedule and the ability to assist your clients at a deeper level. When you have the freedom to shape your practice, you move away from feeling like you're just processing patients.

If this overwhelms you, do not worry; it did me at first, too. Until I started to invest in getting into rooms of successful professionals. Most of us feel we are not worthy or able at first. However, that feeling simply means you want to offer quality to people and nothing less. If you feel unqualified, it is likely because you have that drive for excellence, and that is exactly the type of person who needs to be called to heal others at an elevated level. Just remember, God does not call the qualified; he qualifies the called.

You can build very successful programs; you just have to have a strategy to build these out, like our E.L.E.V.A.T.E.D. Method, which I teach in our Passive Clients course. You can grab access to the next live training for free with the link below (just add your email for notifications when we go live to teach it)!

Chapter 6

Neurologic Disease and Repair

CASE STUDY: WHEN CELLS ARE UNDERNOURISHED AND SUBJECTED TO FOOD TOXICITY, THE NERVOUS SYSTEM SUFFERS

A 75-year-old male presents with severe Parkinson's tremor for the last 10 years. Tremor at rest, worse with increased stress. Patient reports wanting to stop levodopa/carbidopa. Gram-negative bacterial overgrowth and elevated zonulin were revealed on a comprehensive stool analysis. Intervention included eliminating gluten and toxins, liver detox, rebalancing and healing the gut microbiome, and an anti-inflammatory protocol. At the 3-month follow-up, tremor decreased from severe to mild.

Discussion

The concept of neurological decline as we currently classify it is obsolete. It combines categorical misclassification with etiological imprecision. In functional medicine, we have discovered that the same underlying issues can affect different people in unique ways. This means that although we classify certain conditions as mental or neurological disorders, they might actually stem from the same root causes, and different root causes can lead to the same disorder.

We need to ask ourselves what the real issue is. Are we more focused on managing symptoms, or are we committed to identifying the underlying causes so we can reverse them? This is the key difference in functional medicine. There is significant overlap here, particularly in the neurologic mental health sector, as these conditions can impact people differently. Ultimately, our goal is to focus on the person rather than the disease, right?

Back to the Gut-Brain Axis

Let us refer back to the bidirectional route between our brain and the central nervous system and the gut. A healthy gut will decrease risk for neurological decline, while a gut with gram-negative bacteria (for example) will produce neurotoxins and inflammation caused by their LPS, which is a part of the outer membrane of these pathogenic bacteria. Symptoms include impaired memory, tremors, agitation, and decline in neuro functioning.[219] Identifying their presence is just as significant in neurological health as they are in physical and mental health. They act as neurotoxins that can cross the blood-brain barrier and directly affect the nervous system. They also release pro-inflammatory mediators and cytokines, which will lead to further neuronal damage.[119]

We know that they can influence anxiety and depression, as well as repetitive behavior and obsessive-compulsive disorder (OCD). Furthermore, these neurotoxins are implicated in conditions like Alzheimer's, Parkinson's, and autism spectrum disorder. They trigger inflammatory cytokines, such as IL-6 and TNF-alpha, activate our immune system and can lead to complications, including autoimmune diseases.

The process also inhibits the breakdown of dopamine. Dopamine is a neurotransmitter that plays a crucial role in motivation. However, excessive dopamine can lead to agitation and more. Research indicates a correlation between the presence of gram-negative bacteria and this inhibition, as they block the enzyme that breaks down dopamine in the brain.[220]

Autism Spectrum Disorder (ASD)

ASD used to have an occurrence of 1/1000 just a few short decades ago. That occurrence rate has now increased to 1/31 children being affected by the disorder. This is a dramatic increase, and one that many of us are eager to understand why and how to possibly reverse the effects of in as many clients as possible. From a personal standpoint, I can say that while it is difficult to completely reverse all symptoms, decreasing the severity of the disorder is very possible in many cases. I have seen children go from completely nonverbal to speaking several words. I have seen children go from continuous rages to being calm the majority of the time. While the story on ASD is not completely written and there are still many questions to be answered, I can tell you that there is hope and progress, and functional medicine is at the forefront of that progress.

To begin our root cause discussion on ASD, it is most important to note that a thorough review of the literature quickly reveals that it is a complex and multifactorial condition. It has been found that the same syndrome is likely occurring in different people for different reasons. Some reasons being some are more opportunistic, and others hold a strong genetic predisposition. Time spent in research and working with clients clearly demonstrates ASD develops as a result of a combination of a "perfect storm" consisting of several different exposures. Because of its diversity in evaluation, it is important to note that, while this text will delve into some of the most significant findings currently in literature, it must be remembered that this subject is diverse enough for an entire textbook in and of itself, and not everything can be fully discussed here in one section of a chapter.

Biochemistry & ASD

While ASD is associated with over 600 genes, MTHFR polymorphism is particularly showing a strong correlation as a piece of the puzzle for causation. Folate deficiency and MTHFR genetic mutation trends suggest that the C677T polymorphism has a significant link to ASD, while the A1298C polymorphism is less likely associated. There is significant data to back up that folate deficiency in ASD is significantly correlated, as is a mother's deficiency and even excess in diet during the gestational time frame of the affected child.[221]

A study of 49 participants with ASD found that after twelve weeks of supplementing folate, improvement was seen amongst all of those in the intervention group.[221] Another study of 55 ASD children found statistically significant and impressive improvement in their double-blind, placebo-controlled, randomized study administering 2 mg/kg to 50 mg of a daily dose to the intervention group. No changes were noted in the control group. The results indicated a moderate improvement in inappropriate speech and stereotypic behavior and a more than 2x improvement in hyperactivity and noncompliance, then seen in the rate of improvement of the other symptoms.[221]

B12 (cobalamin) is additionally observed as a nutrient of importance in the development of and the exacerbation of symptoms in ASD. It is essential for neurotransmitter metabolism and production of serotonin and dopamine, which regulate mood, cognition, and behavior. B12 is also essential in neuronal myelination to ensure correct signal transmission within nervous system communication. A deficiency is also known to influence and lead to gut dysbiosis, which is known to further dysregulate the microbiome and contribute to the development and symptoms experienced in ASD.[222] There is also a significant effect from the lack of B12 being methylated, causing an increase in methionine, which is neuroinflammatory in and of itself.

A reduction in the methylation and redox capacity found in ASD patients even leads to a predictable reduction in methionine and SA with ASD compared to thirty-three controls in one study. These results represent impaired redox capacity, and these initial findings have even been confirmed for consistency in findings across multiple other studies and laboratories. Another meta-analysis of twenty-two studies discovered a consistency of impaired DNA methylation in ASD, which has been positively correlated with mitochondrial dysfunction. This may indicate the need to delve further into identifying and treating an underlying mitochondrial dysfunction in the general ASD population. These biochemical processes have even been suggested as diagnostic of ASD, as a 98% predictive correlated classification rate has been confirmed.[223]

These biochemical processes may be why one meta-analysis of seventeen studies involving the supplementation of methylated B12 found the results that it did. Improvements of associated ASD symptoms were found, including those for speech, life skills, coping abilities, and social skills. The authors concluded that there may be biomarkers to predict responses to B12 in the right population of ASD patients. Other clinical improvements observed included sleep, gastrointestinal disruption, hyperactivity, tantrums, becoming verbal, sight improvements, enhanced eye contact, and nocturnal enuresis (bed wetting). It is important to note that adverse effects were also identified, though with much less frequent occurrences. These included some having worsened hyperactivity, irritability, insomnia, anger, and worsening behaviors. The authors noted that these were in general uncommon and considered of mild statistical significance compared to placebo.[223]

Gut-Brain Axis & ASD

Another correlation demonstrating positive intervention lies within the gastrointestinal microbiome. In studies focusing on autism spectrum disorder (ASD) and gut-brain research, we have identified distinct microbiotic differences between children with autism and those who are not on the spectrum.[224] For example, children with ASD often exhibit an overgrowth of Clostridia, Bacteroides, and Candida, a type of yeast infection in the gut. Research involving both mice and humans has shown that microbiota transfer therapy (MTT) significantly reduces autistic symptoms in ASD patients.[225]

MTT involves transferring a fecal sample from a healthy donor to an autistic child or patient. The studies have reported not only early improvements in symptoms but also significant increases in bacterial diversity and the abundance of beneficial bacteria like *Bifidobacteria* and *Prevotella*, which are typically deficient in these individuals, even two years after the treatment. While more double-blind studies are needed to further validate these findings, numerous studies conducted to date indicate substantial improvements.

Data also suggest that those with ASD tend to have a higher prevalence of gram-negative bacteria and a decrease in *Bifidobacteria*, which is a class of microorganisms known to contain some of the main healthy psychobiotics within a normal gut flora. *Bifidobacteria* play a role in synthesizing gamma-aminobutyric acid (GABA), the main calming neurotransmitter in the brain. A decrease in this microorganism correlates with lower GABA levels, which may explain why those with autism often experience agitation and are easily overwhelmed.

Additionally, research shows that Clostridium levels tend to be elevated in those with ASD, contributing to the production of endotoxins such as LPS that affect the brain. Propionate, another compound associated with the severity of ASD symptoms, is produced by

Clostridia and Bacteroides.[226] It can cross the blood-brain barrier and induce autistic-like behaviors through the modulation of serotonin and dopamine in lab mice. Propionic acid is a short-chain fatty acid linked to autistic behaviors and is found at higher levels in those with ASD. It generates pro-inflammatory cytokines, triggering inflammatory processes and reducing intracellular antioxidants like glutathione, a deficiency of which is independently associated with impaired neuro-functioning.[213]

The gastrointestinal health of these individuals is compromised when toxic metabolites are present, which increase inflammation and affect communication, social interactions, and interest patterns—repetitive behaviors commonly observed in autism. Similar behaviors are induced in mice when they are injected with LPS[219] or propionic acid.[226] Interestingly, pharmaceutical options have been developed to block the effects of LPS on the brain, potentially alleviating symptoms in autistic children without getting rid of the root cause of why these neurotoxins are present in the first place.

Clinical results from fecal microbiota transplants conducted on 18 autistic children revealed that 80% of them experienced improvements in their gastrointestinal symptom rating scale (GSRS). Significant increases in Bifidobacteria, Prevotella, and Peptococcus were maintained for eight weeks. Eight children exhibited greater improvements in their neurobehavioral symptoms even two years after the treatment. The only noted side effect was short-term diarrhea that occurred two weeks post-transplant, but no long-term complications were reported.[227]

GABA is another neurotransmitter that is found to be consistently imbalanced in ASD clients. However, trends for dysregulation can vary from too much to not enough in different areas of the brain. Increased agitation and enhanced tactile sensitivity can result from insufficient levels in the sensorimotor cortex, whereas social development may be affected as a result of an overabundance of GABA in the bilateral visual cortex. GABA production is also associated with gut flora regulation, and it is produced in the microbiome.[228] Such trends are summarized in the following chart, which provides a comparison of some of the microbiome trends identified in ASD clients.

Microbial Trends Found in Autistic Patients

Microbe	Trend in Autism Patients	Psychobiotic Effect / Clinical Relevance
Bacteroides	Increased ↑	Production of SCFAs and their metabolites — particularly propionic acid — is suspected to influence autistic behavior via disruption of the gut-brain axis.
Clostridium	Increased ↑	Production of endotoxins and propionic acid that may be associated with increased severity of ASD symptoms.
Candida albicans	Increased ↑	Overgrowth in the bilateral visual cortex results in excess GABA production, which can lead to the appearance of autistic behaviors and downregulation of social interactions.
Bifidobacterium	Decreased ↓	Synthesizes GABA — a calming neurotransmitter (NT). As levels of *Bifidobacterium* decrease, GABA levels fall accordingly. Decreased GABA in the sensorimotor cortex leads to increased agitation.
Blautia	Decreased ↓	Aids in synthesis of tryptophan and bile acids (precursors of serotonin). Decreased *Blautia* results in reduced serotonin reaching the brain.

Key: ASD = Autism Spectrum Disorder • GABA = Gamma-aminobutyric acid • GSH = Glutathione • LPS = Lipopolysaccharides • MO = microorganism • NT = neurotransmitter • SCFA = short-chain fatty acid

Heavy Metals and ASD

A study of over five thousand individuals found a significant correlation between elevated levels of cadmium and metal exposure. Metal exposure has the potential to induce reactive oxygen species (ROS), leading to epigenetic changes that may be a root cause in the occurrence of Autistic Disorder (ASD). This leads us to examine the possibility that chelation or nanolite therapy for heavy metal detoxification is a possible treatment option. To date, however, the risk of chelation therapy is considered to outweigh the results seen from such intervention in this population.[229]

Zeolites, however, are emerging as an effective way to decrease heavy metals, such as lead toxicity, and are relatively safe without known contraindications. Zeolites are porous chemicals with high ion exchange capacity.[229] This allows them to work similar to chelating agents, without the risk of chelation therapy. While there is a growing number of qualitative reviews demonstrating the potential of zeolites, from a professional standpoint, the peer-reviewed science is only starting to evolve.

While retroactive treatment post-exposure could help with improvement of symptoms, it is important to note that decreasing exposure is essential. In order to decrease exposure, there must be environmental screening for sources like contaminated fish, unfiltered tap water, and avoidance of certain products like cosmetics and supplements. One source of mercury can be found in the form of thimerosal, a preservative in vaccinations, particularly those drawn up from multiuse vials. Legislation is underway to remove this from vaccinations at the time of this writing.

ASD Overview

The associations between ASD symptoms and root causes should be considered based upon clinical presentation, risk factors, and interventions implemented on an individualized basis. Potential testing should include organic acids, comprehensive stool analysis, genetic testing such as MTHFR, and mitochondrial or nutritional deficiency. Lastly, an anti-inflammatory and gluten-free diet should be considered, as inflammatory processes are an important part of managing any chronic disease in functional medicine. The clinician should be cautious to not impart a false sense of potential recovery for ASD, or any chronic neurological disease, as full remission is not expected. However, an improvement of overall quality of life is often the goal and still considerably significant.

Parkinson's Disease Functional Approach

Parkinson's disease (PD) is a neurodegenerative disorder characterized by progressive motor impairments and is the fastest-growing neurological disorder in the world. From 1900 to 2025, the rate doubled, from 3 million to 6 million affected lives, and is expected to double again by 2040. In 1970, approximately 0.0205% of the population was affected; it is now up almost 50x, at 1 in 100, and America accounts for 9% of those affected, despite being a leading economic powerhouse and accounting for only 4% of the world's population.[230] This significant increase in prevalence demonstrates the dire need to discover root causes to increase prevention and decrease occurrence.

Gut-Brain Connection and PD

Recent research suggests that gastrointestinal symptoms may actually precede the onset of motor symptoms. This finding underscores the potential role of the gut-brain axis in the pathogenesis of the disease and highlights an important opportunity for prevention. Gut inflammation, for example, can exacerbate neuroinflammation, disrupt the blood-brain barrier, and lead to the loss of dopaminergic neurons in the substantia nigra.[231]

The substantia nigra is a part of the brain directly associated with the symptoms of Parkinson's disease. It is well established that gut inflammation and constipation are common among patients with this condition, further supporting the idea that gut health may be a root cause of Parkinson's. Studies have shown elevated levels of pro-inflammatory cytokines, such as tumor necrosis factor alpha (TNF-α), interferon gamma (IFN-γ), interleukin 6 (IL-6), and interleukin 1 beta (IL-1β), in Parkinson's patients. These cytokines were analyzed through real-time PCR and mRNA expression in biopsies from the ascending colon of Parkinson's patients compared to healthy controls.[232]

In Parkinson's disease, the protein alpha-synuclein is involved in a misfolding process that is recognized as a key pathogenic mechanism. A growing body of evidence indicates that misfolded α-synuclein can be transmitted from the gastrointestinal tract to the lower brainstem via the vagus nerve.[231] The most convincing evidence of this correlation includes several studies that have found that vagotomy (a surgical procedure that involves cutting the vagus nerve) reduces the rate of development for Parkinson's disease by slowing the spread of misfolded alpha-synuclein to the brain stem. In a study involving gastrointestinal administration of the pesticide rotenone, which is known to induce Parkinson's symptoms in mice, the mice that underwent vagotomy showed a decrease in the development of Parkinson's disease. However, this was not found to be a viable treatment option, as the mice deteriorated more rapidly due to other symptoms resulting from the vagotomy. Nevertheless, this highlights the strong association between the gut-brain axis and Parkinson's disease.[231,233]

Moreover, Lewy bodies (abnormal protein deposits found in the brains of people with Parkinson's) are considered hallmarks of the disease. LPS, discussed previously in the ASD section, emerges from dysbiosis in the gut and is also linked to this neurodegeneration. Two significant factors for treating and preventing Parkinson's disease are oxidative stress and inflammation. Both can be exacerbated by increased intestinal permeability caused by LPS and chronic infections. Remember, LPS also prevents the breakdown of dopamine. Researchers from the Champalimaud Foundation discovered that preserved dopamine in certain brain regions may actually exacerbate tremor symptoms, challenging the parts of the current model. It is suspected that the specific dysfunctional dopamine metabolism itself is a contributing factor to the development of tremors.[234]

There is additionally a compelling association between Parkinson's disease and basic gut dysbiosis, characterized by trends that represent a decrease in beneficial bacteria and an increase in pro-inflammatory bacteria.[235] Those found to have Parkinson's are more likely to have a decrease in abundance of bacteria such as Prevotella and an increased abundance of pro-inflammatory bacteria, such as Enterobacteriaceae or Akkermansia.[231,235]

Mitochondrial Dysfunction and PD

Age-related biological dysfunction is commonly cited as an etiological part of the process for the development of several neurological diseases. Biological dysfunction increases with the aging process, such as telomere dysfunction, genomic instability, epigenetic changes, and ubiquitin-proteasome. As such, it is reasonably suspected that mitochondrial defects may underpin and facilitate neuronal demise. Treatment of mitochondrial dysfunction may include treatment with CoQ10 supplementation as well as several other potential interventions, which should be chosen specifically based upon the individual clients and results of organic acids or NutraEval testing results.

Another etiological intervention suspected to play a part in the metabolic processes of the cell includes the mitochondrial efficiency in clearing damaged proteins, leading to oxidative stress. Studies have also demonstrated a significant correlation between mitochondrial damage promoting the accumulation of oxidized dopamine and reduction in the enzyme responsible for breaking it down correctly, further suggesting the association found between dopamine and α-synuclein accumulation and the cells' digestive and mitochondrial impairments.[236]

PD Overview

The associations between PD and root causes should be thoroughly evaluated upon clinical necessity and done on an individualized basis. Potential testing should include organic acids, comprehensive stool analysis, genetic testing such as MTHFR (for the potential neurological effects of folate and B12 deficiency), and mitochondrial or nutritional deficiency. Lastly, an anti-inflammatory and gluten-free diet should be considered to decrease the inflammatory processes. Gluten is additionally being more thoroughly looked at as a root cause of PD related to its neuroinflammatory properties, and therefore the client may find benefit in implementing a gluten-free diet.[232]

Alzheimer's in functional medicine

Alzheimer's is the most common form of dementia and is demonstrating no signs of slowing down. There has been a staggering 117% increase in Alzheimer's cases over the past 26 years, with only a 1.7% increase in age-standardized prevalence.[237] Projections suggest that this number could nearly double every two years, potentially affecting 78 million people by 2030. If Alzheimer's disease were treated as an economy of its own, it would rank as the fourth largest in the world.

Gut-Brain Axis and Alzheimers

It is once again necessary to evaluate the association of the gut-brain axis, as there are findings in the literature and clinical studies for Alzheimer's, similar to those of ASD and PD. This may be yet another indication of how the same root cause might manifest differently from client to client. Let us begin by evaluating a cross-sectional analysis of 127 patients without dementia. The study was conducted at a memory clinic where the average age of clients was 76. Testing revealed that plasma LPS concentrations were associated with mild cognitive impairment. Whereas higher plasma endotoxin levels were linked to more rapid cognitive decline. The research also demonstrated that this occurrence was more likely to be associated with a balance between Bifidobacteria and Firmicutes to help prevent the overgrowth of harmful bacteria.[238] It is of little surprise to note that research also demonstrates that Alzheimer's patients more often experience this imbalance.

Key Nutritional Deficiencies

Alzheimer's is increasingly being recognized as a condition influenced by neuroinflammation, metabolic dysfunction, and micronutrient insufficiency. Nutritional status plays a significant role in disease progression and exacerbation of symptoms. Incorporating natural sources of vitamins into the diet is important when indicated.

Omega-3 fatty acids play a significant role in brain development and help reduce neurological inflammation, which is essential for alleviating symptoms in people with Alzheimer's or those at risk. Supplementation has even demonstrated efficacy in the prevention and reversal of early-stage syndromes.[239] This is of significant consideration, as the majority of Americans do not eat an adequate amount of omega-3s.

Magnesium is another nutritional deficiency that is important to consider screening for in the assessment of Alzheimer's. Replacement has been found under double-blind studies to correlate positively with enhancing cognitive functioning in Alzheimer's patients.[240]

Vitamin D, known to be anti-inflammatory, is not surprisingly showing up in the discussion for Alzheimer's. However, while treatment in someone who is deficient is important, the data may point towards this being more of a preventative measure than a treatment thereof.

For example, vitamin D deficiency was associated with a 34% elevated risk of the development of cognitive impairment.[241] But treatment for deficiency has not been found to have significant improvement, and individual assessment is advised.

The nutritional treatment plan for Alzheimer's may include the implementation of a ketogenic diet, which is backed by scientific evidence. Cognitive improvement was statistically significant in a meta-analysis of several studies when the ketone levels of patients were increased. While further studies are warranted, this is still a fantastic intervention that may improve the conditions of those who are able and willing to maintain such a diet.[242]

NAD+ is additionally something that is being more thoroughly looked at for enhancing cognitive functioning in Alzheimer's patients, as it is essential to cognitive functioning.[243] In a professional assessment, I have witnessed improved cognition in several patients after implementing mitochondrial protocols and incorporating NAD+ transdermally, with side effects limited to the potential for dermal reaction to the patch.

Heavy Metals & Toxic Exposure in Alzheimer's Research

We cannot conclude our discussion on Alzheimer's disease (AD) without addressing mercury (Hg). Research has consistently shown a correlation between AD and mercury exposure. This is evidenced by significantly higher levels of mercury found in the nerve tissue of cadavers who suffered from neurodegenerative disease compared with those who did not. The neurotoxic properties of mercury (Hg) alter messenger ribonucleic acid (mRNA) expression, inhibit mitochondrial function, and cause oxidative stress.[244]

Moreover, a strong connection has been established between mercury in dental fillings and an increased risk for Alzheimer's. It is also crucial to educate patients about thimerosal, a mercury-containing preservative found in some vaccines. Not all vaccines contain thimerosal, and it can be avoided by checking ingredients. Vaccines that use thimerosal as a preservative are typically multi-dose vials, while single-dose vials do not contain it. To date, measures are being taken to remove it completely. However, older generations have already had significant exposure, as it wasn't until 2025 that the decision was made to remove it from influenza vaccines, and it wasn't until 2021 that it was removed from vaccines indicated for children younger than six.

Addressing environmental toxins is vital for people at risk for Alzheimer's. Toxic exposures can be derived from sources such as mold, which has been directly linked to gut-brain inflammation. Case studies suggest mold exposure may contribute to depression and asthma, further increasing one's risk. Mold toxins can harm astrocytes and microglia, which are critical components of the brain's immune system, thus attacking it directly. An overreaction of glial cells can lead to severe brain diseases.[244] When complete mold removal is not plausible, detoxing begins with limiting exposure to home remodeling or by using water filters and air filters. Other sources of mold that are often overlooked are dried fruit or nuts. While these provide a value of nutrients and even omega-3s that are helpful to brain health, using the freshest foods possible is preferable.

The proliferation and activation of glial cells influence the microenvironment necessary for nerve tissue repair. The overactivity of astrocytes and microglia can form glial scars, restrict microvessels, and trigger the release of harmful cytokines, hindering nerve regeneration and resulting in irreversible damage. This process is recognized in the development of Alzheimer's, Huntington's disease, various demyelinating diseases, and brain trauma.[219]

Additionally, pro-inflammatory conditions can induce calcium imbalances and mitochondrial damage, leading to oxidative stress and neuronal death. While healthy levels of glutamate are necessary for brain function, excessive glutamate can accumulate and damage brain cells. Mycotoxins produced by mold are also known to contribute to glutamate buildup. High levels of glutamate in the brain are associated with various diseases, including amyotrophic lateral sclerosis (ALS), multiple sclerosis, Alzheimer's, Parkinson's disease, Huntington's disease, strokes, fibromyalgia, and chronic fatigue syndrome.[245]

While gluten may not be considered a toxic exposure in general, it is neurotoxic in the right person. The process of deamidation of gluten produces tTG2, which functions as an autoantigen found to be a part of the pathogenesis of several neurodegenerative disorders, including Alzheimer's Disease (AD) and Huntington's Disease (HD).[245] Therefore, there is significant evidence in suggesting the avoidance of gluten as a beneficial intervention. While some studies indicate no link between gluten and Alzheimer's, many do. Either way, if there is uncertainty, a gluten-free diet is worthwhile.[245,246]

Alzheimer's Conclusion

I was able to help a severely advanced patient with Alzheimer's who recently started to forget her son and had become much more agitated right before she came under my care. While the family rightfully did not feel that strict dietary interventions and advanced stool testing were appropriate at her stage, we were able to address some microbiome and nutritional rebalancing. I started her on ashwagandha mostly for its adaptogenic effects, got her vitamin D to optimal levels, and started omega-3 EPA and DHA.

After just a few weeks, she was able to remember who her son was again and was much calmer for the final days of her life until her passing. That family, no doubt, became a very special part of my memory. While her PCP certainly had reservations about me starting alternative treatments, he obliged, and it became very much worth "going against the grain." That small improvement in her memory (which was huge to the son) is now something that I am honored to have been a part of and one story where I am so very glad to have started this journey into functional medicine.

Schizophrenia

Schizophrenia is a disorder evidenced by the experience of delusions, hallucinations, disorganized speech, incongruent behavior, and cognitive impairment. It is a very complex disease, and this will be a brief overview of the most convincing areas of intervention, not a comprehensive analysis.

Biochemistry, Nutrition, and Schizophrenia

The association between gluten and schizophrenia is quite developed. The viability of this intervention was first evidenced by the discovery that schizophrenics are fifty times more likely to have pathogenically elevated levels of anti-gluten antibodies, including anti-TTG and anti-gliadin antibodies. With continued research, preliminary findings found improvement in positive, negative, extrapyramidal, attentional, and gastrointestinal symptoms in patients.[247,246]

There is also evidence suggesting an association between the implementation of a ketogenic diet and reduction of schizophrenic symptoms.[248,249] A pilot study done in 2024 by Stanford University found a 31% improvement in the overall symptoms of patients with advanced mental illness, including schizophrenia and bipolar disease. No other interventions were implemented. Symptoms showed improvement in energy, sleep, mood, quality of life, and hopefulness. These clients followed a diet consisting of 10% carbohydrates, 30% protein sources, and 60% fat sources. Calories were not counted, and all participants lost weight. The researchers attributed the improvement in metabolic health to being the cause for improved brain functioning.[249]

One study demonstrates that the risk for schizophrenia may begin in utero. Researchers found that niacin deficiency during pregnancy increases the risk of schizophrenia in offspring, further emphasizing the importance of proper nutrition in mitigating the risk of neurological decline.[250]

As happens often in the research, it is found that there is often more than one root cause, and medical interventions truly should be individualized and not just focused on symptoms.

The next root cause to investigate is the potential for vitamin deficiency. Several studies demonstrate that schizophrenia is associated with vitamin B12 deficiency, and when combined with folate and vitamin D, supplementing with vitamin B12 (methylated when necessary) has been found to be a useful intervention for improving symptoms of cognitive decline or even hallucinations.[251,252]

Another meta-analysis that reviewed fifty cases found that a quarter of them involved therapy-resistant hallucinations that fully resolved with the treatment of cobalamin replacement alone, and 60% of cases had neuropsychiatric manifestations that "disappeared." Only 32% of cases also demonstrated pernicious anemia.[252] These, along with other studies, are quite incredible results that underline the power of simple interventions in treating severe cognitive decline.

Step 1 in Healing: Remove

Limiting Environmental Exposure & Removing Toxins

The first step in ensuring that our clients are detoxing effectively is to remove their exposure to harmful substances. This is a top priority but is sometimes limited in what can be done. Remember that this might include heavy metals, toxins, dietary (such as added chemicals or gluten) or environmental chemicals, harmful gut bacterial overgrowth, or pathogens. Toxins and heavy metals might be found in paint, consumer products, and cleaning products. Promising case studies have shown that Alzheimer's patients can significantly reduce their symptoms simply by removing old mercury-containing dental fillings.[253] While this process can be cumbersome, it can lead to substantial improvements and help prevent further issues.

Chelation therapy has been proven effective for the removal of heavy metals; however, it does come with risk and should only be performed by those certified to do so. Less invasive and risky interventions include zeolite spray or using natural binders that pull metals out of the body. These include cilantro and chlorella in combination with modified citrus pectin (MCP). MCP is most effective for lead, cadmium, and arsenic. Activated charcoal (also used in the Herxheimer reaction) will help with decreasing overall toxic burden and will allow the body to better focus on natural detoxification processes.[254,255] Zeolite clay or spray is also known to bind heavy metals in the body. I have seen great results with this intervention.

Another simple intervention is the use of a sauna. While detoxification may be minimal with each session, a healthy and regular practice has been shown to help to remove toxins and metals via the natural sweating process and is beneficial for reducing aluminum, cadmium, cobalt, and lead toxicity.[255] This is compared to the use of exercise to excrete toxins through sweat, which tends to be effective for nickel, lead, copper, silver, and mercury.[255]

If mold is suspected in a client's environment, it is crucial to have it treated. In cases where clients can completely avoid a mold-infested environment, that is strongly recommended, as it can greatly influence mental health and neurodegeneration. The use of air purifiers can also be beneficial.

Detoxification to remove mold from the body can be supported by binders such as activated charcoal and clay, alongside liver support from supplements like milk thistle, alpha-lipoic acid, glutathione, or N-acetylcysteine (NAC). It's essential to first address any gut inflammation before implementing these strategies. In some cases, cholestyramine has been shown to have binding effects that can help reduce inflammation, but it should only be used when clinically appropriate.[229] I would not suggest starting the client on every possible intervention, but only the ones that make the most sense for the person. Removing gluten and dairy products can also help the nervous system heal, as does maintaining a low-glycemic diet.

Gut Detox

During screening, always check for gut symptoms due to the strong evidence linking bacterial gut overgrowth with neurological conditions. Identifying root causes goes beyond merely alleviating symptoms; it's about uncovering and addressing what is harming each patient. Not every patient will have all potential exposures; it could be one main issue or a combination of factors that have pushed their neurological systems to their limits. The gut can be a source of LPS, other bacteria, yeast, or parasites that can be impacting neurological health.

Step 2: Replace and/or Supplement

Potential interventions to consider on an individual basis:

- Methylated folate and B12 if MTHFR genetic polymorphism is identified in testing
- Nutritional deficiencies that may have been found upon nutrition or OATs testing
- Omega-3s are often essential for neurological treatment, as most do not get enough in their diet, and higher doses have proven beneficial to healing.
- Treatment of any hormonal imbalances found
- Mitochondrial support with CoQ10 (100–300 mg/day), acetyl-L-carnitine, alpha-lipoic acid, or methylated B12 and folate
- Curcumin for inflammation (500–1000 mg/day)

- N-acetylcysteine is notably important, especially since many cases are linked to inflammatory processes.
- Adaptogens or nootropics for enhancing cognition and decreasing the experience and expression of stress
- NAD+: Schizophrenia is repeatedly associated with oxidative stress, impaired mitochondrial respiration, and reduced ATP generation.[256] NAD⁺ is central to electron transfer and mitochondrial efficiency, so depletion worsens neuronal energy failure.[250]
- Repairing the gut microbiome is also necessary, along with introducing proper probiotics.
  - Refer back to the GI chapter as needed for a thorough intervention.

Other supportive treatments may involve inositol, which can bind to serotonin and promote a calming effect. This has been found to be helpful for those experiencing anxiety symptoms or neurological diseases. With many options available, it's necessary to determine proper treatment on an individualized basis.

Business Practice Pearl

Back to discussing practice growth, one of the biggest (and most common) mistakes I see practitioners make when starting to market their functional medicine programs is going into excessive detail about the services and components involved. They will plug in a crazy amount of "things" so they feel like their programs are "worth it," such as food services, health devices, or extra time with the provider. It is not that adding more can't be beneficial; just refrain from adding for the sake of bulking up a program. Each "piece" should have a calibrated value, and the truth is, people don't want the pieces; they want the payoff.

I often compare this to someone purchasing a vacation package. They don't think about the flight, going through TSA, the process for checking into the hotel, or any other logistical details. They focus on the payoff—the enjoyable vacation experience. So, instead of selling them a plane ticket, we should be selling them the vacation experience itself. They want the payoff that will improve their lives, and a functional medicine package is more valuable than a vacation—this is their life and quality of life for every day they are alive. While a vacation may cost relatively the same, a vacation is gone in 5-7 days, while they are with their body (and symptoms they suffer with) day in, day out for the rest of their lives, unless they get help.

Furthermore, you are not just prescribing a medication that they might have to take forever while the root cause of their illness remains unaddressed and the damage continues to accumulate. Your goal is to identify that root cause and help them overcome it, empowering them to become their own health advocates. This is one of the most vital aspects of the work we do. In the long run, they save money with you, as the average person spends around $10,000 a year managing illness, and they are being given the opportunity to be liberated from that life.

Emphasize the cost of inaction, because if they don't know the risks they are facing by not undergoing treatment, they may soon reach a point when it is too late. When considering neurological diseases in particular, time not healing a root cause of illness truly equates to loss of brain function. The longer the body remains under attack and inflamed, the greater the risk of irreversible nerve damage, which diminishes the likelihood of reducing or reversing symptoms.

Contrasting this with conventional intervention, we see that some symptoms may be alleviated, but they fail to address the root causes. Even if a patient feels somewhat better, the underlying issues will likely worsen over time, and other issues are likely to develop. There's no definite timeline. However, once that happens, they often realize that there was nothing greater they could have invested in than their health. Sometimes we are the only ones in their immediate circle to save them from the mindset of denial and warn them that the time to take action is now.

Regardless of the specific root cause, if we can eliminate any contributing factors of illness, patients can expect to function better and experience fewer symptoms, which is simply invaluable. It's essential to communicate that the costs of inaction are far greater than investing in one's health, particularly when addressing mental and neurological diseases.

BONUS TRAINING:

Free Neurological Health Functional Medicine Training from our fully accredited Board Certification Course.

SCAN ME

SCAN THE QR CODE

or visit functionalmedicineunlocked.com

Chapter 7

Endocrinology: From Hormones to Weight Loss

CASE STUDY: The Invisible Ceiling When Weight Loss Plateaus

This case study involves a thirty-eight-year-old male who had been working hard to lose weight but had reached a plateau. It serves as a fascinating example of how the simplest changes can lead to significant results. Sometimes the ceiling that keeps us stuck isn't difficult to break; we just have to know how to see it. In this example, actions that might seem minor can actually have a major impact.

He had been engaging in high-intensity interval training (HIIT) and was putting in a lot of effort. He was following a mostly healthy diet and was frustrated by his lack of progress. For this patient, all I did was remove chemicals such as BPA (found in plastics and epoxy resins) from his diet and environment. As a result, he was able to break a one-year weight loss plateau.

The most significant dietary change I made was advising him to stop heating his food in plastic containers and using topical products that had potential xenoestrogens (chemicals that act as extra estrogen in the body). These products included lotions, deodorants, and colognes. After evaluating his routine, I couldn't identify any major issues with his diet. His macros were balanced, and he was eating whole foods. In fact, the only chemicals in his diet that I could identify came from a tablespoon of ranch dressing each day for his vegetables and salads, which I advised him to start making on his own to eliminate other chemicals. I did make a slight adjustment to his workout timing, but it didn't prove to be as impactful as removing the exposure to xenoestrogens.

By making these changes, he finally broke through his weight loss barrier. He called me a "genius," which was amusing since the solution was so simple. The underlying issue was that exposure to xenoestrogens had been negatively affecting his testosterone levels. We will further explain xenoestrogens in this chapter. This case highlights the significant impact that dietary and environmental changes can have in terms of hormonal balance.

Root Cause Investigation: More Than Just Hormone Replacement

Hormonal regulation refers to the rebalancing of hormones, such as progesterone, thyroid hormones, testosterone, insulin, and cortisol, to optimal levels. Common symptoms of hormonal imbalance include fatigue, weight gain, low libido, mood swings, and sleep disturbances. Women may also experience symptoms such as hot flashes and irregular menstrual cycles. A comprehensive and unbiased patient history is essential to gather real insights and personal experiences.

The first step is to identify the root causes of hormonal disruptions prior to supplementing or replacing. Root causes may include toxins in the body, gut imbalances, stress, or even nutritional deficiencies. Nutrients such as vitamin D, B vitamins, minerals like magnesium and zinc, and antioxidants can significantly impact hormonal balance. However, first, we must know which imbalances we are targeting, and that begins with testing.

DUTCH Testing

If the client is female, it is best to assess with a DUTCH test around day 19–20 of the woman's cycle. This may become difficult to determine if periods are irregular, such as with polycystic ovarian syndrome (PCOS), or when she is entering the perimenopausal phase of life, because estrogen levels become erratic and cycles are no longer predictable. Results include the measure of cortisol, DHEA, estrogen, progesterone, testosterone, melatonin, and their breakdown products over the previous 24 hours.

It provides insights into hormone production, metabolism, and circadian rhythm as well as cortisol and cortisone levels. Total cortisol assesses adrenal function and the stress response, while cortisol rhythm evaluates the lack or presence of a healthy diurnal pattern. A normal rhythm will demonstrate peaking in the morning and decreasing at night. Samples are collected by the patient at specific times of the day. The pattern presented can indicate whether a person is experiencing adrenal dysfunction or if the body's adrenal response is functioning normally.

Next let us delve into a summary of the key factors of this test. Please note that this is simply a summary to serve as a user-friendly entry into hormone evaluation, not a comprehensive course.

Overview of the Cortisol Section of the DUTCH Test

Cortisone is a metabolite of cortisol, so it can give us insight into how well our body is clearing itself of cortisol. Measuring both free cortisol and cortisone levels with metabolized cortisol gives a better picture of the body's cortisol clearance rate (CCR). Cortisol levels should decrease at night, accompanied by a spike in melatonin. However, when there are dysfunctions, melatonin production may not be triggered properly. For example, chronic stress, hypothyroidism, liver disease, obesity, sleep deprivation, and certain medications, such as corticosteroids, can lead to a slow CCR. On the other hand, a fast CCR may be the result of Addison's disease or adrenal insufficiency.[257]

Cortisol levels should exhibit a normal daily wave pattern. Cortisol should start highest in the morning and gradually decrease throughout the day. If cortisol levels are consistently elevated above normal production levels, it may indicate an HPA-axis imbalance, as happens in chronic stress or sleep deprivation, potentially leading to chronic fatigue and a lack of compensating. In this state, people often feel wired and tired, waking up to high cortisol levels that persist throughout the day but are unable to shake brain fog and a feeling of fatigue. As people progress to later phases of dysfunction, cortisol may not spike in the morning, suggesting that the body is no longer overcompensating for stressors.

Overview of Sex Hormones

The test also analyzes specific sex hormones, including the three main estrogen types: estrone (E1), estradiol (E2), and estriol (E3). The convenient part of each name is that the number reflects the name (i.e., estrone is estr-one, "di-" means "two," and "tri-" means "three"). Estrone is the primary estrogen produced after menopause and is also produced in fat tissue via peripheral aromatization. Consequently, individuals with more adipose tissue tend to have higher levels of estrone. Elevated estrone is of particular concern because this has been linked to an increased risk for endometrial and breast cancer.[258] For patients who are overweight, weight loss can help regulate these hormones. E2, or estradiol, is the most potent estrogen and primarily serves as the main female sex hormone during a woman's reproductive years. Estriol

(E3) is the primary form during pregnancy and is produced primarily by the placenta.

Xenoestrogens, if you recall from Chapter 3, include substances like BPA, propylparaben, phthalates, plastics, and pesticides. They bind to estrogen and androgen receptors, thereby disrupting normal endocrine signaling, driving up levels of sex hormone binding globulin (SHBG), and leading to symptoms such as decreased sexual drive, weight gain, mood swings, and even potentially increasing potential risk for cancer.[259] Testing for SHBG can give additional insight but must be added as a blood test apart from DUTCH testing.

Estrogen metabolites are measured to assess the body's estrogen metabolism and risk factors, including breast cancer. 2-Hydroxyestradiol is a metabolite of estradiol that is formed by the hydroxylation of estradiol. It serves as a "less potent" form of estrogen. When interpreting estrogen metabolites, it's important to note the protective role of 2-OH estrogen, which is associated with reduced cancer risk. In contrast, 4-OH (4-Hydroxyestradiol) is potentially harmful and linked to DNA damage and increased cancer risk.[258] Elevated 16-OH (16-Hydroxyestradiol) estrogen indicates increased estrogenic activity, known in functional medicine as estrogen dominance, which can contribute to symptoms such as PMS, fibroids, and endometriosis.[257, 260] The ratio of 1-OH and 16-OH can be associated with an increased risk of breast cancer.

Strategies to decrease unfavorable estrogen activity can include supporting estrogen elimination as well as supporting testosterone and progesterone levels. Eating sufficient cruciferous vegetables, regular exercise, hydration, and maintaining a clean environment and water source are all important interventions to consider. In addition, DUTCH testing evaluates progesterone metabolites to assess luteal phase efficiency or deficiency in women. Androgen levels, such as testosterone and DHEA, are tested. These hormones directly affect libido, mood, and muscle mass.

It is also essential to determine if testosterone is being functionally reduced by xenoestrogen binding, which can prevent it from interacting normally in target tissue. A person may have normal testosterone levels but insufficient free testosterone, indicating altered bioavailability.[261] While DUTCH does not measure free or total testosterone directly, a normal DHEA-S with low testosterone can indicate that this phenomenon may be present. Free testosterone is important because it is the "active" form, meaning it is not bound to protein and, therefore, can exert change and help the body function correctly when present in healthy amounts.[261] Free and total testosterone is another blood test that may be considered in addition to DUTCH testing for a more complete evaluation. Lastly, melatonin, a neurotransmitter, and nutritional markers are also included on some versions of the DUTCH test and can aid in a more comprehensive evaluation of a client's health status.

Optimizing SHBG & Decreasing Estrogen Dominance/Sensitivity

As previously discussed, testing for SHBG is an additional test that can be ordered and can give a clearer clinical picture. If found to be elevated, the goal to decrease SHBG can help with unbinding estrogen and testosterone so that they can become bioavailable in tissues. These treatment approaches will focus primarily on natural and root-cause correction. However, when necessary, hormonal replacement therapy (HRT) can be explored for those to whom it is appropriate and desired. When SHBG is elevated in men, free testosterone availability drops, and it leads to decreased libido, irritability, decreased muscular mass, fatigue, and even erectile dysfunction.

Women will experience similar symptoms, such as fatigue, decreased libido, irritability, and decreased muscular mass when SHBG is elevated. They will also often have vaginal dryness and mood swings. If

SHBG is found to be elevated, it is important to screen for underlying contributing factors, such as thyroid dysfunction, insulin resistance, elevated stress, dietary causes, medications, detox issues, or liver disease. A full assessment also includes free and total testosterone, estradiol, fasting insulin, HbA1c, fasting glucose, liver function tests, and four-point cortisol testing.[259]

Next, let's dive deeper into the main ways in which hormones can be naturally influenced under the functional medicine model by identifying and reversing root causes. It is important to emphasize that under the Functional Model of care, we do not follow a specific set of protocols but rather do an investigation to find underlying disturbances that should be corrected. The interventions chosen do not follow a "first, second, or third line protocol" method as we see in the conventional model. Interventions chosen will depend upon the client's needs based on lab and assessment findings.

Thyroid Disease

Symptoms of hypothyroidism may include unexplained fatigue, weight gain, cold sensitivity, dry skin, constipation, and possibly a goiter, which is an enlargement of the thyroid that's visible as neck swelling. Other symptoms can include a slowed heart rate, depression, thinning hair, puffiness in the face, slowed speech, a coarse-sounding voice, droopy eyelids, tingling or pain in the hands, muscle cramps, thinning eyebrows, confusion, brain fog, irregular menstrual flow, and hair loss.[262]

The thyroid produces 20% of the body's circulating triiodothyronine (T3) and all of the thyroxine (T4), with the help of iodine. The body makes the rest of the T3 by converting T4 into T3, which is the more bioactive thyroid hormone that impacts metabolism and virtually every cell in the body. TSH is not produced by the thyroid but by the anterior pituitary of the brain, and it then stimulates the thyroid. When evaluating labs, a low TSH (thyroid-stimulating hormone) indicates that the thyroid is working overtime and may represent a state of hyperthyroidism. Conversely, a high TSH with a low T4 indicates hypothyroidism, meaning that the thyroid is underactive.

A helpful analogy is to think of TSH as an accelerator. When the thyroid is overactive (hyperthyroidism), the body reduces TSH production because it needs the thyroid to "slow down." In contrast, when the thyroid is underactive (hypothyroidism), the brain increases TSH levels to stimulate the thyroid to produce more hormones. When the thyroid is active, it produces T4. So, that is why in cases of high TSH, we often see low T4 levels, and when TSH is low, T4 is typically elevated.[263] A high TSH with a normal T4 is indicative of subclinical hypothyroidism. This is a less severe clinical presentation where the thyroid is showing signs of being underactive, but the T4 levels are not yet low enough to cause symptoms. Conversely, a low TSH and a normal T4 may indicate subclinical hyperthyroidism.

The situations can become more complex with primary or secondary thyroid disease, but that detail goes beyond the scope of this overview and is covered in our full program. However, for a brief overview, in instances of primary hyperthyroidism, the thyroid is not functioning correctly. The thyroid produces excessive amounts of T4 (and therefore T3, as long as there are no issues with T4-to-T3 conversion, like in cellular inflammation), and the negative feedback suppresses TSH secretion from the anterior pituitary.

In secondary hyperthyroidism, the anterior pituitary produces excessive levels of TSH, and the thyroid therefore overproduces T4. While very rare, this is most often due to a TSH-secreting pituitary adenoma.[264] In primary hypothyroidism, the thyroid gland does not produce enough thyroid hormone (T4 and, consequently, T3). This typically triggers a compensatory rise in TSH from the anterior pituitary as it attempts to stimulate the thyroid to produce more hormone.

In early or mild cases (subclinical hypothyroidism), T4 levels may remain within normal limits while TSH becomes elevated. In overt hypothyroidism, both T4 and T3 are low and TSH is high.

This is just one example of how the causes of hypothyroidism and hormone imbalances in general are multifactorial and why accurate diagnosis requires clinical correlation beyond lab values alone. In developed countries such as the United States, the most common cause of hypothyroidism is Hashimoto's thyroiditis, an autoimmune condition in which thyroid peroxidase (TPO) and thyroglobulin antibodies target the thyroid's follicular cells, leading to inflammation and gradual glandular destruction. Globally, however, iodine deficiency remains the most common cause of hypothyroidism and goiter,[265] though it is less prevalent in nations with iodized salt programs.

Hashimoto's is the leading cause of hypothyroidism in the U.S. It occurs when antibodies attack the thyroid, impairing its ability to produce the necessary hormones. This autoimmune disorder occurs ten times more frequently in women than in men, likely due to hormonal and immune system differences, including the influence of estrogen, and is most prevalent in individuals aged thirty to fifty. If untreated, it can lead to complications such as hyperlipidemia, infertility, constipation, depression, and even myxedema.

Free Versus Total T3 and T4

"Free T3 and T4" is the small portion that is unbound from proteins. "Total" includes both free and protein-bound. An easy way to understand this is to view total hormones as money in your savings account. They become "free" when they become cash in your hand. Subtle cues to the underlying root cause can be identified when the trend between these two readings is carefully assessed. Binding proteins can change as a result of hormones, liver function, or illness. For example, when total is low but free is normal or elevated, this pattern can result from decreased thyroxine-binding globulin levels, which can occur with low estrogen, menopause cues, high androgens (as is seen in PCOS), steroid use, or liver dysfunction. TSH and estrogen interact indirectly, as estrogen balance influences thyroxine-binding globulin synthesis and clearance; consequently, excess estrogen can influence elevated TBG levels in downstream processes. Addressing estrogen imbalances may help optimize thyroid hormone availability.[266,267] Assessment should be included as clinically warranted.

Normal free and high total could indicate estrogen-driven increases in binding proteins, such as during pregnancy. Normal free T4 and low free T3 can indicate poor conversion or nutrient deficiency, such as seen in selenium, zinc, or iron deficiency, or stress. Low total and low free are most often consistent with true hypothyroidism as a result of the thyroid not producing enough hormone, and, when both are elevated, this may indicate Graves' disease or other thyroid overactivity.[273]

Trace Minerals and Thyroid Disease

Iodine deficiency is another significant factor, especially in regions where it is not supplemented. A shift from table salt to sea salt or pink Himalayan salt, while having its benefits, can lead to iodine deficiency if table salt is the main or only source of iodine, as these alternative salts typically contain less iodine. Consequently, insufficient iodine intake can result in hypothyroidism. Iodine and tyrosine are the key components required for the synthesis of T3 and T4. Iodine uptake is regulated based upon a concentration gradient to maintain balanced hormone production, which is why one should never assume a client needs iodine and should instead test for deficiency.

Selenium deficiency can additionally impair thyroid health by reducing the production of active thyroid hormone (T3) and weakening antioxidant defenses. This can lead to increased thyroid inflammation, damage, and potential autoimmune conditions, as it is crucial for converting

T4 to T3 and protecting the gland from hydrogen peroxide-induced fibrosis. Screening for selenium levels in thyroid disease is advised.

Medical History

As a thorough clinician, be certain to screen for all causes of thyroid dysfunction. Certain medications, such as iodinated contrast agents, amiodarone, interferon alpha, and lithium, can contribute to thyroid dysfunction. Thyroid surgery or radiation treatments can lead to hypothyroidism, impacting the treatment plan.

Congenital hypothyroidism is a rare but severe condition present at birth, affecting the infant's brain and nervous system. Pituitary or hypothalamic disorders can cause secondary hypothyroidism by reducing TSH or TRH secretion, preventing adequate thyroid hormone production.[268]

Last to note is that while genetics influence the risk for thyroid disease, environment and lifestyle often determine expression. As the saying goes, "Genetics may load the gun, but the environment pulls the trigger." People can still make significant lifestyle changes. Ensuring a healthier diet can help regulate thyroid hormones, addressing potential iodine deficiencies as well as levels of iron, selenium, zinc, and vitamins A, B2, B6, and B12, all of which are vital for thyroid health.

Thyroid & Food

There is a growing body of evidence on the negative effects of inflammation from gluten on thyroid disease, particularly Hashimoto's.[269,270] The evidence is significant even in those without clinical symptoms of gluten intolerance. While not every patient may need to be gluten-free, a trial of being gluten-free for an extended period of time (typically around a year) is recommended. Gluten has been proposed to contribute to molecular mimicry, where the gluten proteins closely resemble the structure of thyroid cells. When the body reacts negatively to gluten, it mistakenly also targets the thyroid due to this similarity. This may help explain why there is a statistically significant association between gluten sensitivity and Hashimoto's.[269] Some literature also supports the same phenomenon in dairy/casein ingestion.[271] Vitamin D insufficiency is additionally linked to increased risk for autoimmune disease and should be assessed as part of the client's situation.[272]

Thyroid Lab Evaluation in Functional Medicine

Thyroid Levels

For a comprehensive assessment of thyroid health, you should include a full thyroid panel that consists of the following tests:

- TSH (thyroid-stimulating hormone)
- Free T4 (to measure the bioavailability of unbound thyroid hormone)
- Free T3 (to assess active thyroid hormone levels and peripheral conversion of T4 to T3). Low levels can indicate hypothyroid function or conversion issues, potentially due to gastrointestinal issues, stress, or high toxic burden
- Reverse T3 (to assess diversion of T4 toward inactive reverse T3 pathways).
- TPO (Thyroid peroxidase antibodies), which is key for identifying autoimmune activity and supporting the diagnosis of Hashimoto's
- Trace Minerals

Now, let's discuss some of the lab results that can help differentiate conditions, as well as the functional ranges, which you can find in the table in Chapter 2. A normal TSH level combined with low T3 typically presents symptoms like cold hands, constipation, and brain fog. This can often be a result of gut dysfunction, since a portion of T4 to T3 conversion is influenced by gut health, though most conversion occurs in peripheral tissues such as the liver and kidneys. Identifying these issues can significantly alleviate symptoms.

Many patients feel better once their TSH levels are optimized, whether through pharmaceuticals or natural methods that target the root cause. It's worth noting that relying solely on TSH will miss a subset of thyroid dysfunction cases, which is why including T3 and T4 levels is recommended when conducting a complete panel.[273]

T3 is the biologically active thyroid hormone that binds nuclear receptors to regulate gene expression. This explains the symptoms experienced, even when T3 levels are sufficient, but inflammation may impair cellular responsiveness to thyroid hormone. Stress and chronic infections can be significant contributors to this issue.[274] For that reason, adding supplements such as ashwagandha, zinc, or selenium for people with thyroid dysfunction may be beneficial to enhance conversion of T4 to T3.

Poor T4-to-T3 Converters

Issues with converting T4 to T3 through the process of deiodinases, where an iodine atom is removed from T4, can be a barrier to balance. This can stem from vitamin and mineral deficiencies, stress, toxicity, excessive carbohydrate intake, or insufficient protein consumption.

At times, the body might convert T4 into the inactive form, known as reverse T3 (RT3). Elevated levels of RT3 may compete with T3 at receptor sites and reflect altered peripheral metabolism, preventing the utilization of T3. Optimizing health, decreasing overall inflammation in the body, decreasing endogenous cortisol and exogenous steroids (when applicable and safe), and improving mitochondrial functioning may help to decrease levels of RT3.[274]

Hashimoto's Root Cause Evaluation: Gut Dysbiosis

Gut health can significantly influence thyroid hormone metabolism, therefore stool analysis is often essential to treatment and correction, as gut inflammation can hinder this conversion and it may contribute to thyroid dysfunction. Gut health also affects thyroid function via chronic inflammation that prevents cells from functioning properly. Mitochondria may deplete their energy stores and, due to inflammation, cells may have reduced responsiveness to thyroid hormone. Thus, some patients exhibit symptoms of hypothyroidism despite having a functioning thyroid and adequate hormonal conversion.[274] Symptoms, such as brain fog, fatigue, and numbness, occur because of a depletion of T3 in the cells of the body as a result of dysbiosis.[262]

The last, and possibly more important, thing to screen for in a patient with Hashimoto's is a parasitic or helminthic infection. This is most commonly found in the gut but can be throughout the body and can contribute to disease in certain cases, despite there not being a focus on intervention for it in the conventional model.[269] A single negative result in stool analysis may be a false negative. Most labs recommend at least three negative readings before parasitic involvement is fully ruled out, as false negatives are common. Elevated eosinophils, without significant allergic symptoms, may raise suspicion for parasitic infection and warrant further evaluation.[275]

Toxin Screening in Thyroid Disease

Screening for heavy metals is critical in assessing thyroid disease. Excessive exposure to fluoride and bromine, highly present in the water supply, is suspected to trigger Hashimoto's and contribute to the inflammatory process, as are substances like bisphenol A (BPA) and perfluorinated compounds associated with nonstick cookware. Teflon, found in nonstick cookware, can leach into food, increasing our health risks.[253] A comprehensive functional treatment plan will include decreasing environmental exposure.

Resistant Weight Loss

Under the Functional Model we examine several areas that could inhibit a person from losing weight, not just dieting and exercise, although these interventions are important and should be incorporated into any comprehensive plan. Interventions specific to functional medicine might include the microbiome, exposure to endocrine disruptors, estrogen dominance, thyroid disease, and insulin resistance. Other issues to address and screen for include sleep apnea, inflammation, nutritional deficiencies, and detox. We will explore each of these in more depth.

Polycystic Ovarian Syndrome (PCOS)

In women, PCOS is a leading cause of hormonal disruption and should be examined for. Root causes may include gut dysbiosis, chemical exposure (especially endocrine disruptors), diet, and lack of exercise.[276] PCOS results from an excess of androgens and leads to cystic ovaries and symptoms that include hirsutism, irregular menstruation, mood swings, and resistant weight loss from insulin resistance. Diagnosis should be by a licensed professional, and root cause treatment begins with identifying and then reversing these root causes while considering hormonal levels and lab results.

Perimenopause

Perimenopause in functional medicine is approached as a systems-wide transition that starts years before the final period. Fluctuating hormones is a natural, though delicate, process. One that can be easily triggered by unnatural triggers that produce effects that ripple through the gut, liver, adrenals, thyroid, and nervous system. This can exacerbate a normal function in life into an experience that is less normal. A functional approach focuses on correcting root causes that are within control and may include impaired estrogen detoxification, blood sugar instability, cortisol dysregulation, micronutrient depletion, and gut inflammation. It is again about supporting the whole system and allowing the body to naturally transition. With that being said, there are times when HRT therapy is still needed depending upon the individual, various health factors, and how soon they make changes before this time. It is imperative to lead with a root cause approach but not fall into an all-or-nothing belief that prescriptions are never necessary.

Low Testosterone

While low testosterone (low T) is a concern most often for men, do not forget that women additionally need testosterone and can suffer from lower than normal levels. Either way, the approach to low testosterone is still to decrease the effects of estrogen dominance or sensitivity and to implement a lifestyle that will naturally boost testosterone, including the interventions we will discuss below. These root causes should all be considered, no matter the formal diagnosis of where we started, whether it is androgen dominance (as seen in PCOS) or estrogen dominance (as is common in low T).

Hormonal Root Cause: Toxins

The effects of heavy metals, pesticides, and plastics found in the environment do not end with increased risk for cancer or neurological disease. They can also act as strong endocrine and hormonal disruptors. As previously discussed in the case study and in more depth in Chapter 3, an investigation into the client's environment, product use, and diet is important to reveal any exposure to chemicals, both those assumed (but not typically proven) to be safe by the general public and those known not to be.

Remember the importance of liver detoxification and methylation, as these processes can impact the ability to eliminate toxins and estrogen.

Supporting the liver with supplements like glutathione or ALA, milk thistle (300–600 mg/day), or NAC (600–1200 mg/day) early on can help to ensure the body is able to detox chemicals properly and utilize the estrogen detox pathways, as the liver is the primary organ responsible for estrogen detox. Detox may also include removing exogenous hormones such as oral contraceptives. By creating the right environment for the body, we can often support its natural detoxification processes.

Hormonal Root Cause: Blood Sugar Dysregulation & Inflammatory Foods

Blood sugar imbalances and insulin resistance are also critical topics to discuss with clients. Elevated insulin levels can disrupt the balance of estrogen, testosterone, and cortisol. It's not surprising that patients with polycystic ovarian syndrome (PCOS) often exhibit insulin resistance, which highlights the importance of glycemic control. Control begins with incorporating exercise (as tolerated) and a lower carbohydrate, though not always keto, diet (typically staying around 150 healthy grams a day) with sufficient high-quality protein and plenty of healthy fats. Simply put, any time there is hormonal disruption, recommend an organic, clean environment and diet.[81] Cinnamon and berberine are an option to help decrease insulin resistance. Berberine is contraindicated in pregnancy. In the right patient, though, these interventions will help to reverse any potential insulin resistance.

Insulin acts as a growth hormone, and high levels can lead to weight gain. Also, insulin spikes lead to hormonal dysregulation and need to be avoided. Regular periods of fasting help to avoid glucose spikes. This is why intermittent fasting can be of great benefit for decreasing insulin resistance. Conversely at times, for those already practicing long-term intermittent fasting, the body may begin to store calories in response to perceived starvation risks. Consequently, these people may end up plateauing. In such cases, I recommend increasing meal and snack frequency to help counterbalance this.

However, a large group of the population has fallen into habits of daily grazing, and intermittent fasting can help trigger the body to release stored adipose tissue because of the periods of time without insulin spikes. The point is that individuals need individual planning. While some may go years on an intermittent fasting protocol and do well, some need to be transitioned off it. It is individualized, as metabolism is based on a complex network of hormones, neurotransmitters, and enzymes.

The second part of nutritional timing is when the client consumes certain macros. For example, eating high-carb meals, especially at night, can disrupt hormonal function and reduce melatonin production. To help "wake up" metabolism, I may recommend that the client switch to eating more protein and healthy fats in the evening and try to eat most of their carbs during the morning and afternoon, when the body more naturally needs quicker sources of energy. It may also be beneficial to suggest longer fasting periods by eating supper earlier in the evening and not eating again until the next day's breakfast for better hormonal balance.[271] Ultimately, achieving balance is crucial, as is understanding each person's unique circumstances and lifestyle factors.

Protein intake should be around 20–30 grams per meal, more specifically around 0.8 g/lb of body weight if sedentary and around 1.5 g/lb of body weight if performing endurance training. Protein is important for maintaining insulin resistance control. A high-protein diet will tend to negate the body's desire for carbs, helping the patient follow a lower-carb diet. This is beneficial for hormone regulation as well as decreasing inflammatory processes. This is evidenced by studies that show a higher-protein diet results in lower inflammatory markers, such as high-sensitivity C-reactive protein (hs-CRP), tumor necrosis factor-alpha (TNF-α), and interleukin 6 (IL-6).[277] A high-protein diet also decreases the risk of diseases such as diabetes, osteoarthritis, sleep apnea, cardiovascular disease, and even cancer, which are just a few of the hundreds of diseases with an inflammatory basis.[278]

Removing inflammatory foods, such as ultra-processed and sugary ones, is nonnegotiable when re-regulating hormones. Trans fats and refined sugars both impair liver function, increase inflammation, hinder hormone balance, and prevent toxic detoxification. Advertising will often boast that a food is "low carb" to attract health-conscious people, but the consumer often does not realize that these foods are chemically altered and not naturally low-carb. The "food" will often do more damage than good. A common error is eating a low-calorie, low-carb, or low-fat diet but ignoring the quality of food. The belief that it's not what you eat but how much of it you eat only goes so far. You might lose weight in the short term, but if chemicals are still disrupting your hormones and causing inflammation, you will experience issues with health and weight loss at some point.

Decreasing the amount of ultraprocessed foods is helpful, but we unfortunately also cannot always trust even whole foods sold in the mainstream groceries, as they are often injected with chemicals that are not always put on an ingredients list. Even whole chickens are often injected with tenderizers, potassium, sodium benzoate, and flavor-enhancing chemicals. Red meat naturally does not retain its bright red color for long. As it begins to break down, it will naturally take on a grayer appearance.

To counteract this, manufacturers add chemicals and dyes to meat to make it look more appealing and redder, thereby enhancing its marketability. From my personal experience, many clients who seem to benefit from extreme diets continue to do well when the food group is reintroduced in its healthiest form. For example, if someone comes to me on the carnivore diet and we add organic vegetables and gluten-free grains, from my experience, they maintain the results they had on the carnivore diet. Likewise, adding farm-fresh or wild game to a vegan diet could possibly still yield the same benefits simply because the chemicals in the store-bought protein sources were not added back into the diet. Unfortunately, the literature is not yet developed around this idea.

Even a presumably small amount of these toxins can lead to toxic overload and cause chronic damage. I once met an individual who started their small business, an organic farm, because they threw up every time they ate chicken. Believing it to be an allergy, they avoided the meat altogether until they tried a locally farm-raised chicken.

The results blew the person's mind when they were able to eat without vomiting. This is another example of how individuals can be sensitive to things in different ways. Some have more obvious symptoms, while most have more subtle issues that lead to chronic disease that "sneaks up" on them. Either way, harm is likely ensuing at some level. I believe that to be the case for the majority of the population, and that is why cancer and autoimmune diseases are particularly on the rise.

Either way, we grossly underestimate our exposure to the tens of thousands of "approved" chemicals. It takes extra effort and often a certain investment, but being careful to choose foods that are fully chemical-free can reduce inflammation, lower insulin spikes, aid in weight loss, and lead to better cortisol and hormonal balance, ultimately saving thousands of dollars and hours of being unwell. Promoting anti-inflammatory whole foods is essential, especially cruciferous vegetables, which aid in estrogen metabolism. Healthy fats and omega-3s are also necessary for hormone production. Studies have tied adequate amounts of omega fatty acids to an improved transition into menopause, and they act as critical components in cell membrane structure, hormone production, and reducing inflammation that can disrupt endocrine function when not present.[279]

Another way foods either enhance or disrupt hormonal balance is by altering gut flora. Healthy foods will help to ensure a balance of healthy microbiomes that help to break down excess estrogen to maintain balance. Conversely, an imbalance in the microbiome can prevent the proper breakdown of hormones, aiding in the development of estrogen dominance, which we'll discuss in relation to autoimmune diseases.[280] When the gut is imbalanced, the body struggles to metabolize hormones effectively.[100]

Also, certain foods contain endocrine disruptors, such as BPA, phthalates, and pesticides, especially non-organic meats, produce, and packaged foods. These substances can mimic natural hormones and contribute to estrogen dominance. There is conflicting evidence that high amounts of milk consumption in young women lead to an earlier onset of menstruation, two to three years earlier than in the past. However, there is considerable consensus that moderate probiotic yogurt intake and extended periods of breastfeeding as an infant decrease this risk. High sugar and high carbohydrate intake, on the other hand, increase the risk, and many of those products are high in sugar, and homemade selections are best.[98]

While food experts will likely never come to a complete agreement on most topics, a safe goal is to focus on balance and implementing foods in their original form as best as possible. From the practitioner's standpoint, I believe in considering patient preferences and what they are most likely to adhere to. Two things (or studies) can be true at the same time. More than one diet can be healthy. Maintain that nothing is ingested in excess, and if all other controls are accounted for, always recommend progress over perfection.

The nutritional approach for patients experiencing hormonal imbalances should include dietary plans tailored to their specific hormonal levels, nutritional deficiencies, and genetic predispositions. Additives often include preservatives to extend shelf life in foods such as broth solutions, corn syrup, or concentrates. Many foods from fast-food or regular restaurants may contain similar additives that are not always listed online, making it appear that one is eating whole foods while actually consuming excess sodium and other chemicals.

To identify specific food triggers, IgG (not IgE) testing can be performed. Although there can be discrepancies in the accuracy of these tests—leading to possible false negatives or false positives—they can still serve as a helpful starting point. It's crucial to focus on the person rather than solely on the test results. With that said, for those suspected of having a hormonal imbalance, some literature is strong to support the benefits of avoiding dairy, gluten, and especially soy, as soy acts as an estrogen in the body. At the same time, meta-analysis shows many good studies that support milk as beneficial and strongly backs yogurt without high amounts of sugar as beneficial.[93] If kept within the diet, raw or A2 milk is recommended, and again, the focus is the individual and how their body responds. Glucose monitoring can reveal this at an individual level. High glucose spikes after ingestion are unlikely to be beneficial for hormonal rebalancing.

Tapping into the Power of the Mind for Healthy Habits For Weight & Hormonal Balance

Dietary changes are an important part of healthy change. However, as sufficient providers, we must acknowledge that simply telling clients what to eat is not sufficient in and of itself. Learning how to make healthy changes is also a learned skill that I recommend you help your clients achieve. It's important for clients to recognize that their minds hold a powerful influence on health choices. When making healthy dietary changes, I help educate them on how to take control of their decisions, not just "willpower" through it. If negative thought processes are an issue, they must be empowered to know that they hold the power to take thoughts captive; it is simply that we were not often taught the necessary tools to do so. Once they realize this and are equipped with the skills required, it's like turning on the lights to expose the "enemy," and darkness cannot exist in the light. They can reclaim their power. A practical way I guide people in this process is by applying Maslow's hierarchy of needs to help them identify what they truly need.

At the very bottom of this hierarchy are our basic needs: what we need to survive. I encourage clients to focus on what their bodies need rather than just what they want. If they experience cravings, I help them identify which unmet need they're trying to fulfill through food.

For instance, the need for social connection is fundamental. People often go to great lengths, such as buying expensive purses, to gain social status. This psychological drive can additionally lead people to eat unhealthy foods simply to fit in. I challenge clients to find other ways to fulfill that need at social events without relying on food. If they feel down or sad, instead of turning to food, we discuss alternative strategies, including journaling, exercise, breathwork, prayer, and self-reflection. Although when food is used to console, that is a cue to recognize that they require much deeper work that is past the scope of this text.

Journaling and leaving notes of inspiration to themselves can additionally be a powerful trick to stay on track. During my transition to a healthier lifestyle, I wrote down the reasons for avoiding unhealthy foods. My motivations weren't solely based on weight loss; they revolved around not wanting to feel anxious, preventing depressive episodes, and avoiding IBS flare-ups. I found that cravings can hijack your brain and make you forget your goals. But when they are written down and kept in plain view, they are not as easily forgotten. Often, places to write these down could be in the notes section of a phone or written down and left in cupboards or refrigerators. In moments of temptation, it's easy to lose sight of your goals and the negative consequences of certain foods.

Many people tend to adopt an all-or-nothing mindset when it comes to their diet. For instance, if they eat one donut, they might think, *Oh, I failed. My behavior is shameful, and there's something wrong with me.* However, the reality is that they simply ate a donut. It's important to avoid spiraling into negative thoughts like *"I shouldn't have done that"* or dwelling on the "should've, could've, would've" mentality. A common phrase is "Don't *should* all over yourself." Instead, it's beneficial to recognize that there's usually a reason behind choices. Maybe we ate the donut because we were stressed or had a craving. Understanding the reasons for actions is key, rather than feeling guilty about them. We can use these experiences as a source of empowerment for the future. By approaching life with the mindset of striving to be just 1% better, we set attainable goals that are not overwhelming.

At times, when it is right for the patient, suggest trying healthier (not always the healthiest) options first, as a way to break food addictions. Examples may be lower sugar, whole food, and granola bars over candy bars, for example. Less sugar and at least some fiber is a win over straight processed, chemical-laden sugar. If cravings persist, recommend drinking a full glass or bottle of water, which can help curb them. It's also important to avoid sustained times of feeling deprived. Allowing occasional treats—rather than calling them "cheats"—can make the process more enjoyable and easier to stick to. Also, when treats are scheduled in, clients don't feel like they have "failed" and can prevent the all-or-nothing self-sabotage that occurs. I help clients understand that this journey is a process with no strict end goal. It's not about perfection; it's about progress.

It's crucial to realize that we are human and that this journey is a process. If making these changes were easy, we wouldn't be facing the obesity epidemic we see today. Our food environment has been engineered in a way that makes these challenges more difficult. However, that doesn't mean we can't empower ourselves to improve little by little.

One of the key areas I focus on with my clients is reframing and understanding triggers when it comes to food. Many are not aware of the psychological cues we tend to have when it comes to eating and dietary choices. I implement cognitive behavioral therapy when appropriate. However, it's equally important to educate that cravings and food addictions are not always personal; they're often related to the way food is ultra-processed. Most commercial foods have been modified extensively to make them more addictive. These modifications can alter our moods and hormones and even change the chemical signals in our brains. For example, high-sugar and high-carb foods, like a delicious piece of cake, are considered "highly palatable."

This is a combination that is not typically found in nature. High-fat foods are not high-carb, and vice versa. The chemically modified and sweetened foods trigger a dopamine release in the brain and our "reward transmitter," giving us a pleasurable spike in emotion that lasts momentarily. However, after that initial high wears off, people often feel sluggish and irritated as they withdraw from the unnatural spike.[280] This cycle can lead to an imbalance in hormones, contributing to issues like estrogen dominance in both men and women. Feeling sluggish prompts many to seek more dopamine hits through such addictive foods.

Hormonal Dysfunction Root Cause: Nutritional Deficiency

It's not just about the negative components in our diet; it's also about the lack of essential nutrients. Numerous vitamins and cofactors are necessary for the synthesis of serotonin. For example, tryptophan is a precursor for serotonin, but for this conversion to take place, the body needs cofactors, such as iron, magnesium, calcium, B6, folate, vitamin C, and zinc.[281] Without sufficient tryptophan, we cannot make enough serotonin. This leads to increased stress and hormonal disruption. However, it doesn't just stop there because serotonin is also necessary in regulating estrogen and progesterone, circadian rhythm, and thyroid hormones.[282] Nutrient deficiencies, such as in zinc and protein, can also cause an inverse relationship with SHBG, while for every twofold increase in fluoride, estrogen and testosterone decrease by over 8% and 7%, respectively. While these numbers represent a small cohort of studies, they represent the impact that optimizing protein and micronutrients can have on overall hormone health.[283]

This is important to note because clients need to know that food is not just calories. In an honest attempt to be healthy, many opt for a chemical-laden, nutritionally devoid diet to avoid calories, which is not beneficial. At times, having deficient cofactors may be why a supplement is not producing the desired effects. Addressing only the deficiencies without considering the cofactors is inadequate. This disconnect contributes significantly to health issues in our society, yet it is often dismissed as insignificant. Nutritional evaluation testing, such as NutraEval, may be of benefit to discover underlying root causes of imbalance.

Maintaining a balance of healthy carbohydrates, fats, and proteins is much more effective than maintaining a certain caloric range. Meals should be planned based on addressing gaps in macro balance and nutritional needs, rather than simply relying on cravings or seeking low-calorie options. One way to simplify the process is by aiming to get the same macros per meal and then simply switching out types of foods daily to ensure a balance of nutrients. For example, aim to always have a couple of servings of vegetables each evening, but rotate the type of vegetables daily or every few days to ensure nutrient balance.

Prioritize whole-protein sources, such as grass-fed meats. Grass-fed beef is particularly important because animals raised primarily on grain tend to have an unhealthy ratio of omega-6 to omega-3 fatty acids. A healthy omega-6 to omega-3 ratio is typically around a one-to-one and no more than a four-to-one ratio. This is also why I recommend game meats, such as venison. These animals consume a completely natural diet, producing one of the most nutrient-dense protein sources available. Unfortunately, many modern diets, including the standard American diet (SAD), often have ratios as high as thirty-to-one.

Keeping a diversity of protein sources is also something to consider, as it is yet another example of why "lower calorie" does not always indicate better health. While all food groups should be kept in moderation, red meat in particular has been demonized for some time despite it having a better omega ratio than lower-calorie meats like chicken. Despite chicken being lower in calories, it often does not provide the beneficial omega-3s we need, which are found in abundance in oily fish sources such as salmon. Another option is to source chicken from farms that feed the animals a balanced diet of flaxseed and other sources of omega-3s.[284]

Another important source is organ meat, which is rarely consumed but is much more abundant in micronutrients.[285] Lastly, consider the amount of micronutrients, essential and nonessential fatty acids (like L-carnitine, which is predominantly sourced from meats), and other microcomponents of food that are diversely a part of all food groups.[286] When considering a strict "trending" diet, consider that the studies that fuel these trends cannot ever take into consideration all of the different variables that affect health, even when performed scientifically, rigorously, and without bias. Furthermore, the studies often do not account for lower-quality sources and sources that are devoid of natural balance. Just notice how the outcomes of studies that measure grass-fed beef consumption compared to grain-fed are vastly different. That is where balance and going back to basics are key. While too much of any food group is most often not good, not enough of the food can also cause issues. A diverse diet also positively affects levels of prebiotics and probiotics and their impact on gut health. Strict diets that restrict entire food groups completely ignore the lack of natural prebiotics and probiotics that are necessary for health.

Also, it is important to note that macros from different sources change in bioavailability and specific health benefits. For example, the proteins in plants are not processed or utilized in the body in the same way as those from whey. Plant proteins differ from those found in meat and dairy products and are absorbed differently by the body. Meat protein lends to more abundant production of lean muscle mass.[287] It again demonstrates how important it is to maintain a balanced diet and supplement with the right amino acids, rather than just focusing on broad categories.

Hormonal Dysfunction Root Cause: The Estrobolome and Microbiome

In both men and women, it is equally important to consider the estrobolome axis, which is where gut bacteria and estrogen interact. Specific microbes in the gut break down excess or old estrogen, but are not able to do so effectively if dysbiosis exists. A portion of the microbiome carries genes for the expression of enzymes to break down estrogen, altering the levels of estrogen in the body. When dysbiosis exists, not as much estrogen is being broken down. This effect is so profound that it is even being investigated as a root cause for estrogen-sensitive breast cancer.[288]

While we know that chemicals can directly impact reproductive and hormonal health, it is often overlooked that chemicals, such as BPA, are also known to negatively affect the estrobolome.[289] This highlights how chemicals can affect not only our hormones but also our gut health, exacerbating nutritional deficiencies and leading to the development of even more issues. This is why a comprehensive stool analysis is essential to most hormonal workups.

Almost any time there is weight loss resistance or hormonal imbalance, we need to know what is going on in the client's gut, not only for hormonal balance but also to assess digestive components of the microbiome. Part of the microbiome's job is to help break down certain foods. For example, Bacteroides spp., Blautia obeum, and P. copri all aid in carbohydrate metabolism and maintaining insulin sensitivity.[290,291] This means that if a person has more of the microbiome that helps to break down and store carbohydrates, and they are on a high-carbohydrate diet, they will gain more weight than someone who does not match that microbiome.[292]

The same is true for microbiomes that store fat and high-fat diets. It's a remarkable discovery, and it makes a lot of sense as part of the reason why some diets work for some and not others. It may also give insight into rebound weight gain that occurs in most who stop their extreme diets. Extreme diets that severely restrict macronutrients will induce pronounced shifts in microbiome composition.[111] This can lead to rebound weight gain with the reintroduction of carbohydrates and a disruption in metabolism.

Some bacterial species, such as Bacteroides spp., are titled as being a part of the "lean" microbiota, while others are associated with an increased risk of obesity. This association is so strong that they have even done fecal transplants, inoculating healthy-weight mice with the gut flora of obese mice, and the mice will gain weight without any dietary changes.[293] The reverse was also found to be true. Therefore, rebalancing the gut is often a key part of the treatment of weight loss resistance.

Estrogen-Based Food

Another potentially relevant impact may be a result of diets that contain phytoestrogens, which are plant compounds that are found in a variety of foods, like soybeans. After ingestion, the microbiome can take inactive phytoestrogen foods and make them into metabolically active aglycones, which will enter the circulation and bind to the body's estrogen receptors. While phytoestrogens can lead to estrogenic effects, the formation of aglycones can also allow them to compete for binding sites, exerting anti-estrogenic effects. This may be the cause for findings demonstrating high levels of phytoestrogens leading to a reduced breast cancer risk. These phytoestrogens are then conjugated in the liver and deconjugated by the microbiome.[294,295]

However, phytoestrogens, like soy, are identified as potential endocrine disruptors.[295] Furthermore, they can negatively affect the endocrine system by working on the hypothalamus to trigger the pituitary to make more follicle-stimulating hormone, promoting the secretion of estrogen and progesterone, or trigger the secretion of testosterone by the testes or ovaries, and can disrupt levels of SHBG.[294]

In human studies, 60 mg/day of soy product consumption was found to directly increase levels of SHBG and decrease free testosterone (the bioactive form). It is suggested that human variability in a person's capacity to produce equol, which is a nonsteroidal estrogen produced by the gut for the metabolism of soy, may be one determining factor in whether soy raises or lowers estrogen levels.[296] Other variabilities include the type of phytoestrogens and the amount of circulating endogenous estrogens.[294] Again, one diet does not fit all.

Lastly, it is always worth remembering that over 90% of soy products (not meaning whole foods like edamame) are genetically modified organisms (GMOs), and even a 10% increase in soybean oil has been associated with liver, spleen, pancreatic, and kidney disease.[297] Furthermore, glyphosate is often used in soy and other GMO foods and poses a known risk for several diseases, such as neurological disease and cancer.[298] Therefore, even with some health benefits being a potential, studies still support that GMO soy carries risk.

Hormonal Dysfunction Root Cause: Medications

Many medications can affect our hormone balance, both directly and indirectly. Even so, this is not to say that we will always discontinue medications or that the patient should not be on the medication. However, understanding the full picture is nonetheless important.

Risk for thyroid and hormonal imbalance increases if the client has a history of taking oral contraceptives (OCs) because they directly alter sex hormone levels. Oral contraceptives have additionally been found to enhance the risk for developing intestinal hyperpermeability ("leaky gut"). A hyperpermeable gut will directly affect hormones, as dysbiosis can affect the part of the gut flora that is meant to metabolize hormones.[288] As for OCs affecting thyroid function, one study found a 46% higher risk of hypothyroidism in this population.[266]

The medications we need to watch out for go past the obvious ones, such as oral contraceptives, metformin, or spironolactone, which are used specifically for their impacts on sex hormone influence and insulin resistance. SSRIs, for example, like fluoxetine and sertraline, have been found to negatively affect libido.[299] Statins don't just lower cholesterol; they can also cause key sex hormones to plummet (including testosterone), because cholesterol is the precursor to these hormones.[300] Corticosteroids suppress the pituitary-adrenal axis and lower testosterone and progesterone, which can suppress ovulation and thyroid functioning.[301,302] Beta blockers can lower testosterone, leading to fatigue and even erectile dysfunction.[303,304] PPIs work to decrease stomach acid and can thus impair the absorption of zinc, B12, and magnesium, which are all necessary for the production of endogenous hormones, and can contribute to hormonal dysregulation and hypothyroidism.[305,306]

Hormonal Dysfunction Root Cause: Environmental Exposure

Screening household products may reveal endocrine disruptors that are influencing hormonal changes. Most commercial lotions, perfumes, shampoos, laundry detergents, soaps, and so forth also contain chemicals that disrupt our natural rhythms and can be absorbed through the skin or even breathed in. There are even those in the water and the air that we cannot completely avoid. Trying to eliminate all that we have control over will help decrease the profound effects of those we cannot completely avoid. The effects of some of these products extend beyond that of hormonal disruption and are even tied to increased risk for cancer and cognitive decline, including delayed learning in children.

Hormonal Dysfunction Root Cause: Genetic Variations

Additionally, you will want to check for MTHFR and COMT polymorphisms, as these can disrupt women's hormones by decreasing the client's ability to methylate, which is a part of estrogen detox.[307] In one study of 980 MTHFR polymorphisms, a correlation for increased risk of some breast cancers was found in those with the polymorphism, highlighting the significance.[308] COMT and MTHFR are genes that provide biological directions for enzymes that are instrumental in key metabolic and biochemical processes, such as the methylation of nutrients. But also recall that an important byproduct of this process is DNA repair and neurotransmitter regulation, which do not happen if methylation cannot be completed. Potential polymorphisms and their effect were discussed in more depth in Chapter 5, which you may refer back to.

Cytochrome P450 variances are another genetic predisposition to consider. With some of these variants, known as inhibitors, people retain too much of a medication, impacting their hormone metabolism. For example, a person with a cytochrome P450 inhibition may not break down medications efficiently, causing the medication to remain in the body longer. In contrast, someone with cytochrome P450 induction can eliminate medications more quickly. These variations can influence overall health and hormone regulation, highlighting the complexity of this system. These systems can be tested, lending to a very comprehensive plan.

Hormonal Dysfunction Root Cause: Stress

Stress is a critical component to hormonal balance, or imbalance. Prolonged stress can have a considerable impact on the hypothalamic-pituitary-adrenal (HPA) axis, which may additionally play a role in memory loss and neurodegenerative conditions like Alzheimer's disease. Activation of the HPA axis over chronic periods of time disrupts cortisol regulation, leading to the decline of both physical and mental health by interacting with inflammatory pathways and generating oxidative stress. This additionally contributes to cellular damage and neuroinflammation in addition to decreasing sex hormone production.[309,310] If stress is an issue, consider an adaptogen like ashwagandha, as stress can lead to hormonal imbalances by triggering the pregnenolone steal.

To further assess adrenal health, a four-point cortisol stress test that uses saliva samples taken four times throughout the day may be added to the evaluation if DUTCH is not ordered. This test helps identify adrenal dysfunction, previously referred to as "adrenal fatigue," which is a misleading term. Instead of the adrenals "giving out," the body stops compensating for prolonged stress, leading to a situation where it no longer spikes cortisol to help with alertness and focus. Other metabolic effects of sustained stress, such as depleted nutrients, further contribute to symptoms of fatigue. This is vastly different from adrenal insufficiency and Addison's disease, which should both be a differential diagnosis for low cortisol, and advanced assessment and diagnostics (or referral as necessary) may be required to safely rule them out. When compensation of extended periods of stress ceases, many people experience what is colloquially termed "burnout." Clients may describe the experience as a lack of energy or having emotional numbness, even to things that once would excite the person. It is also often accompanied by significant hormonal disruption and, often, weight loss resistance.

Pregnenolone Steal

DHEA is a crucial hormone produced by the adrenal glands and serves as a precursor to both testosterone and estrogen. It's important for various functions, including energy production, fat metabolism, mood regulation, cognitive performance, immune resilience, and healthy aging. However, an increased demand for cortisol, often driven by stress or insufficient sleep, can deplete pregnenolone. This phenomenon is often referred to as the "progesterone or pregnenolone steal."[311]

Dysregulation of the HPA (hypothalamic-pituitary-adrenal) axis can impair DHEA rhythms and its conversion, along with disrupting cortisol transport, which is necessary for DHEA synthesis. Because pregnenolone is excessively needed for the pathway to produce cortisol in order to cope under stressful situations (toward the right, in the diagram that follows), less is diverted to the alternative pathway, which leads to less DHEA. and, therefore, less estrogen and testosterone, leading to hormonal disruption. This phenomenon is referred to as the "pregnenolone steal," as pregnenolone is taken away from producing these essential hormones.

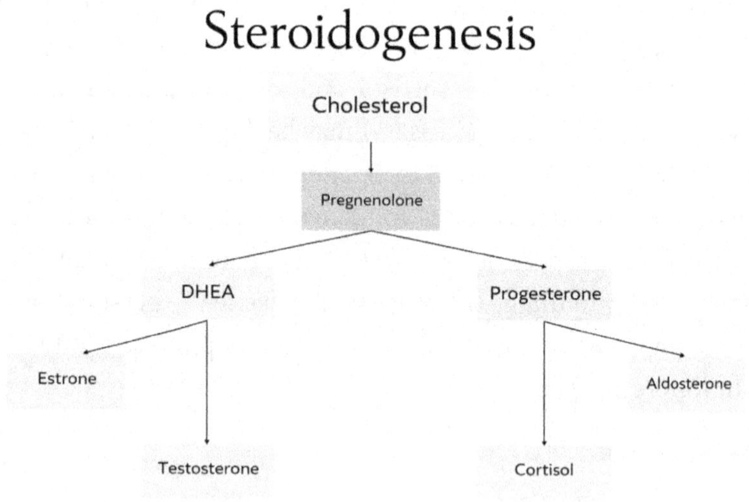

Relationship Between Cholesterol and Hormonal Balance

There is also a direct correlation between low cholesterol and various symptoms. Whether it is a result of diet, genetics, or medication, if the client does not have enough cholesterol for all body functions, they may struggle to produce the hormones they need. Steroidogenesis is the production of hormones via cholesterol. The previous diagram shows its importance and how it flows.

This correlation is one reason why people with very low LDL cholesterol (less than 40 mg/dl) frequently report feeling fatigued, lacking focus, and experiencing a diminished libido.[312,313] Cholesterol is also essential for neurofunctioning. This connection underscores the need for balance and screening for overprescribing statins.

Finding Balance Means Finding Freedom: Stress Management

Stress management is essential to help regulate hormones and is greatly underestimated in our society. Using practices such as breathwork, meditation, or mindfulness can help reduce cortisol levels. Furthermore, sleep optimization is critical for metabolism and cortisol balance, as inadequate sleep can disrupt hormonal pathways and the circadian rhythm.[314] The practitioner may recommend adding adaptogens, such as ashwagandha, rhodiola, or Cordyceps. These plant derivatives and mushroom blends, are known to help regulate the HPA axis, decreasing the physiological and psychological effects of stress, as well as the need for excessive cortisol production.[218,315]

Supporting adrenal health through proper nutrition is also beneficial to stress management. Zinc and magnesium can play significant roles here, with magnesium often providing a calming effect, making it more suitable for evening use, and deficiency can have the opposite effect.[316] For those experiencing considerable estrogen dominance, supplements like DIM, magnesium, and B vitamins can be useful, especially when combined with detox support and adaptogens. The goal here is to start with what is applicable and right for the client, not every intervention possible. This is when relying on testing and clinical presentation is important to know which of these interventions is right for the client.

Sleep & Hormonal Balance

Sleep deprivation is a common cause of the body overcompensating with excessive cortisol. Sleep is quite literally paramount for several reasons, as it is when the brain detoxifies itself.[316] Patients need to understand the deep impact sleep has on their hormones. Many people survive on just four to five hours of sleep when they should be aiming for six to eight hours each night. Consistency is key, so maintaining a regular sleep pattern is important. Growth hormone, which aids in tissue repair and muscle growth, is released during sleep. This is crucial not only for children but also for adults, as it helps maintain healthy body weight, regulate BMI, and ensure proper metabolism.[318]

Hunger signals are also negatively influenced by sleep deprivation because of its effect on leptin and ghrelin. Sleep deprivation can decrease leptin, the hormone that signals fullness, making individuals more prone to overeating—especially if they work night shifts. When leptin levels chronically drop, the body may increase the desire for energy, leading to heightened hunger due to elevated ghrelin levels, which can ultimately result in weight gain.[318] This is why some people experience increased hunger signals that are difficult to overcome, often leading to increased carbohydrate consumption. The body has an increased need for a quick energy supply to compensate for the deprivation and triggers cravings for such a source of energy. This dietary habit directly feeds back into the hormonal and circadian disruption.

Insufficient sleep can also disrupt thyroid function, potentially affecting TSH levels and leading to thyroid dysfunction and metabolic issues. While the body may initially overstimulate TSH, it will eventually stop overcompensating and resort to a lack of stimulation.[25]

It is imperative to encourage healthy sleep habits, maintain a regular bedtime routine, and reduce late nights to ensure overall well-being. Sleep interventions to do so include avoiding blue light exposure from screens, using dim yellow lights in the evening, avoiding late-night television, and rebalancing the gut microbiome, which can be beneficial in helping cases of insomnia. Avoiding late-night carbohydrate consumption, as it can inhibit melatonin production, helps rebalance the natural circadian rhythm. In the morning, it's beneficial to get sunlight exposure as soon as possible and to minimize the use of sunglasses throughout the day, helping to establish a natural contrast between morning and evening light.

These interventions also benefit conditions such as PCOS, estrogen dominance, and adrenal fatigue by helping to regulate the hormones that are all interconnected. The body operates like a web of hormones, meaning that you can't affect one area without impacting others. That's why it's crucial to adopt a whole-body approach when helping our patients.

Supplements in Hormonal Regulation

DIM at 100–200 mg/day is the most commonly used supplement to help support the 2-OH pathway, decrease estrogen dominance, and help to regulate SHBG. Calcium D-Glucarate is another popular supplement used to manage estrogen dominance. It works by supporting the liver's detoxification of excess estrogen and inhibiting the enzyme beta-glucuronidase, which prevents reabsorption of these hormones in the gut. Supplementing zinc at 30–50 mg/day, as indicated by deficiency, can help to reduce SHBG because zinc has an inhibitory influence on SHBG production. Boron, 3–6 mg/day, is also proven to decrease SHBG and increase free testosterone, and vitamin D needs to be optimized as well.[320] Cruciferous veggies (if tolerated and no active SIBO is present) help the body detoxify excess estrogen and xenoestrogens. Alternatively, sulforaphane can be taken in supplement form. It is the extract from broccoli sprouts and other cruciferous vegetables that is responsible for their strong detox, antioxidant, and cancer-protective properties.

Intervention Overview

Hashimoto's is an autoimmune disease. While it received special attention in this chapter as a thyroid disease, please note that interventions in the next chapter on autoimmune disease may very well apply as well. Remember, in true functional medicine, you are looking for the root cause of disease, and that may be different from person to person, despite them having the same disease. Therefore, whether it is classified as thyroid or autoimmune is not of most importance. The important thing to focus on is the root cause.

Overall, in the process of rebalancing hormones, as with any functional protocol, your first step should be to remove underlying causes of inflammation. Screening should include dysbiosis of the gut, including bacterial overgrowth or parasitic infection, as well as day-to-day chemicals and nutritional imbalances. Xenoestrogens and endocrine disruptions in the toxins chapter are additionally important to screen for. Common sources include topical chemicals in body lotions and soaps that are absorbed via the skin, aromatic chemicals also sprayed onto the skin (perfumes), or those sprayed into the air, breathed in, and absorbed via the pulmonary system. Others are found in processed foods and sugars.

Business Practice Pearl

Sharing testimonials is a key aspect of building your program. It's where the real magic begins. In our program, we implement a proprietary system that allows our students to specifically apply this framework. I have already developed a program, the Mindset Academy, that my students can use for their advertising as they are trained under my model of care, complete with proven testimonials.

You can create your own version based on how you want to empower your clients. Essentially, we help our students guide their patients in overcoming mental barriers and making healthy changes. We believe that while the root causes of disease may stem from unhealthy foods and chemical-laden products, the true root cause lies in the mindset that enables these indulgences. By empowering the mind, we can motivate any actions needed for change.

Our approach involves helping clients reframe and restructure their mindset around food and eating, as well as their perceptions of shame and guilt. This mindset shift supports their ability to make lasting changes. Practically speaking, when patients adhere to a program, they achieve results, which naturally leads to testimonials. It is essential to focus on delivering measurable outcomes rather than simply enrolling patients.

Part of this process involves helping patients remain steadfast in pursuing their goals until they reach them. In functional medicine, the approach is not just about prescribing a pill and sending patients home; it is about facilitating life changes and ensuring that clients can sustain those changes. This is how they achieve genuine results and, consequently, how you garner testimonials. This method not only helps you build your business but also creates a truly impactful functional practice that drives meaningful change.

It's crucial to have a comprehensive program that goes beyond a brief consultation. Clients benefit from a holistic approach that includes stress management, accountability, and mindset, as these elements significantly influence hormonal balance and overall physiological health. By additionally incorporating mental and spiritual healing, we help clients stay on track as they begin to heal naturally.

BONUS TRAINING:

Power of Testimonials Reels. See our testimonial reel as an example of how building an authentic testimonial empowers you to believe more in what you can do by seeing others like you doing this.

SCAN ME

SCAN THE QR CODE

or visit functionalmedicineunlocked.com

Chapter 8

Autoimmunity in Functional and Integrative Medicine

Case Study: A Forty-Two-Year-Old Female with Hashimoto's

Patient presented with a history of Hashimoto's, fatigue, diarrhea, joint pain, and mood swings. She had been on a high dose of Synthroid for most of her life and had a history of chronic diarrhea and hypertension. Patient reported coming home exhausted and would spend much of her time off work lying on the couch, which greatly affected her relationships with her children, as she often missed their sporting events. She expressed concern that they might not understand how much she loved them because she lacked the energy to show it, and she was happy to no longer have that concern.

Her husband was very supportive and expressed his understanding of her struggles but also shared that it had become difficult for him, as he was managing all the cooking and cleaning. Both were devoted Christians who supported each other, but the demands of parenting their three very active boys were taking a toll on them.

Labs

TSH was the normal limit (on Synthroid). T4 was in the normal range, but T3 was low, indicating poor conversion. CBC and CMP were unremarkable. Positive for TPO antibodies. Stool analysis showed bacterial overgrowth and the presence of parasitic infection. Found to be heterozygous for MTHFR. Iodine, selenium, and folic acid levels within normal limits.

Intervention

The patient was placed on a gluten-free diet, and liver detox with milk thistle was initiated. Once genetic testing resulted, she was found to have MTHFR polymorphism and was started on methylated B12. Chronic diarrhea was found to be linked to parasites revealed on stool analysis. Treatment included using artemisinin. Bacterial overgrowth was addressed with oregano, allicin, and berberine. Within a few months diarrhea resolved, her joint pain completely stopped, and her mood swings and fatigue greatly improved. Synthroid was weaned off, and repeat TPO levels at 9 months were within normal limits.

Discussion

There are hundreds of autoimmune disorders, and more are being identified as autoimmune on a regular basis. These include Hashimoto's, Graves' disease, celiac, multiple sclerosis, systemic lupus erythematosus, rheumatoid arthritis, IBS, psoriasis, Addison's, Sjogren's, type 1 diabetes, pernicious anemia, and myasthenia gravis. Studies indicate autoimmune disease occurrence is compounding at a rate of 3-12 percent annually. Occurrence is most prevalent in industrialized Western nations, with the highest rates among those in North America. It is not an understatement to say it is an epidemic.[321]

It is important to acknowledge that conventional medicine plays an important role and that some patients will still require traditional treatments despite the best efforts of functional medicine. However, in many cases, clients have even better results than when they were on prescriptions, as many are able to wean clients off of them altogether. This is of great benefit because these medications pose a high risk for illness. For example, many immunologics work by suppressing the immune system to avoid symptoms, but this can increase the risk of infections and certain cancers because the body is less able to mount a full defensive response against cellular damage.[322]

On the contrary, the functional medicine approach helps clients experience a higher quality of life by focusing on overall health. Decreasing damage from chronic inflammation and disease by alleviating the root cause improves longevity and overall health. Functional medicine is the ultimate health leverage; by addressing one issue, we can improve many other aspects of a patient's life. In many instances, treating the root cause can feel like getting a second chance at life.

Autoimmune Risk Factors & Root Cause Analysis

Identifying and treating the root cause of autoimmune diseases starts with proper screening. This may include screening for methylation polymorphism, gut dysbiosis, parasitic infection, and other causes of chronic physiological inflammation, as discussed in Chapter 1. However, the main approach to addressing autoimmunity in functional medicine can be summarized by the most common tetrad that involves four key elements: genetic factors, root causes of chronic inflammation, hormonal imbalance, and recognizing environmental triggers. Unlike conventional medicine, which typically follows a step-by-step medication protocol, functional medicine acknowledges that the same disease can be caused by various factors in different individuals. This is why the practitioner must take into account the summation of physiological insult, known as allostatic stress load.

Allostatic Stress Load

Under the Functional Model, AI assessment goes beyond examining individual risk factors to understand how the cascade of illness unfolded. We want to fully understand what triggered the body to start breaking down. We do this by examining what led to the accumulation of stressors, often referred to as allostatic load. The underlying mechanism of autoimmunity can differ or can be the same across different autoimmune diseases. Often, the symptoms differ depending on which tissues are affected. I reference the "allostatic stress cup" analogy here. If a person has a genetically smaller "cup of resistance" in a certain system, it indicates that the organ system is more vulnerable to insult. For example, symptoms of multiple sclerosis may develop once the nervous system has endured enough exposure that symptoms start and tissue damage occurs. This is when the cup is "overflowing." Conversely, if the thyroid is more vulnerable, conditions like Hashimoto's thyroiditis may develop. Essentially, the condition affecting the "weakest link" in the body will manifest the most noticeable symptoms.

In a stressed body, this often starts with disruption at the cellular, microbial, and mitochondrial levels from chemicals, genetic polymorphisms, or pathogens. At this phase, there are sometimes few, if any, symptoms, and they tend to be vague, such as chronic fatigue. Then, as inflammation continues to grow in the body, metabolic or hormonal dysfunction occurs at the tissue and then the organ level. As the cascade continues, other organ systems are affected by coping mechanisms, such as impaired detoxification pathways.[323] Influential factors may include genetics, an inflammatory diet, nutritional deficiencies, gluten intolerance, mast cell activation syndrome, gut dysbiosis, past viral infections, parasites, chronic stress, or toxic exposures. For instance, environmental triggers could include exposure to mold, heavy metals, food toxins, or hormonal imbalances.

As an example, chronic inflammation might start with gut imbalances. Or another example could be the body's inability to process histamines in certain foods. Those who struggle with histamine breakdown may have genetic predispositions, such as DAO polymorphism, affecting how they metabolize histamines. Foods high in histamines include avocados, wine, chocolate, eggplant, eggs, aged cheeses, tomatoes, and processed meats.[324] When the body cannot effectively break down histamines, they accumulate and provoke an inflammatory response, leading the body to react as if these substances are harmful invaders. This cycle can result in a chronic inflammatory state, ultimately contributing to autoimmune disease.[325] This is not an exhaustive list, but one to get started with.

The Mind-on-Body Impact

Psychological trauma is known as a risk factor contributing to the overall progression of disease, especially autoimmunity. If this goes unaddressed, it is like keeping a fire burning in one room of a house while deep cleaning the rest. This is something that is not often discussed in conventional medicine, and when you start opening those "closed doors" in medicine, not everyone is ready for what's inside. In my transition from conventional medicine to functional medicine, I have had my fair share of "naysayers." So, I tend to be a little "on guard" when addressed by practitioners who are only trained in the conventional model. One time, right before taking the first big stage I had ever spoken on, I had a matter-of-fact, one could say "gruff," retired rheumatologist approach me. After seeing my presentation title, he firmly asked, "Now, what is this that you're teaching?!"

After I explained that my goal was to help with the impact of psychosocial trauma to improve performance and health from a root-cause approach, I braced for criticism about being a "woo-woo practitioner." He said, "Doctors these days SUCK!"

Yikes, here it comes, I thought.

He went on to explain that with every autoimmune patient he saw while in practice, he would ask, "*When* did you experience big-T trauma?" He emphasized that he would ask *when*, not *if*, because all of them had encountered it at some time. That is how convinced he was of the correlation. He finished by saying, "If we really want to help people, we have to start looking at the complete picture and not just what a bunch of labs tell us!"

I exhaled a sigh of relief, as I was already nervous to step onto the stage, and smiled.

He was right. A significant history of PTSD is associated with a 2.70- to 8.23-fold higher risk for the development of autoimmune disease.[326] Therefore, a full treatment plan should address this in the proper patients.

Family & Personal History of Autoimmunity As Risk Factors

Having a first-degree relative with an autoimmune disease is a risk factor, as there is a hereditary component. However, it is known that the disease progression and expression thereof can be eliminated with functional medicine. For example, there can be several genetic patterns of the gut, which is the mainstay of our immune system, that can be directly correlated to the development of autoimmune disease. While gut patterns can be hereditary, they can still be altered post-birth.[327] This demonstrates that just because it "runs in the family" doesn't mean we have to submit to acceptance as if it's unavoidable or irreversible. Put another way, even with genetic predisposition loading the proverbial gun, we can prevent pulling the proverbial trigger by avoiding or reversing exposure to root causes.

Personal history is also a risk factor for additional autoimmune diseases. Approximately 34% of autoimmune patients go on to develop a second one. Realizing that autoimmune disease often stems from things outside of the affected organ helps us make sense of why having one autoimmune disease increases a person's risk for a second, irrespective of the organs affected.

Gender as a Risk Factor

Females are twice as likely as males to develop an autoimmune disease.[328] This is thought to be related to estrogen dominance.[329,330] Estrogen dominance is a key factor in the development of most autoimmune diseases, which may shed understanding as to why women are 80% more susceptible to this development. Further increasing risk is the direct correlation that estrogen has on the immune system.[329,331] Estrogen directly suppresses the generation of T and B cell lymphocytes, and high doses are correlated with suppression of the thymus, which is paramount in immune function and T cell formation.[329] Research indicates a complex relationship between hormonal birth control use and the rising incidence of autoimmune diseases exists, particularly since the introduction of the pill.[330] Correcting estrogen dominance, whether the client has taken estrogen in the past or not, is often a key factor in the treatment of autoimmune disease, depending on the individual. Next, let's dig deeper into these hormonal imbalances to understand their origins.

The Estrogen Autoimmune Connection

Hormones also play a critical role in autoimmune conditions. Shifting hormones can act like the hidden switch that turns a smoldering imbalance into a full-blown fire. Estrogen, in particular, plays a powerful role, which is why many autoimmune conditions flare during times such as puberty, pregnancy, postpartum, and perimenopause. Understanding this connection is key to understanding symptoms and how to finally calm the allostatic storm. Cholesterol is another part of the hormonal equation, as it is the precursor for pregnenolone, which then converts into progesterone and DHEA, the latter of which further converts into estrogen or testosterone. Progesterone then proceeds to either cortisol or aldosterone.

Understanding estrogen in relation to autoimmune disease requires a closer look at its receptors, A and B. Receptor A functions like an accelerator; too much stimulation can lead to negative health outcomes, such as an increased risk of breast cancer. In contrast, receptor B acts like a brake. It is associated with lower cardiovascular risk and improved bone health, but it can easily convert into estrone, which is the estrogen most suspected to be associated with risk of further illness.[331,332] Another way estrone can become elevated is through oral estrogen, as it is converted into estrone after being metabolized in the liver.[333]

Estrone stimulates at a ratio of five to one. This means that estrone has five times the stimulatory effect compared to its inhibitory effect. On the other hand, estradiol stimulates B receptors, with varying effects depending on tissue type, but is inhibitor on A receptors.[334] These different ratios may contribute to why some individuals, particularly those with certain receptor sensitivities in their cells and tissues, are at higher risk for conditions such as breast cancer.[335] However, estrogen, in general, does not need to be demonized. Even estrone is vital for mental health, bone density, and, of course, sexual health. Issues arise when estrogen detoxification is impaired, when estrogen balance is inappropriate for the phase of life, and/or when environmental factors contribute to imbalance.

Lab Testing for AI

Basic Labs

To evaluate autoimmune diseases, essential laboratory tests include a full thyroid panel, CMP, CBC, and screening for infectious diseases such as Epstein-Barr virus and H. pylori. Other tests may include autoantibodies such as TOP, ANA, RF, and tissue transglutaminase. Inflammatory markers, such as CRP and ESR, help to evaluate sustained inflammation. Metabolic nutrient markers of importance include vitamin D, iron studies, B12, and folate levels. Elevated eosinophils (a type of white blood cell) can provide valuable insight. Elevated eosinophils are often associated with allergies, such as seasonal allergies, but they can also indicate a parasitic infection, particularly in the gut.[349] This idea may seem far-fetched, but those of us in clinical practice have frequently observed it in patients. Gastric parasitic infection has been found to contribute to a root cause in the development of AI, particularly Hashimoto's, which is not a part of basic labs but should be included under the functional treatment plan.

DUTCH Test: Hormone Testing

An underlying, almost hallmark, part of autoimmune disease is estrogen dominance, where the estrogen has surpassed its normal levels in comparison to progesterone and/or the body is too sensitive to the estrogen in the body.[331,336] Supplements such as DIM and calcium D-glucarate can help correct this. However, another key aspect is adopting a low-stress, low-carb, low-tox life to help decrease estrogen dominance. Additionally, if imbalanced hormones are coupled with a gut imbalance, unaddressed polymorphisms, or nutritional deficiencies, oftentimes correcting such issues first will allow the body to self-correct the hormonal imbalance. It's remarkable how often this approach works. Allowing the body to heal on its own can be a powerful process.

Sex hormones function somewhat like children: if one receives too much attention, the other may not get the support it needs, leading to an imbalance. Cortisol, our stress response hormone, can be one of those "noisy children" that kick off dysfunction. Typically, when this happens, the first hormone to become depleted is progesterone, which can directly result in estrogen dominance. When we facilitate healing and rebalance progesterone levels, we often observe a corresponding decrease in estrogen levels. Therefore, a baseline DUTCH test is a great way to assess whether this is occurring in the body, as it compares both cortisol and sex hormones, as well as the different types of estrogen, including testosterone and progesterone.

As discussed earlier, LDL is low-density lipoprotein cholesterol, while HDL is high-density lipoprotein, considered the "healthy" cholesterol. High levels of LDL and very-low-density lipoproteins (VLDLs) are associated with increased cardiovascular risk.[337] Chronic stress and inflammation can disrupt the HPA axis, lowering DHEA and testosterone, and may contribute to elevated LDL and VLDL, particularly in the setting of impaired thyroid function. This is due to a lack of thyroid hormone lowering the liver's metabolic ability to clear the body of LDL in a hypothyroid state.[338] Insulin resistance and increased cortisol output decrease the size of lipoproteins and alter oxidation, leading to an increase in atherosclerotic formation.[339.340] These changes contribute to a metabolic environment where hormonal balance becomes harder to restore and provide some insight into the treatment of hyperlipidemia under the functional medicine model.

LDL concentration only tells part of the story.

Shifts in cardiometabolic risk result largely from changes in LDL particle size:

- Small, dense LDL particles are highly atherogenic—more likely to oxidize, penetrate the endothelium, and drive inflammation, as seen in insulin resistance.
- Large, buoyant LDL particles are far less harmful and often rise in metabolically healthy patterns (e.g., low-carb states or optimized thyroid function).

When LDL levels are elevated on standard labs, don't assume equal risk across the board. Best practice includes ordering a calcium scan, lipoprotein profile, or ApoB, to differentiate particle size and number.[341] Conversely, if small, dense LDL is discovered on assessment first, this may warrant screening for insulin resistance, chronic inflammation, thyroid dysfunction, high cortisol with low DHEA patterns, or impaired mitochondrial capacity. Additionally, when elevated LDL is an issue, calcium scans should be ordered to monitor actual risk for atherosclerotic disease, not simply relying on LDL alone. When appropriate, cardiovascular referral is recommended.

Furthermore, in high-stress situations, cortisol takes priority in hormone production, which can lead to what is known as the "pregnenolone steal." This occurs when the body fails to produce DHEA (the precursor to sex hormones) and instead prioritizes progesterone to produce cortisol.[354] This highlights the importance of stress management as part of a comprehensive plan of care.

While the acceptance of this concept is controversial in some schools of thought, I have personally observed significant improvements in patients' hormonal balance simply by helping them regulate their stress response. Ultimately, my focus is on patient outcomes rather than on which theorist is correct in the details of pathophysiological debates.

Please use the following diagram for a visual explanation of this phenomenon:

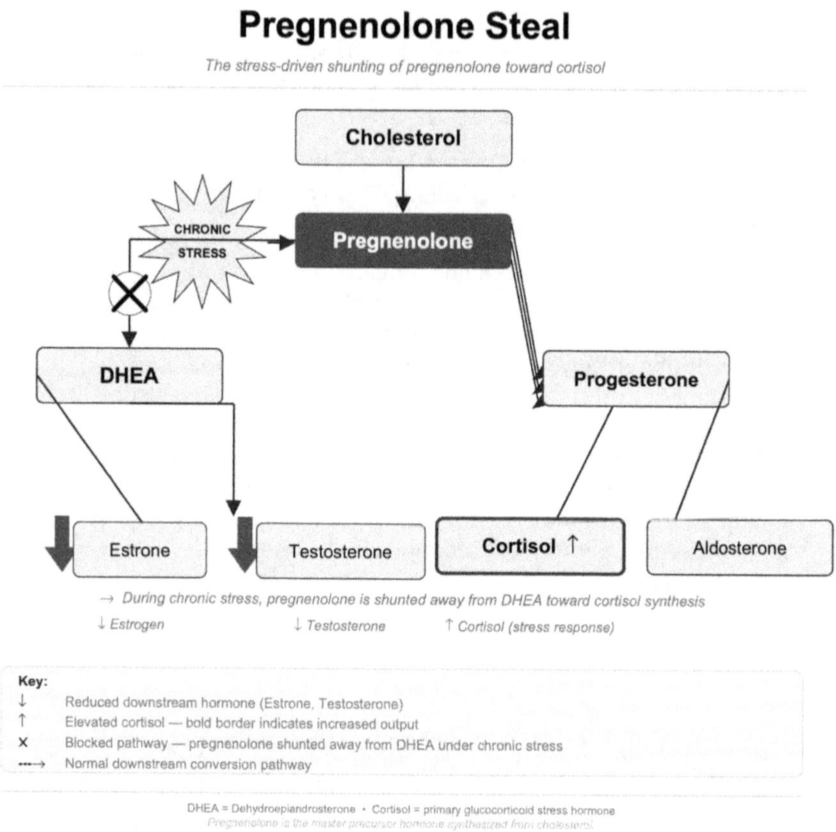

Liver Function Tests (LFTs)

Lastly, liver enzyme levels are also an important factor to monitor in this context. This can be done by a basic CMP to evaluate AST and ALT levels.

Liver function and cholesterol levels are closely connected. It's essential to monitor cholesterol levels because they directly impact our hormones. We need to ensure that liver function tests (LFTs) are within a healthy range. If the liver isn't functioning properly, it can't produce essential proteins, such as glutathione, which plays a crucial role in managing inflammation and neutralizing free radicals in the body.[222]

To maintain liver health, address any potential insults, such as the use of statins, certain medications, over-the-counter drugs like Tylenol, and alcohol consumption (which is known to deplete the body of essential glutathione). Screening for such risk factors is especially important if there are indications of liver damage, as indicated by elevated LFTs.

Four-Point Cortisol Testing

The four-point cortisol test assesses cortisol levels and rhythm. Testing is done four times during the day: morning, afternoon, mid-evening, and evening after brushing teeth. Cortisol testing is the gold standard for addressing adrenal function and the body's ability to handle stress. It is important in autoimmune disease because chronic stress will negatively impact the body's inflammatory and hormonal balance. In the presence of adrenal disruption, adrenal support can be obtained by starting adaptogens, such as ashwagandha. This test will reveal how well the client's cortisol level follows a normal circadian rhythm and can also be used to assess for Cushing's or adrenal dysfunction.[342]

It is worth noting that there is controversy about acknowledging "adrenal dysfunction." The accepted terminology used to be "adrenal fatigue," but this term has come under controversy. From my experience, addressing a person's response to chronic stress (regardless of the terminology used) is a key factor in achieving patient results. Critics argue that the adrenals are not "burned out" or "dysfunctional." While that is likely accurate, the body, when under long periods of stress, undeniably taps into compensatory systems that are maladaptive, so fighting over semantics is silly. We are here to help patients, and the bottom line is that addressing the stress response is important, regardless of its title.

Comprehensive Stool Analysis/GI Mapping

Screening for dysbiosis, pathogenic overgrowth, or infection is crucial in the treatment of AI, as it is often a root cause of the disease. There are, in fact, specific strains that, when deficient, like Akkermansia, are directly associated with a high risk of developing AI.[343] Additionally, a stool analysis can help identify sources of chronic inflammation. For instance, pancreatic elastase levels should be no less than 200 μg/g and optimally greater than 500 μg/g. However, this enzyme tends to decrease in individuals who are prediabetic or insulin-resistant, which can be a red flag for early intervention. When levels are not sufficient, malabsorption is additionally an issue.[344,345]

Supplementing digestive enzymes can help with such insufficiency. Pancreatic elastase plays a crucial role in the digestion of food. If the body fails to break down food adequately, it can lead to various downstream issues past that of malabsorption, such as increased gas, bloating, irregularity, steatorrhea, and chronic inflammation. Fecal elastase-1 is a marker found on the comprehensive stool analysis that measures exocrine pancreatic function.[344,345,346]

Important markers to screen for in patients at risk for ulcerative colitis, cancer, or Crohn's disease include calprotectin, lactoferrin, and lysozyme. SIG-A is another significant laboratory finding on a comprehensive stool analysis. An elevation in SIG-A levels indicates increased intestinal permeability, while very low levels suggest that a patient may have lost their mucosal membrane, which is supposed to separate the intestinal cavity from the intestinal lumen. In these cases, healing the gut lining will be a priority to decrease allostatic load within the entire system.[37,347]

Organic Acids Testing

As discussed in Chapter 2, the OATs test provides an evaluation of metabolic functioning, gut health, cellular health, neurotransmitter balance, and detoxification pathways, as well as a secondary check for yeast and fungal overgrowth. It can be a very effective tool for assessing root causes in AI.

Organic acids reveal several important intricacies—more than what we go over in this discussion. However, there are a few markers that you want to focus on specifically for the AI patient. Oxalic acid and glyceric acid, for example, are important because they signal the presence of oxidative stress and are a measure of mitochondrial dysfunction. Mitochondrial function is also measured by succinic, fumaric, and malic acid. Detox pathways can be assessed by pyroglutamic acid, orotic acid, and 2-hydroxybutyric acid. This assesses their ability to undergo Phase II detox.

Arabinose can indicate yeast overgrowth, and hippuric acid, benzoic acid, and phenylacetic acid will be elevated in the presence of bacterial overgrowth, which can be a root cause of AI. Organic acids can also help assess B12, folic acid, and B6 status to indicate if further genetic testing might be necessary. Lastly, neurotransmitter imbalance can be assessed using vanillylmandelic acid, homovanillic acid, and quinolinic acid, as well as their ratios.[189] Neurotransmitter imbalance leads to stressors in the body beyond just anxiety or mood disorders.

Food Testing

Testing a panel of various foods that align with the patient's typical diet can be helpful in identifying potential sensitivities that add to the allostatic stress load. The goal here is to decrease the underlying causes of inflammation that may have contributed to “filling up” the allostatic stress load, causing the proverbial spillover. Here, I am referring to our cup analogy to disease, and "spillover" refers to the point at which symptoms begin to appear.

In this context, it's essential to differentiate between IgE and IgA/IgG reactions. IgE reactions are immediate and can lead to severe conditions, such as anaphylactic shock, as seen when someone is stung by a bee or is allergic to peanuts and experiences a severe allergic reaction. In functional medicine, we focus more on IgA, which can cause gastrointestinal symptoms like gas and diarrhea, and IgG, which is associated with delayed hypersensitivity reactions.[35,348] For instance, gluten can trigger delayed hypersensitivity, leading to significant inflammation over time. IgA and IgG food testing should be interpreted as a potential guideline for starting a specific elimination diet, as the tests do not tend to have high specificity or sensitivity.

When assessing for reaction, it is best to wait at least one month, but up to three months, before reintroducing a food to see if it can be tolerated after being eliminated. Do this one food at a time. If intestinal hyperpermeability was present and treatment is effective, foods that were once assumed to be a trigger may be newly tolerated. This needs to be patient-specific and a slow process. Gluten and dairy products are nonetheless common triggers as a root cause for autoimmune disease.

Genetic Testing

MTHFR testing (discussed in more depth in the mental health chapter) is essential in root cause analysis for autoimmune disease as well. There is an elevated risk for genetic polymorphisms in the autoimmune population, which leads to high homocysteine. This prevents the body from functioning properly under stress, along with inhibiting other essential factors crucial for healing and preventing autoimmune diseases. Low levels of methylated B vitamins can hinder detoxification pathways, increasing inflammation and triggering the immune system, so it's vital to ensure that patients have adequate levels of methylated

B vitamins. Additionally, liver function and glutathione levels are also critical. The COMT genetic polymorphism is additionally more common in the autoimmune population and should be screened for and treated accordingly, as it can be a significant cause of chronic pain when not addressed. While these are by far not the only genetic tests that could be considered, they are among the most commonly studied in this population.

Viral/Bacterial Testing

Chronic viral infections, such as those caused by the Epstein-Barr virus, can be a significant trigger for AI flare-ups and contribute to overall allostatic stress load. Many people have been exposed to Epstein-Barr at some point, which can be noted by a history of mononucleosis (or simply known as "mono"). However, many go undiagnosed as children, so do not rule this out because the client does not remember a diagnosis of mono. Other viruses that can add to the overall allostatic stress load include hepatitis C, herpes simplex, or Lyme disease. Lyme disease is bacterial, but it can cause chronic infection and issues, just as viruses do. It can be a very serious issue that most carry undiagnosed for years and commonly present with weakness, fatigue, brain fog, and a slew of vague symptoms that can be very severe. This is a disease that is addressed under the Functional Model.[349]

Toxicity Testing

Testing for toxic exposure, including mold and heavy metals, is advisable. There are several connections between myotoxin exposure and the contribution to and/or exacerbation of autoimmune disease as antibodies to mycotoxins can form adducts and stick to human tissue, thought to attribute to the development of autoimmunity.[350,351] This is one of the many things that can overload a client's immune system and prevent it from "quieting" down. While the accuracy of mold testing varies, if exposure is suspected and tests are positive, there are several steps to mitigate mold effects. Using HEPA air purifiers and activated carbon filters, and ensuring proper ventilation, is helpful for decreasing exposure when remodeling, if completely leaving the environment is not possible. Maintaining humidity levels around 50% in living and work spaces can help to prevent mold growth. In the interventions section, we will discuss some options, but please refer back to Chapter 3 for the full treatment protocols.

Kidney Function

Maintaining a glomerular filtration rate (GFR) above 90 is also vital. Inflammation and dehydration can negatively impact kidney function, leading to a reduced GFR. Improvements can often be observed through the treatment of chronic infections and inflammation. If, however, conservative measures do not improve GFR, referral to nephrology is warranted. Precautions for associated risks with supplements are additionally advised as risk increases with impaired clearance.

For patients with a GFR below 90, consider starting N-acetylcysteine (NAC). However, a simple increase in fluids and a possible decrease in protein (if being overconsumed) can do wonders for most people without chronic kidney disease or heart failure. Increased fluids are contraindicated in these patients, and clinical training in determining a differential diagnosis between chronic and acute kidney disease versus dehydration is indicated.

Autoimmune Interventions

Detox

Cholestyramine can help detoxify the body of mycotoxins.[352] Over-the-counter options, like activated charcoal, bentonite clay, zeolite spray, and chlorella, are also effective. However, it's crucial to get chlorella from a reputable brand, as it can become toxic if not properly sourced.[353]

When detoxifying, remember to support the process with supplements such as glutathione, N-acetyl cysteine, alpha-lipoic acid, milk thistle, or broccoli sprout extract. Supporting mitochondria during detoxification is additionally vital. Options besides CoQ10 include L-carnitine, which aids in transporting fatty acids into the mitochondria. People on a vegan diet, especially, may require supplementation since carnitine is primarily found in meat sources.

Vitamins & Supplements

Selenium is important for helping glutathione function through the peroxidation processes, while magnesium activates glutathione. Glutathione, as a supplement of its own, is a great intervention for decreasing the inflammatory processes, supporting the immune system, and healing properties of the body.[354] These nutrients also assist in liver function and self-detoxification. Milk thistle, dandelion, and alpha-lipoic acid are good supplements to support liver detoxification, whether individually or in a combination supplement.

Vitamin D is another critical component of overall health and an essential lab to screen for. It functions as a pro-hormone that influences nearly every system in the body, from mental health to hormonal balance to autoimmune risk. It is an essential element, as it helps inhibit the growth of breast cancer cells and supports the immune system. In functional medicine, the vitamin D goal is to keep levels higher than 50, ideally closer to 80, to achieve optimal health.[355] However, there are conditions where even with high-dose supplementation, levels do not easily rise. One such scenario is in the presence of gut dysbiosis; the ability to absorb vitamin D may be compromised. For patients who are resistant to vitamin D or supplementation, consider conducting a zonulin test to assess for gut inflammation, which may be a root cause of the issue.

Magnesium, methylated B-complex vitamins, and D-ribose are important deficiencies to screen for. Supplementing with them can aid in the restoration of ATP—the body's primary energy currency. Magnesium is essential for reducing inflammation and is a crucial component of our immune response, so deficiency should be screened for. There are also several studies that associate low magnesium with increased severity of autoimmune disease, and therefore aiming for optimal, not excessively high levels may be beneficial. One study looked at low magnesium diet in rats, and the rats had a 70% decrease in severity.[356]

Zinc is also essential to our immune response and can lead to deteriorated immune functioning when levels are chronically low. However, excessive supplementation is associated with worsened autoimmune development and should therefore be monitored and only recommended in reasonable doses.[357]

CoQ10 is crucial to mitochondrial functioning. If mitochondria are impaired due to inflammation or deficiencies, the body cannot function optimally. Our program includes a comprehensive education module on mitochondrial dysfunction, but this is a general starting point for correction of this potential root cause. Omega-3 fatty acids can additionally help balance the immune system and reduce inflammation. Incorporating curcumin while avoiding a high-inflammatory, high-histamine diet can also be crucial for these people.

If MTHFR polymorphism is detected, the client will require methylcobalamin B vitamin supplementation. Typical dosing is around 1,000 to 2,000 mcg daily for one to two weeks for a loading dose and then decreasing to 100 to 1,000 mcg daily to maintain, titrated based upon lab values to stay within an optimal range of 500 to 900 mcg. Some may feel better at higher doses, and you may find that the levels are more of a guideline. This is especially true if they have the more severe polymorphism, homozygous (TT), versus the less severe heterozygous (TC) polymorphism. Remember, "T" stands for trouble. More "T" (as in the homozygous polymorphism) means more trouble. While most studies demonstrate little to no risk for B12 levels that are too high, there are rare occasions when oversupplementing with B12 can cause heart palpitations, insomnia, anxiety, and other symptoms, so monitoring blood work is best practice.[207]

Iron & Ferritin

In autoimmune patients, it's crucial to monitor ferritin levels. Inflammation triggers the release of hepcidin, which is a hormone that blocks iron absorption by sequestering it into storage sites. Chronic inflammatory processes, such as those seen in autoimmunity, trigger the release of hepcidin. Chronic exposure can lead to iron deficiency and subsequent weakening of the immune response.[358] Low ferritin additionally impairs oxygen transport to tissues, leading to increased pain, as seen in patients with sickle cell anemia, where pain is directly related to oxygen deficiency.[359]

Approach to Stress/Adrenal Dysfunction:

One way to decrease cortisol and stress—and subsequently aid in correcting DHEA levels—is to consider adrenal adaptogens. Even when cortisol levels are in a normal range, if a patient mentions stress of any kind, adaptogens should be considered as part of the treatment plan for the proper patient. Ashwagandha is a common adaptogen that is found to be generally safe for daily consumption, especially for up to three months. After six months, the data is lacking, but there are some very rare cases of chronic use being associated with liver failure and irregular heart rates. To date, true double-blind studies are lacking to prove the correlation of these observations.[315]

Normal cortisol levels found on 4-point testing can sometimes be masked during a state of pre-burnout. While the body may still be compensating physiologically, without intervention, this state can lead to dysfunction, causing cortisol levels to drop while the patient goes from experiencing a state of "tired and wired" to complete exhaustion. Taking steps to prevent that include rebalancing sleep, avoiding (or, at a minimum, decreasing) caffeine, and decreasing stress levels.[315] Once an exaggerated fight-or-flight response is addressed, cortisol has the opportunity to return to a healthy level. This optimally opens the opportunity for hormones to begin rebalancing and the liver to decrease overproduction of LDL cholesterol.[360]

When the body is stressed, it signals the liver to produce extra LDL, or low-density lipoprotein.[360] Therefore, as stress decreases, LDL may decrease. This also diminishes the pregnenolone steal, discussed in our hormones chapter, helping to regulate estrogen dominance, which tends to be a key factor in AI. In conventional medicine, while we may address dietary interventions, we often prescribe statins without even considering stress levels, which is surprising, knowing this correlation.

L-theanine is a natural amino acid that helps in regulating stress and another option that can be added to a treatment plan for autoimmune clients who have associated anxiety.[217] Interestingly enough, there is research that demonstrates a strong effect of L-theanine in preventing ulcerative colitis, another autoimmune disease, by regulating CD4 immune cells via their effect on the gut microbiome.[361] Dysregulated CD4 cells also play a significant role in autoimmune disease.[362] While there are limited studies in L-theanine directly affecting autoimmune disease, there is theoretical basis for the benefit of it over, or in conjunction with, other supplements, especially if stress support is a part of the treatment plan.

Finding Purpose to Uncover Healing

The evidence is clear that the perceived amount of purpose people have in their lives dictates their level of happiness, much more than a bank account does. While it may seem off-topic to discuss this in the autoimmune chapter, it is not. It is, in fact, important. Numerous studies indicate that people who feel they are making a meaningful impact in their world experience less stress. When people are engaged in activities they are passionate about, their work doesn't feel burdensome, and stress is not such a big issue. Work feels encouraging and purposeful. Work itself is not inherently negative; the challenge arises when we take on too much, and our bodies can't cope. A truly comprehensive treatment plan will explore a person's true happiness, not just use supplements as a Band-Aid.

Recall that autoimmunity is significantly tied to a history of stress or trauma. While that may not be every client's experience, it is so common that you would be harming more people than helping by removing this aspect of care from your treatment plans. Throughout this text are tips for helping with the mind and spirit, not just the body, but one that has not been discussed yet may be the most important of all: finding purpose. I encourage my clients to incorporate a routine into their weekly, if not daily, practice that helps them lock in purpose.

This is an area where I practice what I preach, as purpose is exactly why I left conventional medicine to pursue functional healing. I realized that I wasn't where I wanted to be in conventional medicine. I felt burned out and overworked. I was tired of simply treating numbers and titrating medications, and I didn't feel I was having the impact I'd originally sought when entering health and medicine.

This disillusionment, coupled with extremely long hours in the clinic away from my family, led to bitterness, stress, and resentment over my student loans and the long hours I worked for a relatively small paycheck compared to my effort in running the clinic. Eventually, I decided to prioritize what I was truly passionate about.

I know that functional medicine is where I am called, and that purpose gives me a passion that never burns out. My life has transformed, and work no longer feels like a job; it has become something I am truly passionate about. I feel excited about helping others, which is how I expected to feel when I first entered the medical field. Whenever I have a treatment plan to send to a patient, I look forward to it because I am fulfilling a purpose. I am helping patients who were often seen by many providers before me without results and were left feeling desperate. I've seen how my patients have navigated the conventional medicine system and often felt let down by it.

I am motivated to help because I know I can address the root causes of their issues and correct them in ways that align with my principles. It no longer feels like work or a mere checklist; it feels impactful. This shift has significantly reduced my stress, which, in turn, has helped regulate my hormones. It's astonishing how focusing on this can benefit not only my clients but also myself if I find myself in a similar situation.

Approach to Estrogen Dominance

Estrogen detoxification is essential in the presence of estrogen dominance, as it often contributes significantly to increasing overall stress and irritability. Additionally, if or when progesterone is depleted, anxiety tends to further increase.[363] This heightened anxiety can disrupt cortisol levels, causing further hormonal imbalances and creating a vicious cycle for patients. This, again, highlights the importance of focusing on stress reduction.

When our bodies successfully metabolize and detoxify excess estrogen, estrogen dominance is reduced. DIM (diindolylmethane), found in cruciferous vegetables, aids in this estrogen metabolism. Some studies suggest that DIM may also have the ability to destroy cancer cells and reduce inflammation, making it particularly beneficial for people who may be prone to estrogen-dominant cancers.[364,365] DIM is the most commonly used supplement for rebalancing estrogen dominance. Some studies even report that it might reduce inflammation, further benefiting an autoimmune condition, when clinically appropriate.[364]

Another supplement used in rebalancing estrogen dominance is calcium D-glucarate. This substance promotes biotransformation, making estrogen molecules more water-soluble, which facilitates easier breakdown and excretion.[373]

Removing Free Radicals/Toxins or Imbalances

Milk thistle is known to help protect the liver by providing a robust source of hepatoprotective compounds. It also increases antioxidant enzymes and reduces proinflammatory cytokines.[366] Dandelion is a phytochemical option for helping to detoxify the liver and is proven to be hepatoprotective.[367] Alpha-lipoic acid (ALA) for liver detoxification is another great option to optimize the liver before estrogen and chemical detox. ALA has been proven to protect against the effects of hepatotoxic drugs.[368]

Glutathione is a primary anti-inflammatory agent (known as the "master antioxidant") in our bodies and plays a crucial role in eliminating free radicals. Other antioxidants, such as acetylcysteine and resveratrol, are also important for reducing the formation of estrogen and preventing chronic inflammation, which is often a major contributor to autoimmune conditions.[369]

With all of that being said, be sure that your clients are also drinking around 8 eight ounce glasses of purified water a day. As basic as hydration is, do not miss screening for this. It's also important to ensure daily movement and exercise as medically tolerated (which moves the lymphatic system). Hydration and movement are equally important for detoxification as protocols are.

Prescriptions

Most clients come to a functional practitioner because they don't want to take as many prescriptions due to the potential risks they are associated with. For example, corticosteroids will decrease inflammation but increase the risk for diabetes, weight gain, and even Cushing's disease.

Disease-modifying anti-rheumatic drugs (DMARDS) increase a person's susceptibility to infections, can be hepatotoxic and nephrotoxic, have adverse effects on bone marrow, and even lead to a 1.15-fold increased risk for cancer.[370,371] Biologics increase the risk for infections, heart problems, and cancer.[372] Therefore, our goal is often to either decrease the need for these medications or decrease the effects and risks of the medications when they cannot eventually be discontinued, not necessarily discontinue them initially.

I never advise someone to stop their medications before interventions. If they are on any of these medications, work with the specialist to wean down, evaluate treatment, and monitor labs with the provider. That is beyond the scope of this book, but please be aware that initiating a functional plan does not immediately replace traditional treatment. As the body reverses disease and inflammation, which is the ultimate goal, it will take time for it to heal, and the level of healing will vary from patient to patient.

That said, in functional medicine, prescription medications are used selectively, and not every practitioner will adopt this approach. In truth, I have successfully helped many clients with autoimmune diseases without resorting to medications, and I have case studies to illustrate these successes. Many clients had completely normal markers and were able to avoid immunologics altogether, often greatly surprising their rheumatologist. One such case was a student of mine who put herself into full remission, and her doctor subsequently started placing referrals to the student out of her own clientele. What a fantastic way to start a clinic!

However, one prescription that is accepted under the functional medicine model is low-dose naltrexone (LDN). Some people may benefit from LDN, and it can be particularly helpful in accelerating the healing process if you have a license to prescribe it.[373] LDN, which is primarily used for opiate withdrawal, functions as an immunological modulator.

It helps rebalance the immune system's set point and can treat pain and inflammation effectively. Severe fibromyalgia and cancer pain have also been found to be responsive to this medication.[374]

LDN helps in the treatment of autoimmune disease by modulating innate and acquired immune responses.[375] It also helps regulate T-regulatory cells and reduces inflammation by decreasing the amount of TNF-alpha and IL-6 present.[375] It may also assist with weight loss and has a positive impact on brain function. The starting dose is usually 1.5 milligrams taken orally at night (you can microdose at <1 mg daily if the client does not tolerate that dose). After that, you can increase the dose by 1.5 milligrams every one to two weeks until you reach a goal of 4.5 milligrams. If the medication isn't well tolerated, you can reduce the dose or titrate more slowly, or just keep the patient at a lower dose.[376,377] Potential side effects include headaches, GI upset, fatigue, insomnia, vivid dreams, mood swings, and, rarely, a flare-up of autoimmune symptoms.[379]

Risk in Stopping Immune Modulators (Especially Too Soon)

When we discuss autoimmune diseases, it's important to acknowledge that these diseases can and often do cause irreversible damage, especially without treatment.[380] For example, rheumatoid arthritis, or neurologic diseases like multiple sclerosis, can cause lasting harm to joints and the nervous system, respectively, that we may not be able to reverse. It's crucial to convey to patients that they might have only one opportunity to address their health effectively, and stopping or delaying medications can contribute to this, as much as delaying functional intervention. This is important when discussing options for the patient pertaining to the discontinuation (or delaying of) prescription medications. It's a balance of risk versus benefit where there is not often a clear, perfect choice.

Autoimmune Dietary Connections

Diet is crucial in managing autoimmune conditions. One of the few instances where I will insist that someone avoid wheat or gluten is in cases of autoimmunity. There is often a delayed reaction to gluten, so patients might say that they've consumed it their entire lives without issue, but that doesn't mean it isn't causing long-term effects.

Clinical and scientific evidence consistently grows to support the theory that gluten plays a significant role in immune responses, especially central to causing inflammation in the gut.[381] Therefore, we must reduce gluten intake, especially for those with autoimmune disorders. Many patients may not notice an immediate change, although some experience instant benefits. Changes may take up to four to several weeks to notice as the body eliminates gluten. This is especially relevant for those with conditions like Hashimoto's.

If you recall, gluten in the body can lead to molecular mimicry.[381] This means the body sometimes confuses gluten with its own cells. The thyroid cells are particularly susceptible to this confusion because they share a similar chemical structure with gluten, but this issue can affect the entire body. When the body begins to attack gluten, it may inadvertently target its own cells/antibodies as well, mistaking them for gluten.

The leading diet for autoimmunity is by Dr. Terry Wahls, who used her protocols to control her own multiple sclerosis (MS) symptoms. The diet is Paleo-based and consists of an abundance of vegetables, quality protein, healthy fats, and the elimination of grains, legumes, nightshades, dairy products (except ghee or clarified butter), sugar, and processed food.[382]

If you notice, this diet is low-carb and good for controlling glucose and insulin spikes. Fasting blood sugar levels trigger insulin release, a critical hormone in our body. For reference, any fasting blood sugar reading above 84 mg/dL indicates an increased risk of developing diabetes over the next ten years. (Although "normal" lab is <100, optimal is <84.) This measure is a vital indicator of inflammation and insulin regulation in the body.

Example Autoimmune Protocol

Phase 1 Cleanse: Eliminate or decrease exposure to triggers (1–2 weeks) while you wait for stool analysis, genetic testing, OATs, DUTCH, or any other testing ordered.

- This may include triggers not discussed here from our toxins chapter.
- Avoid any triggers mentioned here.
- Initiate liver cleanse.
- Avoid sugar, gluten, dairy, seed oils, alcohol, and GMO soy, and start an anti-inflammatory diet.
    - If the client is stopping sugar and carbs for the first time, they may have a Herxheimer reaction. This is a flu-like reaction that results from the yeast or bacterial die-off, as the pathogens are no longer being "fed" their carbohydrate/sugar source. If the reaction does not occur in this phase, it might occur in Phase 2. Binders like charcoal can help to reduce the risk of an AI flare-up. Clinical judgment is necessary here. Working with a clinician who has experience detoxing AI patients is recommended for the new practitioner.

Phase 2 Remove:

- Treat any underlying gut issues according to the proper GI protocol.
- Treat estrogen dominance when present.

- Move on to any detox or heavy metal protocols as indicated.
- May add anti-inflammatory and immune-modulating supplements, such as curcumin, resveratrol, or Boswellia.[383]
- May add adaptogens, if appropriate.
- Consider IG or IV immunoglobulins (IV has to be administered with a trained specialist)
    - Throughout this phase, continue to monitor for Herxheimer reactions.
- Consider low-dose naltrexone as appropriate.
- Consider myo-inositol for Hashimoto's.[384]

Phase 3: Rebuild

- If the client wants, you can try to reintroduce any foods that were eliminated but are still anti-inflammatory.
- Establish a health routine with exercise, spiritual, and mental components.
- Replace vitamin deficiencies, like B vitamins, vitamin D, or omega-3s.
- Heal the gut with glutathione/NAD.

Business Practice Pearl

Functional medicine emphasizes individualized care. There is no one-size-fits-all approach; you won't follow a single route with every patient. That's why it's essential to have a supportive team around you. It can be easy to overlook critical aspects, especially when trying to shift your mindset to identifying root causes rather than simply following established protocols.

A valuable piece of advice is to ensure that you have the support you need as a practitioner. Surround yourself with people who are also focused on making a difference in the world. This community should uplift and encourage each other, aiming for total impact rather than competition. I am proud of the supportive group we have at the Academy of Functional Medicine and the Institute of Functional Nurses. We are here to heal, and we do not view each other as competition. Collaboration, not competition, happens at the top, and locking arms with other incredible practitioners serves to help you elevate your life, practice, and impact faster than ever imaginable! That is why we have private social channels that are safe places to support one another as clinicians. You can meet many of my colleagues and other peers in our Skool community and try it free for 7 days by going here: https://www.skool.com/functionalmedicine/about.

We view each other as part of the same army, fighting to reclaim what the enemy has stolen from us: the health of our nation. This should never have happened, but unfortunately, it did because evil exists in our world. Surrounding yourself with people who share this mission will significantly increase your chances of success. It's no coincidence that they say your level of success, your mindset, and your potential are often an average of the five people you spend the most time with.

This principle is crucial for ensuring your success in your practice and the positive impact you are called to have. You wouldn't be reading this book right now if you weren't meant for something greater, so surround yourself with people who share this mindset.

When designing programs for your clients, make sure you infuse the same level of passion into your work. Personalize each program by incorporating their spiritual and emotional needs alongside their physical health. Avoid viewing this as simply a matter of trading time for money on a one-to-one basis.

Instead, we strongly recommend creating comprehensive packages for individuals. This approach is not about running countless people through a system; it's about genuinely helping the few people we are called to serve at a higher level. It means empowering them to take charge of their health and make their own decisions, rather than relying on the medical community for their core health needs.

The way you build and present these programs to your patients should focus less on the individual components and more on the overall payoff they'll receive from the investment in their lives. Have them consider the feeling of "parenting from the couch" or what it is like to come home at five o'clock, when their kids are eager for their attention, but they are too exhausted to engage. Ask them directly, "How does this affect your long-term health and happiness?"

Have them consider longevity and the joy of seeing either their future or current grandchildren. Help them see the bigger picture and the true benefits of their health journey—not just enduring hardships but thriving in life. Avoid overwhelming your clients with too many options. Instead, deliver what they truly need. By personalizing your approach, you'll create a greater positive impact in their lives.

BONUS TRAINING:

The Power of Finding Your Why.

This is the why and vision of our team!

SCAN ME

SCAN THE QR CODE

or visit functionalmedicineunlocked.com

Chapter 9

Functional Medicine Approach to Long COVID

Case Study: A Twenty-Eight-Year-Old Woman with Long COVID Symptoms

A twenty-eight-year-old woman stopped working due to fatigue and persistent diarrhea that she found embarrassing. It has developed after contracting COVID-19. She felt extreme guilt about having to leave her job and considered applying for disability. This situation was both a familial concern and a social stigma for her, which intensified her distress.

Her mental health suffered greatly during this time. She felt isolated and believed others were judging her, especially since many people who had COVID experienced milder symptoms. There was little support or answers from healthcare providers, which compounded her feelings of hopelessness.

To help her, I focused on rebalancing her gut microbiome. We were able to address her chronic diarrhea, and I also started her on CoQ10, methylated B12, and a high-dose probiotic. Within about three months, her symptoms began to improve significantly, and it took roughly six months for her to feel more like herself again.

In addition to these functional medicine interventions, I recommended a short course of Benadryl—50 mg at bedtime for two weeks—which is not typically classified as functional medicine but may aid in recovery. It has been found that Benadryl may help modulate histamine-related symptoms and improve sleep for those suffering from Long Haulers. (Mashauri, 2023).[385]

Discussion

Acute COVID typically lasts about seven to ten days, although it can sometimes be shorter—around three to five days—depending on the individual's age, overall health, and the state of their microbiome and vitamin D levels at the onset of the infection. Long COVID is identified as symptoms that continue to develop or persist for more than twelve weeks post-initial infection and are not part of another cause of illness.[386] It's important to note that a client doesn't need to experience all the symptoms that were associated with their initial COVID-19 infection.

For example, a person may have symptoms such as coughing, shortness of breath, fatigue, body aches, and brain fog during their acute COVID-19 infection. However, their long COVID symptoms might only include body aches and brain fog, while their coughing may have resolved. Conversely, they might still have a persistent cough but no longer experience muscle aches. Thus, it's not necessary to have all the original symptoms from the acute phase.[386]

Understanding what drives long COVID is essential as it continues to evolve and new information emerges. Long COVID is triggered by viral persistence within the body and associated T-cell abnormalities.[386] Other contributing factors include amyloid-inducing metabolites, immune dysregulation, platelet hyperactivation, potential coagulopathies, and microclots in various tissues, such as the brain, kidneys, and muscles. These disruptions can lead to decreased oxygen delivery to tissues and impaired mitochondrial function.[386]

Furthermore, oxidative stress often results from gut dysbiosis triggered by viral infections, including COVID-19. Such infections can cause chronic diarrhea and significantly impact the gut microbiome.[387] This, in turn, can lead to autonomic dysfunction and the development of autoimmunity. There's also abnormal metabolism of tryptophan, which affects the pathways of serotonin and melatonin, potentially leading to depression and anxiety as common symptoms of long COVID.[386]

Chronic inflammation in the body directly affects neurotransmitters that influence mood, as approximately 90% of serotonin is produced in the gut. The protein misfolding caused by viruses such as COVID leads to disruption that may cause central nervous system symptoms, dysbiosis, disruption of the blood-brain barrier, endocrine dysfunction, altered circadian rhythms, and depletion of serotonin that reaches the brain.[386] Other symptoms include chest pain, breathlessness, fatigue, and conditions such as postural orthostatic tachycardia syndrome (POTS). POTS can manifest as dizziness, lightheadedness, fatigue, and easy fainting, along with heart rate irregularities, and is commonly associated with long COVID.

Gut Dysbiosis and Immune Hyperactivity in Long COVID

A stool analysis can reveal specific needs for rebalancing the gut microbiome, which is vital for recovery when present. Chronic diarrhea, abdominal pain, and bloating are common post-COVID-19. Studies are now revealing that patients with higher zonulin levels suffered more severe COVID reactions, leading to hospitalization.[388] This connection indicates that those who had a current dysbiosis upon initial contraction of COVID were at higher risk for severe acute illness as well as more prone to chronic dysbiosis and symptoms. Next, let us explore some other pathophysiological occurrences that can complicate long COVID.

Histamine Involvement

In some individuals, research indicates that Long COVID results from immune hyperactivity (which leads to insufficiency) alongside mast cell hyperactivity. Mast cells produce histamine, an inflammatory substance that the body uses to fight viruses and bacteria. It can additionally be found naturally in food,[389] which supports the implementation of a low-histamine diet in long COVID sufferers.

Gaining control over the systemic antiviral response and the pro-inflammatory cytokines plays a crucial role in managing various symptoms. Dysregulation can lead to sleep disturbances, increased agitation, and even delirium. This is where antihistamines that stabilize mast cells can be beneficial for improving sleep. However, it is important to note that taking diphenhydramine for more than a couple of weeks is not recommended, and chronic use is tied to increased risk for cognitive decline.[390]

Adopting a low-histamine diet for at least a few weeks to months can additionally help to re-regulate the immune system. If dietary changes are too difficult, diamine oxidase (DAO) is a supplement that helps to break down histamine. There is also genetic testing for the DAO enzyme, which can reveal further reasons for histamine sensitivity. Both approaches help to decrease the amount of histamine in the body.[391]

Hypercoagulability of COVID

COVID can also lead to hypercoagulability, where neutrophils, T cells, monocytes, and macrophages bind to platelets, increasing the risk for thrombotic events. This process can lead to tissue hypoxia and vascular inflammation, raising the likelihood of heart attacks and strokes.[392] While the goal is to resolve the hyperactivity of the immune system caused by the initial infection, garlic, ginseng, and ginkgo biloba are known to be anticoagulant and antiplatelet.[393]

Caution must be taken with these supplements, and a good health screening and medication checklist are necessary. These supplements are not recommended for those with a history of hemorrhagic stroke, thrombocytopenia, spontaneous bleeding, or other bleeding risk factors, or if they are on any prescribed blood thinners, as they can cause a significant, sometimes fatal, risk of bleeding when combined with other medications or in combination with one another.[393] Caution should also be taken for those who additionally are on SSRIs, NSAIDs, and other supplements (such as fish oil). Ginkgo biloba can additionally lead to severe headaches, so it would be contraindicated in clients with a known history.

Chronic Viral Infections

The reactivation of dormant chronic viral infections, such as Epstein-Barr or herpes simplex, can exacerbate long COVID symptoms. When exposed to COVID, acute flares of chronic viral infections, such as hepatitis or Epstein-Barr Virus, are possible, leading to an intensified expression of the immune response and disease severity, and even negatively impact long-term outcomes, including post-acute sequelae of COVID-19.[394]

Microcirculation

Microcirculation plays a vital role in COVID and long COVID reactions. There are approximately 60,000 miles of blood vessels in the body, and research has shown that even at the micro-level, these vessels are incredibly important and literally touch every part of our body. Experiments have been conducted using cadavers, where all tissues were dissolved except for the vessels, and the body outline is still perfectly visible as if the skin were still present. The vascular endothelial cells in just one human could wrap around the world four times. This highlights the extensive role of the vascular system. Most of the endothelial surface is found in the vascular bed, and it plays a crucial role in tissue nourishment, oxygen delivery, and the removal of carbon dioxide. Microcirculation is essential for these processes, which is why the damage that COVID-19 causes to the endothelial cells affects virtually every part of the body. Small arterioles are present throughout the body and our lymphatic system, collecting ducts, and venules. The eye, inner ear, brain, liver, and skeletal system are all affected. This yields insight into the widespread symptoms seen in long COVID and the varying groups of symptoms that arise.

Lab Testing

Lab testing will depend largely on the client and symptoms but will most often include a complete stool analysis, organic acids testing (OATs), and genetic testing. Determining whether an individual has an MTHFR polymorphism can aid in healing, as those affected may require supplemented amounts of methylated B12. The abundance of homocysteine and a lack of methionine that occurs as a result of an inability to methylate properly may contribute to long-term inflammatory processes.

Treatment and supplementation should be guided by symptoms and lab findings. Discussion of supplements to follow should not be considered as a prescription to start all listed supplements, but rather as a list of potential options to consider, which are appropriate for the individual.

Mitochondrial Dysfunction

Mitochondrial dysfunction is common in long COVID. OATs testing will reveal the necessity for treatment and proper supplementation, which may include several options, but the most common supplements include CoQ10 and alpha-lipoic acid.[395] Interestingly enough,

CoQ10 is also relevant for people on statins who experience muscle cramps and related issues and represents an example where the effects of CoQ10 on the mitochondria can be directly witnessed. Fatigue, brain fog, and myalgia associated with statin use (medications designed to lower cholesterol) are often due to the depletion of CoQ10 in the mitochondria.

Potential Supplements to Consider in Long COVID

Melatonin

Supplementing with melatonin can reduce dysautonomia, alleviate muscular fatigue, enhance glycolysis, and improve mitochondrial integrity, ultimately increasing levels of ATP, which provides energy to our cells. This, in turn, helps decrease brain fog and neuroinflammation. High doses of melatonin have been shown to improve these conditions. It also has an impact on hormonal balance, making it a valuable option for people dealing with long COVID.

Melatonin may also help mitigate the interaction between SARS-CoV-2 and ACE2 receptors. The SARS virus uses ACE2 cells to enter the body, which is why studies have found a connection between the use of lisinopril and an exacerbation of symptoms during an acute COVID-19 infection.[395] This interaction is intricately linked to the cytokine storm that COVID is infamous for causing, where an overabundance of IL-6, IL-2, IL-8, IL-1β, IL-1b, and IFN-γ are produced. Melatonin and a low-histamine diet aid in suppressing this overreaction. While the evolving data for mechanism of action continue to grow and adjust, clinicians should be aware of the potential interactions between COVID and ACE inhibitors and stay current as the literature develops, taking into consideration clinical presentations.

Vitamin D

Early in the COVID epidemic, it was noted that people deficient in vitamin D often experienced more severe illness,[383] likely because vitamin D is crucial for many cellular and immune functions. It helps with regulating mast cell storms, supports ACE2 modulation, and enhances microbial properties (Sumantri, 2023).[396] Optimizing vitamin D is an essential part of helping clients recover from long COVID.

Monolaurin

Monolaurin may be a consideration for viral recovery. Higher serum levels of monolaurin have been found to help decrease the severity of COVID and viral infections in general. Monolaurin is a naturally occurring monoglyceride found in human breast milk and coconut oil that can additionally be supplemented over the counter to help support immune and digestive health.[397]

Adaptogens

Adaptogens, such as Cordyceps, have been found to be beneficial post-COVID. It is suspected that they affect adrenal re-regulation. They are also commonly known for their overall immune-boosting properties.[398] Further adrenal support may be necessary, as defined by a client's 4-point cortisol testing, and should be ordered if fatigue is an underlying issue. Cordyceps is particularly beneficial as it inhibits platelet aggregation—a symptom of long COVID—thus decreasing the risk of blood clots and strokes. Furthermore, Cordyceps has anti-tumor, antiviral, and antihypertensive properties, and it improves mitochondrial activity. Mitochondrial dysfunction is common in long COVID patients. Ashwagandha and rhodiola are other options.

Probiotics

Proper probiotics should be chosen based on the client's comprehensive stool analysis. Research indicates that even six months after contracting COVID-19, many people continue to shed viral RNA. A study of COVID-19 sufferers found that 63% of participants experienced persistent COVID-19 symptoms, and 37% progressed to long COVID. These prolonged symptoms often correlate with significantly elevated levels of certain microbes known to trigger inflammation, specifically from the genera *Proteviola* and *Valonella*. Dysbiosis is often how long COVID affects the gastrointestinal tract, increasing the risk of diarrhea and impairing the immune system, which further contributes to inflammation in the body. Notably, these genera produce lipid polysaccharide (LPS), which can adversely affect the nervous system, causing symptoms like brain fog, memory loss, and anxiety. Recall from our neurological chapter that LPS is a neurotoxin associated with cognitive decline. Also interesting to note is that the overall microbiome composition of long COVID patients closely resembles that of people with chronic fatigue syndrome.

Anti-Inflammatory Support

Other supportive agents include liposomal glutathione or black cumin seed with curcumin, both of which are known for their anti-inflammatory properties. Glutathione deficiency is common in patients who react severely to COVID, and supplementation has been found to help reduce oxidative stress by supporting the redox process. Clinical improvement has been documented with the supplementation of glutathione.[354]

Another anti-inflammatory polyphenol that can help reduce chronic inflammation in the body is grape seed extract. This extract acts as a vasorelaxant, protecting the endothelial lining from oxidative stress and reducing vascular permeability. Studies have demonstrated an up to tenfold decrease in viral concentration versus controls in adding this supplement to the treatment plan.[399]

Ginkgo biloba contains flavonoids and acts as a vasodilator to help relax blood vessels, which is vital for increasing microcirculation that can be impaired in long COVID syndrome. Ginkgo biloba protects the vascular endothelium and inhibits inducible nitric oxide synthase (iNOS), reducing the breakdown of telomerase activity. This is important for gene health and preventing genetic damage.[400] Additionally, it inhibits the oxidation of LDL, which can contribute to inflammation in the body.

Mango extract, specifically *Mangifera indica, is another* option to help decrease general inflammation. This fruit is rich in polyphenols that support endothelial function and have anti-inflammatory properties. It also aids in metabolism and is vital for maintaining the endothelial lining of the vascular system. Mango improves fatty acid oxidation, hepatic fatty acid oxidation, and lipid homeostasis. It also promotes mitochondrial biogenesis, which is the body's process of creating more mitochondria. Its use may enhance energy levels, especially in overlapping cases of mitochondrial deficiency or dysfunction.

Palmitoylethanolamide (PEA) is a compound derived from fats, naturally found in foods like egg yolks and peanuts, and produced in the human body. It binds to cells to reduce pain and swelling and is an endogenous lipid mediator. PEA has analgesic, immunologic, neuroprotective, antipyretic, anti-epileptic, and anti-inflammatory properties. It may help with anti-convulsions, neural pain and has antibacterial and antiviral effects, contributing to enhanced muscle recovery, improved cognition, mood, and sleep. PEA is indicated for various conditions, including anti-aging, brain health, allergies, and joint health. The usual dosage ranges from 300 to 1200 milligrams per day in divided doses and can help alleviate long COVID symptoms.[401]

Detoxification & Diet

Another important aspect of treating long COVID involves incorporating detoxification. Detox should begin with the proper diet, including the encouragement of as many green leafy vegetables as possible. These vegetables aid in detoxification and are high in various B vitamins and folate needed for effective detoxification. A full liver detox may be considered prior to implementing full treatment.

An antioxidant-rich diet is advised for long COVID recovery. This may include berries, such as blueberries, strawberries, raspberries, and blackberries. Turmeric, garlic, ginseng, and ginger also demonstrate strong anti-inflammatory properties and can be consumed in pill form or incorporated into cooking. Green tea may help reduce inflammation and can be an easy addition to a diet where caffeine is not contraindicated.

Excessive alcohol consumption should be avoided for several reasons. To begin, it depletes CoQ10, as our mitochondrial cells work harder during intoxication, requiring additional energy and oxygen. It also depletes the immune system, induces neuroinflammation, increases dysbiosis, and triggers inflammatory markers, among other issues.[402] These are all factors that are essential to being in peak performance and enhancing recovery from long COVID. Patient education to decrease alcohol use, especially during recovery, is an important focus.

Chapter Conclusion

Recovery from long COVID can be a multifactorial process, and education for patient expectations should be set prior to starting intervention. While some may recover in weeks, more complex cases may take months to identify and reverse root causes, as this is an area of care that is still very new. Developments and changes are still rapidly evolving, and care should be taken by the practitioners to stay up-to-date on new research and recommendations as they come out. All interventions should be clinically adjusted and applied on a personalized basis.

Business Practice Pearl

"You don't have to be great to start, but you have to start to become great."
-Zig Zigglar

No one ever actually achieves "perfection," and still the fear of not being perfect stops most before they even start. If perfectionism presents as not wanting to start before feeling ready, you need to realize the truth that getting started sooner is your only shot at feeling prepared. None of us feel "ready" to do something we have never done until we've done it a while. And while we will never actually attain perfection, we still strive to be the best we can, maybe even *the* best. The only way to attempt that is to get in more proverbial reps in than the competition. Grit and expanded comfort zones win over natural talent, always. Only then will the goal actually become plausibly attainable.

Extensive preparation and waiting on perfect timing is nothing more than busy work disguised as playing it safe. It does nothing more than help your conscience hide from reality: you are dodging your calling. Telling ourselves that we don't have what it takes to just get started is always self-deception, and self-deception is the worst deception because it is the inception of the very thing that we least desire.

An obsession with perfection often translates to a reluctance to act. Don't let the fear of starting hold you back. Do what you can now. Begin making an impact, even if it's just by sharing small pieces of information on social media or with current patients, as I did when I first got started.

If you believe that God expects you to be perfect, remember that this was never His goal. In fact, we are reminded that He desires growth rather than perfection in our Christian journey in Philippians 3:12–14. The Apostle Paul, a man called so strongly by God that God called him to write a significant portion of the Bible, even admitted that it has never been that he "arrived" at perfection but that he keeps pressing forward, forgetting the past and simply striving for the future goal. Additionally, 1 Corinthians 2:6 tells us that God has chosen the weak and the simple to accomplish great things.

As a new functional practitioner, the obstacle that many focus on is that they are not perfect in their own journey and therefore fear that they should not be counseling others in health. However, it should not deter you from helping others. To begin, sometimes it's even *more* powerful to join others by saying, "Hey, we're in this together." You may find that your clients relate to your experience better, leading to a more significant impact due to this transparency. But also, the majority of us do not start out being perfect in our health. I often share with my patients that while most of my current lifestyle choices are healthy, I didn't start that way at all. I openly discuss the unhealthy habits I had and explain that I reached my current state through gradual progress. This serves as inspiration and removes shame for them where they currently are. This shared experience can have a profound impact and highlights that no matter what stage of your journey you are in, there is value to be had. Also, being transparent about your own path can help eliminate feelings of imposter syndrome for yourself. As long as you are not trying to pose as someone or a status you are not, you can rest assured that you're doing the right thing, and everyone knows that we all start somewhere.

There is a movie called *Catch Me If You Can*. The main character, portrayed by Leonardo DiCaprio, goes through various scenarios where he pretends to be a pilot and a professor, among other high-level professionals. When he was caught, the police stated that they understood how he managed to pretend to be in some of the professions. For example, he simply put on a pilot's uniform and claimed to be a pilot. This allowed him to enjoy free rides from one place to another. However, they are stumped by the fact that he taught an entire room of college-level students while pretending to be a professor. He explained that it was easy—he just stayed *one step ahead.*

I want to encourage you by saying that you are also ahead of the game simply by reading this book. You might only be one step ahead, but more often than not, you are further along than you realize. This does not mean you can't make a significant impact, even through small actions.

Think about the story of David and Goliath. David was much smaller, yet that makes his victory even more impressive. If you find yourself starting from a disadvantaged position, like David facing Goliath, it only amplifies your potential triumph, and the great thing is that God desires to use the underdog to glorify His strength and greatness. This is a common theme in the Bible. For example, in 1 Corinthians 1:27, God shares that He deliberately chooses the weak and foolish things of the world to shame the wise and strong, ensuring no one boasts in themselves but in God. Then in 2 Corinthians 12:9, we are told that God's power is made perfect in weakness, as His grace is sufficient. So if you feel inadequate, rejoice. You're exactly who it makes sense to be called.

If you haven't noticed yet, everything we're discussing involves a form of spiritual warfare. The enemy may be in your mind, trying to prevent you from going for your calling. Disease and mental illness are on the rise, despite billions being spent on health care. Children are targeted from a very young age to eat junk food like candy and cereal that is advertised as "whole grain." It's often said that nothing is more profitable than a sick child, which perpetuates reliance on the pharmaceutical industry. The list goes on, and we are no doubt living in a time of spiritual warfare.

We have known for decades that chemicals affect children's health, yet it has taken too long to address this issue, largely due to money, greed, and evil interests. But be encouraged that we are a part of this movement, and it is gaining significant ground. If you believe in your role, which you do, or you wouldn't have read this far, and if you've found your way here today, then you are, indeed, a wellness warrior. God is on your side, and He will turn your imperfections into strengths, enabling you to make the impact He calls you to achieve. Ultimately, it's not about us; it's about the patients and the positive influence we are meant to create.

Chapter 10

Chronic Pain and Orthopedics

Chronic pain is defined as pain that has lasted for at least three months, and it may or may not be associated with an acute injury. In conventional medicine, first-line treatment for chronic pain typically includes NSAIDs (nonsteroidal anti-inflammatory drugs) and over-the-counter analgesics.[402] As the pain persists and these treatments become less effective, patients often transition to stronger analgesics such as narcotics. A significant concern within the conventional chronic pain management model is the high risk of mortality associated with these medications.[402] To address this issue, recent regulations have pressured healthcare providers to avoid prescribing pain medications. While decreasing pain medications is undoubtedly a great goal for the patient, there is often not a plan to correct the underlying cause of pain, and the method most frequently used is simply weaning them down and encouraging the patient to tolerate a higher level of pain. Unfortunately, this leaves many patients struggling to manage their pain without adequate support, as simply discontinuing medication does not address the underlying causes of their pain. With functional medicine, however, there are effective alternatives for managing chronic pain.

Functional pain management does not simply follow an algorithm for supplements. The goal is to find the root cause (or causes) of inflammation. When the majority of these processes are mitigated, the body can heal, pain can decrease, and hopefully, disappear completely. When inflammation resolves, microtears and even larger traumas are given the opportunity to heal and repair. The body is built to heal itself; our main goal is to optimize the body and allow an environment where it can do what it's designed to do.

Case Study: Forty-Five-Year-Old Female Patient With Fibromyalgia and Rheumatoid Arthritis

One example is a forty-five-year-old female patient I worked with who suffered from fibromyalgia and rheumatoid arthritis. She had been living with chronic pain and depression for many years. While she came to me for pain management, she was still hesitant to start narcotics, though she was prepared to resort to them if her pain could not be improved.

We found relief for her primarily by focusing on her gut health and reducing inflammation in her body through removing the root cause of inflammation. This allowed natural supplements, such as turmeric, to start taking effect. By rebalancing her gut microbiome, neurotransmitter levels were corrected to enhance both mental and neurological health and decrease pain perception. I also used L-theanine to help manage her anxiety and depression. Sometimes, simply improving a patient's mood can have a profound impact on their experience of pain. As our treatment progressed, the patient reported that her pain became manageable, alleviating her need or desire for narcotics. In this patient's case, she also had an MTHFR polymorphism, which we addressed by providing her with methylated B vitamins to lower her homocysteine levels. We also eliminated gluten from her diet, starting her on a low-FODMAP diet. Removing gluten can create a remarkable improvement for sensitive individuals.

I would like to offer a practical tip regarding pain management: while Tylenol (acetaminophen) and ibuprofen are common options, they are far from optimal for long-term use. Tylenol poses risks to liver health, impairing detoxification processes, increasing homocysteine levels, and decreasing glutathione.[403] Ibuprofen, although anti-inflammatory, can cause gastrointestinal issues and disrupt gut flora. In some cases, I may switch a patient from ibuprofen to Tylenol, despite my reservations about Tylenol, to help reset their gut health. Once the gut is in better shape, it can enhance the production of neurotransmitters, positively impacting both mood and pain levels, hopefully leading to no longer needing pain medications.

The power of functional medicine can often be overlooked in extreme cases. However, I want to highlight a colleague of mine, whom I greatly respect. He is an orthopedic surgeon and his name is Dr. Doug Lucus, DO. You can find him on social media. This individual left a successful career in surgery to do functional medicine, as he found that he could have a stronger impact in his purpose to heal through functional interventions than through surgical procedures. This weighed heavily on his conscience, prompting him to leave conventional medicine altogether after he found incredible results helping patients under the Functional Model. He was a lead surgeon in a hospital, but he abandoned that career to pursue functional medicine, driven by a desire to heal.

Ultimately, he built a massively successful business dedicated to teaching and helping patients heal their pain and manage conditions like osteoporosis. So, while he took a significant risk in his career to help people with a clear conscience, it has paid off financially. Leaving the conventional model can be overwhelming and uncertain. I went through this fear personally. I had spent over eight years in school, dedicated to the belief that running a traditional family practice was going to be my end-all, be-all. That is, until it no longer felt morally right to push medications during a short appointment. I knew that, for many, there was a better route to reversing the alignments through functional medicine. But when you follow a true passion and calling to heal and help, I believe God shows up and shows out. We have a plethora of student results to demonstrate this truth.

I myself struggled with chronic pain in my knee, neck, bilateral hips, shoulders, and feet. I received steroid injections, took oral steroids, underwent multiple imaging procedures, including MRIs and CT scans, full blood panels drawn, and everything was "within normal limits." Despite the normal labs and imaging results, the pain in my neck was so severe that I could barely move it on some days. My child would come in for a hug, and I had to explain, "No, no, no, sweetheart, Mommy has a bad neck." This became the turning point for me in fully understanding pain as being more than just a linear connection between the body and the brain. After I had corrected my gut, the inflammation in my body resolved, and I was able to heal. It truly blew my mind when my toddler son hugged me around the neck for the first time, and it didn't hurt. It made me realize how impactful this insight can be.

This also demonstrates one of the key aspects I emphasize to my students about the impact they are making in the world. Overcoming pain (or any root cause) isn't just about alleviating symptoms; it's about helping others reclaim the ability to live life fully. I can't put a monetary value on the sheer joy of hugging my son again or allowing him to squeeze me without fear of pain. He is the type of child who loves to give strong hugs, and there is nothing more emotionally painful than telling him to hold back on that expression of affection. When I no longer had to do that, it allowed me to fully embrace the connection he longed to share with me. It was a moment where he wanted to express his deep love for me, and I was finally able to receive it instead of pushing it away. That's life-changing. That's the power you can wield as a functional practitioner.

As you work with your clients, it's essential to also help them recognize this aspect of their struggles. Often, people become adept at hiding the true impact of lived experiences. By helping your clients see this broader perspective, you can become a catalyst for transformation in their lives that lasts a lifetime. Remember, it's not just about addressing the one issue they initially came to you for; it's about helping them see the bigger picture of their overall well-being and pain management. When we correct one aspect, several others follow. You will see again why I say functional medicine is the ultimate health leverage.

The Joint-Gut Connection

Alterations in the microbial flora of the lungs and gastrointestinal tract of preclinical rheumatoid arthritis (RA) and osteoarthritis (OA) suggest a role for dysbiosis in the progression and protraction of joint disease. Interestingly enough, DMARDs have been known to modify the intestinal microbial composition of the patients who take them and may actually be one underlying reason for their effectiveness.[404]

In some cases of RA, recirculation of innate immune cells from the GI tract to the peripheral joints has been identified as a key factor in the chronic inflammatory process.[404] Similar findings have also been discovered for osteoarthritis, arthritis, and spondylarthritis.[405] Even when considering the known hereditary patterns of autoimmune disease, the science backs this up. The composition of the gut microbiome, reflecting similarities in RA and IBD patients, can be hereditary. Antigens being passed down activate autoreactive T or B cells, triggering an autoimmune mechanism. This is another representation of molecular mimicry.[405]

Osteoarthritis (OA) has long been thought of as a degenerative disease in which the joints simply "break down." That belief is no longer upheld. Instead, OA is recognized as a complex, chronic inflammatory process representing several interactions, including the gut microbiome and generalized inflammation. The inflammatory process associated with obesity may, in many patients, have more to do with joint pain than simply the weight itself. People with OA have been identified as having elevated levels of Actinobacteria and Proteobacteria and reduced levels of Firmicutes compared to those without the disease, adding to systemic inflammation.[405]

The effect of inflammation alone directly affecting pain is something that can be clinically demonstrated but quickly overlooked if not fully understood. I have had clients lose a mere ten pounds from dieting (by removing chemical-laden, sugary, inflammatory foods) and report that their joints felt better, despite still being at least a hundred pounds from their goals. They will naturally perceive that it was the sheer loss of weight, but arguably, it wasn't the small amount of weight loss so much as the decrease in chronic inflammation.

In my scenario, steroids, both oral and injected, Tylenol, and NSAIDs did little to nothing for the pain. However, I experienced a dramatic reduction in pain after fully addressing my gut health, without any other interventions. I had already learned that improving gut health could help with my pain, but I was still amazed when it actually worked for me. Then, because I was able to absorb it through my gut, I also began to feel and see the benefits of taking collagen, whereas prior to that experience, such supplements didn't seem to help at all. This experience highlights an important point: natural treatments may not be effective in chronic disease if the gut isn't able to absorb the necessary nutrients and compounds. Inflammation in the body can block the body's ability to heal itself, and the gut can lack the ability to absorb supplements properly. Therefore, addressing gut health is essential when pursuing long-term relief strategies.

The conventional medical model often focuses on suppressing symptoms. However, suppressing pain without addressing the underlying problem is futile. For example, while narcotics can provide temporary relief, long-term use carries an increased risk of severe side effects, including death. Moreover, frequent suppression of pain receptors leads the body to produce more pain receptors, exacerbating the pain sensation over time, known as opioid-induced hyperalgesia.[406] Consequently, patients may require higher doses of medication, creating a dangerous cycle. Research from reputable sources, including the NIH, supports the connection between chronic pain and inflammation. Chronic pain is often associated with increased levels of inflammatory cytokines, such as TNF-alpha and IL-6.[407] To effectively address chronic pain, it's crucial to investigate why the inflammation is present and target those underlying causes, in addition to gastric dysbiosis.

Other Causes of Inflammation

Other causes of system inflammation may include, but are not limited to, hormonal imbalances, chemicals, nutritional deficiencies, smoking, obesity, chronic disease, bacterial infections, viral infections, parasitic infections, inflammatory foods, allergies, and sedentary lifestyles.[6] The primary goal, then, as a functional practitioner, is to identify any present source of inflammation, reverse it, and allow the body to heal naturally or with supplementation. Fortunately, when systemic inflammation decreases, the associated pain also tends to get much better. This is a fundamental principle in managing chronic pain, which affects 20.9% (or one in five) of the global population.[408] This is all said to note that we don't want to guess the underlying cause of a client's pain. Therefore, an essential part of evaluating pain is determining its source. Understanding this can help guide appropriate treatment strategies.

Assessment

Physical Screening

A good physical assessment will help to differentiate etiologies. For example, does the client have more stiffness in the morning that improves with movement and/or warmth? If so, then it is more likely to be OA. Does the client have nodules that are swollen at the base of their fingers in the metacarpophalangeal joints that are bilateral, erythematous, and swollen? If so, then it is more likely to be RA. Does the client have Heberden's nodes at the most distal interphalangeal joint of their fingers? Then it is more likely to be OA. Does a family history of autoimmunity run in the family, and is the pain bilateral? Then the client should be screened for RA. The etiology therefore dictates the best first approach. For example, if the pain is autoimmune in nature, you will want to reference the autoimmune approach.

These are a few starting points that you should have in your assessment toolbox, not a fully comprehensive outline for ruling out differential diagnoses. Please note this is not a full course for diagnosing, as your degree should have equipped you with that information. If you are unable to diagnose due to license limitations, it is recommended to collaborate with a skilled practitioner who can provide the necessary diagnosis or for the client to present with a confirmed diagnosis when they begin working with you. This is not to downplay those without the ability to clinically diagnose. There is no doubt a great need for all disciplines, but to identify legal "gray" areas so we do not accidentally cross them, which could compromise patient care and put you at legal risk. To identify the proper scope of practice, coaches, nurses, and medical providers need to consult with their proper board and legal team.

Labs To Consider In Root Cause Evaluation

Screening for Key Vitamin Deficiencies

The etiology of pain associated with numbness and tingling can include nerve damage or impingement, diabetic neuropathy, or deficiencies in vitamin B12, as well as an excess of B12 in some people.[409] Each root cause may be different and may or may not be a fit for functional intervention. If B12 deficiency is suspected, it's important to test and not guess, as both too much and too little B12 can lead to numbness and tingling, particularly in the peripheral areas of the body. In the event that symptoms are present and levels are normal, MTHFR genetic polymorphism testing could be considered.

Vitamin D levels may be tested as a root cause. Deficiency is associated with increased pain, and replacement should be prioritized when found.[410] Vitamin D is chronically low in the American population and is something that most often should be considered when pain is an issue. It is also an essential part of the client's overall health.

Calcium and magnesium are both essential for muscular contraction, and deficiencies can additionally lead to muscular cramping and associated myopathy. Testing can reveal if supplementation can help alleviate symptoms before starting medications such as muscle relaxants.[411]

Autoimmune Factors

If the possibility is there for RA, adding a rheumatoid factor (RF) screening as well as an HLA-B27 screening is helpful. A negative result does not necessarily rule out RA. Not all cases will come up positive for RF, and the HLA-B27 should be added, as it may come up positive instead.[412]

Genetic Testing

COMT, or catechol-O-methyltransferase, is an enzyme vital for metabolizing catecholamines, like epinephrine, dopamine, adrenaline, and norepinephrine, in the prefrontal cortex of our brains. This enzyme helps break down these neurotransmitters to maintain a proper balance in the brain and body. Variations in the COMT gene can impede this process, leading to unaddressed inflammation and a deficiency in neurotransmitter production. Consequently, patients may experience an overabundance of catecholamines, which can be catabolic and result in tissue breakdown, inflammation, and pain.[413] This gene influences how people feel and manage pain by regulating dopamine and other catecholamines in the nervous system. Dopamine, a neurotransmitter, is significant in modulating pain and stress responses.

COMT is often found in patients with conditions like TMJ (temporomandibular joint pain), migraine headaches, chronic tension headaches, and fibromyalgia.[414] In terms of COMT variations, there are three types: Val/Val (normal), Met/Met (most concerning and likely cause of severe pain), and Val/Met (intermediate and impacts pain at least some, possibly moderate to severe, depending on the individual).[415] People with the Met/Met variant are particularly susceptible to these conditions, as it amplifies their pain perception due to a lack of dopamine breakdown. The following diagram helps to demonstrate how this happens at the synaptic level.

Dopamine Breakdown

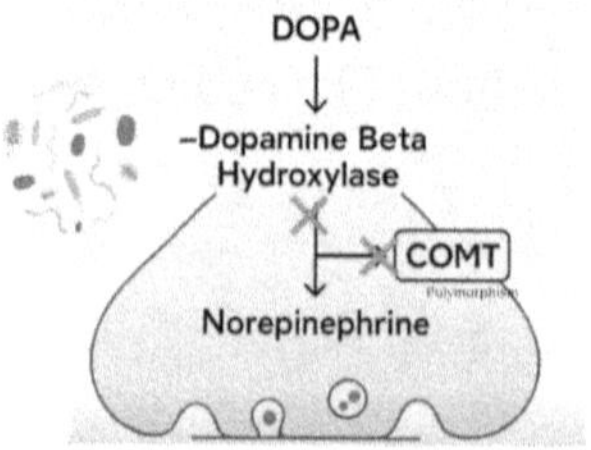

MTHFR is another genetic test that is important to consider in pain management because the polymorphism leads to limited B12 and folate methylation and increased levels of homocysteine, which is inflammatory (previously discussed in depth in the mental health chapter). Deficiencies in methylated B12 and folate lead to the body being unable to repair and can have a direct effect on pain.

Organic Acids Testing

You can observe the breakdown of dopamine through organic acids testing because both gut health and the COMT gene can affect dopamine metabolism. This can be helpful in differentiating the root cause and is evaluated by comparing the proper ratios. Additionally, mitochondrial dysfunction, examined on OATs, may contribute to muscle cramps, so people experiencing persistent muscle aches might benefit from supplements like CoQ10, magnesium, and B vitamins. This allows recognition that the cause of chronic pain is often multifaceted, and organic acid screening can give insight into these disturbances.

Comprehensive Stool Analysis

An imbalanced gut-joint axis should be screened for as a potential root cause of pain.[416] Assessment starts with a comprehensive stool analysis, and treatment depends upon subsequent findings. A source of inflammation can be overgrowth of gram-negative bacteria that produce LPS (lipopolysaccharide), which are proinflammatory compounds that can navigate from between the tight junctures of a hyperpermeable gut and enter into the bloodstream, thereby leading to systemic inflammation and subsequently affecting joints, leading to the possibility of diseases such as osteoarthritis, rheumatoid arthritis, and spondylarthritis. Parasitic infection may also trigger this source and lead to systemic inflammation and subsequent pain.[405]

Thyroid and Hormone Function Tests

Thyroid dysfunction may also contribute to chronic pain. Cells are prevented from correctly utilizing cellular energy, leading to thyroid myopathy. Both hyperthyroidism and hypothyroidism can lead to the symptoms of myopathy.[417] Once the thyroid is rebalanced, after addressing potential root causes, pain may improve or subside.

Toxic Screening

Potential toxins in a patient's body, such as heavy metals, pesticides, or molds, can significantly contribute to chronic pain and headaches. Cadmium and lead can cause an increase in not only joint pain and inflammation but also contribute to the development of OA. Supporting detoxification from these substances can play a crucial role in helping individuals reduce reliance on narcotics and other medications.[418] Lead, cadmium, and chromium are identified as etiologic factors of fibromyalgia and rheumatoid arthritis, as their presence is associated with parathyroid hormone dysregulation and a depletion in vitamin D. Insufficient vitamin D is independently associated with increased pain.[419]

Heavy metal toxicity is especially common in tobacco and vape users. Pain is additionally harder to control in tobacco users, as tobacco reduces opioid receptor effectiveness. For these particular reasons, screening for use of either product should be a planned part of assessment.[420] Moreover, screen your clients for exposure to pesticides. Pesticides can contribute to pain, so opting for organic options may be beneficial.[421]

Water supply should be screened as a potential exposure to harmful toxins, such as heavy metals. Environmental Working Group (EWG) is an organization that screens and reports levels of toxic chemicals and metals in municipal water based on location. Their online resource can be used for assessing potential exposure. It is not uncommon for even many very well-developed and prosperous towns to be burdened with high levels of chromium, specifically chromium-6, which is known to be carcinogenic. Surprisingly, many places do not provide warnings about the safety of drinking water or recommend using filters. Other sources of heavy metals include certain fish, such as swordfish and mackerel, while lower-mercury alternatives include salmon and sardines.[422]

When discussing heavy metals in fish, it's worth noting that fish also contain selenium, which can help bind mercury and mitigate its effects. Research suggests that consuming fish in moderation may not pose a significant risk for most people.[423] However, if someone is particularly sensitive to heavy metals, it would be wise to avoid these fish temporarily and supplement with omega-3 fatty acids that are third-party tested for metals and quality. Lastly, it is always advisable to minimize exposure to heavy metals by reducing the consumption of canned goods, which may contain aluminum, for those for whom that is an issue.

Inflammatory Markers

Ordering labs such as erythrocyte sedimentation rate (ESR) and C-reactive protein (CRP) can be helpful in evaluating if inflammation is present as a potential source of pain.[424] CRP is more effective at identifying acute inflammatory levels, while ESR will help differentiate chronic inflammatory exposure. The addition of both may help in differentiating progress and etiology. Both, however, are non-specific and are general guides for monitoring improvement, should you decide to add them to your treatment plans.

You can use these markers to assess your treatment plan and determine if you're addressing the underlying causes of inflammation effectively. Keep in mind that a normal ESR or CRP does not necessarily rule out inflammation. When patients see tangible data showing improvement, it can significantly boost their confidence and receptiveness to the treatment plan.

Patient History

Lastly, listen to the patient and ask why they think their pain is there. You may find some surprising pieces of information. Screen for hydration status. Even mild dehydration can contribute to pain threshold sensitivity and even be a trigger for severe pain in and of itself.[425] There are cases where patients with chronic pain found significant relief simply by increasing their water intake to five to eight glasses a day. Although this solution may not be an easy fix for everyone, assessing and addressing hydration should be an essential part of evaluating each patient, not only for headaches but also for joint pain. Staying hydrated also helps the body detoxify by keeping the kidneys flushed and well perfused. Dandelion root, with a typical dosage of 500 milligrams taken two to three times a day, and cranberry extract, at 500 milligrams daily, can help promote kidney health and aid in toxin excretion.

General Interventions

Physical Therapy

With all of my pain patients, I incorporate education on physical therapy, stretching, and good ergonomics, especially when sitting or working for prolonged periods. Incorporating physical therapy, specifically tailored exercises, can be incredibly beneficial. While it is beyond the scope of this text to detail specific exercises, identifying which exercises are suitable for individual patients can make a substantial difference. Activities like Pilates and tai chi can be particularly helpful.

Delving deeper into physical therapy is essential when incorporating pain management into treatment plans. Many patients feel that moving worsens their pain, but a lack of movement can actually exacerbate their discomfort. For anyone who's been inactive for an extended period, getting up can lead to feelings of stiffness and soreness.

Finally, screening for adequate sleep is helpful, as sleep plays a significant role in managing pain. Sleep deprivation can lead to muscular cramps and joint pain.[426] Maintaining a regular circadian rhythm and ensuring that the HPA axis and cortisol levels are within normal ranges are vital for reducing stress

Detox

Remember, detoxification methods, including the use of zeolites or chelation therapy, can be effective in reducing heavy metal levels.[427] Optimizing detoxification pathways by supporting liver functioning can be achieved through supplements like glutathione (500 to 1,000 milligrams per day) and N-acetylcysteine (NAC; typically 600 mg daily to three times daily), known for its antioxidant properties and ability to assist in detoxification. Milk thistle is another supplement for detox that supports liver health, typically taken in doses of 150 to 300 milligrams twice a day. Alpha-lipoic acid (ALA) can be effective as well, with a recommended dose of 300 to 600 milligrams per day. Depending on the client's background or the practitioner's preference, one or two of the above supplements can be implemented.

Choosing between detox supplements depends on where the patient's bottleneck is in the detoxification process. If the client has a background of acetaminophen intake or other reasons to suspect that glutathione depletion may be leading to high toxic burden, NAC should be considered as it provides the raw materials to build glutathione and support phase II detox. Directly supplementing glutathione is another option when immediate antioxidant support is desired, especially in neurological or high oxidative stress cases, since it delivers the active form directly. Milk thistle is preferred when the liver itself needs protection or repair, such as with elevated liver enzymes, medication use, a history of alcohol abuse, or hormone metabolism issues. Alpha-lipoic acid (ALA) is most helpful when mitochondrial dysfunction, blood sugar imbalance, or systemic oxidative stress are additionally present, as it helps regenerate antioxidants and support cellular energy.

Additionally, a lack of the correct minerals can block detoxification systems. Functional lab screening to test for deficiencies in certain minerals, like zinc, magnesium, and selenium, may need to be performed. A diet rich in antioxidants, cruciferous vegetables, sulfur-containing foods, and vitamin C is also important for detoxification. Epsom salt soaks can enhance detoxification and relax muscles.

Promoting lymphatic drainage is another key aspect of detoxification. Engaging in lymphatic drainage treatments one to two times a week, particularly during detox phases, can help the body eliminate toxins. Combining lymphatic drainage with Epsom salt soaks can produce noticeable benefits, especially when you're feeling unwell, such as when you have an acute illness producing body aches.

Psychosocial Components to Address

Lastly, cognitive behavioral therapy has been proven to improve pain due to mind strengthening and decreasing the overall stress threshold. Other psychosocial techniques include EMDR (eye movement desensitization and reprocessing), central sensitization, and neurolinguistics. These methods are worth exploring, as I've successfully integrated them into my comprehensive treatment programs and shared them with my students, but they are each full subjects, in and of themselves. Therefore, the purpose here is simply to broaden your awareness.

Sometimes, addressing emotional trauma is relevant for patients, particularly when past traumatic experiences are linked to pain. Research indicates that people with traumatic histories are at a higher risk of developing chronic pain. Neuroplasticity, the brain's ability to reorganize and form new neural connections in response to learning, plays a significant role in pain perception. This adaptability allows the brain to compensate for injury but can also contribute to chronic pain when maladaptive. Changes can occur in pain-processing pathways that may not be helpful, so it's important to assist clients at this deeper level. If you're not trained in these therapies, consider referring patients to specialists in that area for a comprehensive treatment plan or build them into your concierge packages.[428]

Using neurolinguistics, the associations of how the brain processes words and often induces feelings to rewire pain perceptions allow us to adjust how the brain interprets pain. For instance, some people may describe hitting their elbow as merely "weird," while others report it as "extremely painful." Helping patients reframe their understanding of pain can be beneficial without encouraging them to ignore or excuse discomfort. Our goal should always be to identify the cause of the pain and alleviate it.[428]

Potential Joint-Specific Supplements

Just as conventional medicine might use SSRIs, which are antidepressants and have a positive impact on pain, the use of adaptogens can have similar effects on pain. Adaptogens, like rhodiola and ashwagandha, have been found to positively affect pain not only through decreasing overall perception of stress but also to help decrease neuroinflammation. They have additionally been found to be neuroprotective and help decrease the effects of aging on the nervous system, which could additionally help alleviate pain.[429]

Collagen hydrolysate, passion fruit peel extract, Curcuma longa extract, Boswellia serrata extract, curcumin, pycnogenol, glucosamine and chondroitin, and L-carnitine have all been proven to be effective for pain management.[430] Glucosamine and chondroitin are especially helpful in OA. They are thought to work by aiding in the repair of the building blocks for cartilage repair, decreasing inflammation, and slowing cartilage breakdown in osteoarthritis, which leads to pain relief and improved joint function. One patient I had, I started on a liquid form, and she found it more effective than the tramadol she was previously on. Her words were that it was a "miracle." The way she went from walking stiff and rigid to more smooth and coordinated certainly seemed to be something of a miracle. She had very advanced OA. Not everyone will respond that dramatically, but many do. This is not a new intervention, as veterinary medicine has been using this on animals for a long time, demonstrating its effectiveness, as an animal's response could not be from a placebo.

Anti-inflammatory treatments such as curcumin, Boswellia, and ginger can be beneficial for reducing pain as well. Boswellia, in particular, inhibits the 5-lipoxygenase enzyme, which helps reduce inflammation associated with osteoarthritis and rheumatoid arthritis.[431] Ginger, known for its natural anti-inflammatory properties, can also alleviate pain and muscle soreness.[432]

Assessing for GABA deficiency, which may arise from gut imbalances or genetic factors, can additionally be of benefit. GABA is our main calming neurotransmitter, and potential deficiencies can exacerbate the experience of pain, as supported by clinical trials.[433] While GABA supplementation may produce a sensation of being short of breath, no cases of severe respiratory distress have been documented.

Nutrition

For patients with chronic pain, I often recommend a gluten-free diet and typically advise avoiding dairy. There is a growing body of evidence about the connections between gluten (especially that used in the standard American diet) and pain.[434,435] Neurodegenerative diseases are strongly associated with the gliadin and gluten proteins due to their pathological immune response, which can directly trigger pain, fatigue, gastrointestinal issues, and inflammation.[434,436]

Sugar is a "food" product that is very strongly affiliated with inflammation, pain, and a decrease in tissue repair, all of which directly affect pain. A high-fat and high-sugar diet has been found to significantly activate the NF-κB (or Nuclear Factor Kappa-B cells) pathway. This pathway is a key network of cell signaling that regulates genes for immunity, inflammation, stress response, and cell-survival signaling, associated with phosphorylation and COX-2 upregulation.[437] This is all in addition to sugar's propensity to increase yeast overgrowth, leading to gut dysbiosis and thereby causing another potential avenue for pain to be worsened and negatively affected.

Identifying food triggers and other potential sources of inflammation can also aid in decreasing overall symptoms. An elimination diet can be effective, and incorporating bone broth may aid in healing the gut and reducing inflammation. It's essential to provide patients with appropriate probiotics, a diet that is supportive of diverse flora, and treatment based on their comprehensive stool analysis as well.

Chapter Conclusion

The main goal of pain management is to find the root cause of inflammation. In most cases, the root cause is an assimilation of inflammatory processes. When the majority of these processes are mitigated, the body can heal, pain can decrease, and hopefully, disappear completely. When inflammation resolves, microtears and even larger tears are given the opportunity to heal and repair themselves. The body is built to heal itself; our main goal is to optimize the body and allow an environment where it can do what it's designed to do. While this chapter did not cover all the causes of pain, genetics, chemical-laden food, sugar, gluten, heavy metal toxicities, and gut dysbiosis are all some of the main focuses to screen for and eliminate appropriately. Supplements can be added for increased benefit, and even modalities such as red light therapy, cryotherapy, and cold lasers can be added for further benefit.

Addressing the root cause of inflammation can take time, so supporting patients with a positive mindset is essential. Incorporating these techniques into your high-touch programs is a fantastic way to prevent patients from feeling lost or discouraged. It is important to remember that seeing results may take a few months—unfortunately, healing is not as immediate as taking a pill. However, the long-term benefits can be remarkable.

Business Practice Pearl

One effective way to make your offer and program truly irresistible is by creating what we call a proprietary method. "Proprietary" means that your method is unique and cannot be found anywhere else. This is also known as a "unique selling proposition," or USP. It tells patients why your program is exactly what they need, and since they have not had an opportunity to utilize it, it even makes sense why they have not gotten the results they wanted with other programs or treatment plans. In my method, which I allow my students to license if they choose, I integrate mind, body, and soul, but I present it in a way that is entirely distinct. When potential clients see and hear about my method, they immediately understand its value. Remember, the first rule is that a confused mind will not buy, so it's essential to clearly define what you offer and how you can help your patients.

Given the advancements in technology, I find AI incredibly useful for developing unique names for these methods. I employ what I call the "name-mixing method," which involves combining two key elements: what your audience needs and desires (the results they're looking for) and a distinguishing feature of your product.

A brilliant example of this in the marketing world is “Facebook.” They combined seeing one another's “face” with a “book” of names and contacts, like you would have in a contacts book. It represented the feeling they were going for, which was connection, and the need that was to be fulfilled, which was simplicity in connecting with those at a distance that didn’t require stopping life to get “caught up” over the phone. The name represents this.

You can apply this strategy to your products as well. It's important to realize that the notion of "build it and they will come" is misleading. Many skilled providers excel at their craft but struggle with effective positioning and conveying the benefits of what they do differently. You can be the most skilled practitioner on the planet, but if you don’t know how to get your name out there, you can never serve a big clientele. I encourage you to take some time to journal about what makes your approach unique. For instance, I focus on helping my patients with their mindset and spiritual health, and I've incorporated that into my program descriptions. Reflect on what makes you stand out. Often, what distinguishes you is tied to frustrations with what others are doing—or not doing. This frustration can become a source of inspiration, allowing you to articulate the value you provide. For example, does it drive you crazy that gut health is not incorporated into mental health plans? Does it drive you crazy when autoimmune treatment plans ignore the association between AI and trauma? Have your name reflect this and highlight it as your USP that sets you apart from the rest.

Other times, the things you are most resistant to can become your superpower. Take the biblical figure Moses, who initially told God he wasn’t the right person for the task—he couldn't speak or lead and was not intelligent enough. Ultimately, he became the voice of the people, confronting Pharaoh to free them. This highlights that your greatest fears can often be the very things you are meant to embrace. They are also often the things others are afraid of doing, and if you can choose to be the first, you have the opportunity to be very successful. Interestingly, when Moses voiced his doubts to God, the response wasn't gentle reassurance. According to scripture, God "burned with anger" for Moses' reluctance. The message was clear: do not settle into complacency; pursue your true calling.

Scripture teaches us that if we are lukewarm, He will spit us out of His mouth. You need to have passion for whatever you are doing. It's important to get past the things you perceive as obstacles because, more often than not, they are actually where your true strengths lie. For instance, when I first graduated as a nurse practitioner, I had a strong aversion to psychiatry. I thought, *I'm not going to treat psych paitents. I'll just refer my patients to specialists*. I was excited about performing procedures like removing cysts and doing joint injections, things that many people find intimidating, but I was firmly set on avoiding anything related to psychology.

As fate would have it, I started working in a small, rural area where there were no psychiatrists available for referral. Many of my patients lived in a very poor area and didn't have cars, making it impossible for them to travel an hour and a half to reach the nearest city. So, I had no choice but to learn everything I could about mental health to be the best I could to help them. I studied the pathophysiology behind different medications and immersed myself in cognitive behavioral therapy to better assist my clients. This journey led me to write my first published book, *Living Between the Lines*. The insights I gained became central to my practice, as I witnessed the significant impact it had on my patients. I realized that understanding psychology had to be integrated into everything we do with clients.

My point is this: keep your mind open and try not to resist where you see a need based on your own feelings. Sometimes, the very thing you resist the most may be where you are meant to grow. This could be a clue for you as you develop your unique method. Just remember to differentiate yourself and avoid becoming just another voice in the crowd, while also ensuring that your clients aren't confused.

BONUS TRAINING:

Chapter 10 Book Bonus: Building a Foolproof Plan with A LIA SYSTEM

SCAN ME

SCAN THE QR CODE

or visit functionalmedicineunlocked.com

Conclusion

The most important idea that I want you to take from the book is not to fear implementing it. As we discussed, there will be "kiwis"—those who might discourage you from taking action. While many kiwis peck at you from behind, remember that the most influential ones nest in your mind. Often, our biggest enemy is the self-doubt we create for ourselves.

I frequently observe this mindset among even the most intelligent and educated people: they don't feel ready, or they are afraid to start implementing functional medicine. If you find yourself in this position, I encourage you to seek out a coach. Whether our program is the right fit for you or not, it's crucial to find someone who can support you through this process, because taking action while you're passionate is vital. If you do want to explore our program, you can set up an appointment with one of our advisors or me here:

To Book a Call

SCAN ME

SCAN THE QR CODE

If you reflect on the biblical story of Exodus, the Jewish people were promised a land flowing with milk and honey. God performed great miracles before them, such as parting the sea. However, when they reached the Promised Land and sent spies to scout ahead, the spies returned with reports of giants, claiming that they felt like grasshoppers in comparison. Only two people believed they could conquer the land. Even after God had led them through all they had done, doubt still infiltrated their minds. They doubted themselves, even when others knew their favor was strong and their God was stronger.

Rahab, a flawed Canaanite woman from Jericho, recognized the provision God had for them, even being outside of their inner circle. While God's people were doubtful that they could claim the land He had promised them, she saw their provision and feared the Lord. Because of that, she risked being caught as a traitor to help them. Sometimes, we are too close to our own skills and abilities to see our true potential. While others are waiting, you may be hesitating.

It's also important to note that when the Jews first hesitated to claim their land, they wandered for forty years. This is a struggle I often see in people: they become excited and motivated to start something but then freeze, feeling the need to be perfect. However, God does not call the qualified; He qualifies the called. As stated in James 1:25, the perfect law sets us free. You are already called to this purpose in a significant way. If your heart focuses on helping, healing, and serving others, you are on the right path. However, James reminds us that we must not forget what we've heard; we must be doers to truly change lives. James 1:22-25 (ESV) commands believers to be "*doers of the word, and not hearers only, deceiving yourselves.*" Too often, people let their fears hold them back before they even have a chance to make a positive impact. Don't let the start stop you.

Functional medicine is about incorporating knowledge and practices and getting better in your skills with practice, even if that means starting with your own health as a case study. I encourage you to pursue this because it can be transformative. However, it will likely still be a journey of self-discovery. Even after healing myself and several others, I still struggled with self-doubt. I encountered skepticism from others who dismissed the efficacy of herbs and functional medicine. But I knew what I had experienced. It took me many successes in healing others before I was unwavering in my belief. But I had to start somewhere. With my first client, I was very transparent that I was new to all of this, but they still proclaimed, "Please, I know nothing is promised, but can you just try?" As Zig Ziglar famously said, the beautiful truth is, "You don't have to be great to start, but you have to start to be great."

There's a fascinating study I love to share with my students. Researchers took a group of kindergartners and split them into two groups. One group was taught by first graders, while the other group was taught by certified teachers. Surprisingly, the kindergartners who were taught by first graders scored better than those taught by the teachers. The first graders remembered what it was like to be in that earlier stage, which enabled them to help their peers identify and break through barriers more quickly. This demonstrates the power of being *just one step ahead.* Never underestimate the power that each step of your journey holds, especially the first step.

While there are benefits in developing skills, gaining experience, and becoming a more knowledgeable practitioner, there are also significant advantages to being at the beginning of the journey. You can help others heal and grow right from the outset. I often tell my students that sometimes, those who are called to help are meant to engage with others right at the start. There is a unique gift in locking arms with them and saying, "Hey, we're doing this together." Rather than being at the finish line and cheering someone on with a distant "You can do it." You become closer to them in their journey, which fosters a deeper understanding and often reignites your passion for the work.

Getting started has its own set of benefits. Don't let anything or anyone (including yourself) discourage you from taking that initial step. I want you to join this movement, but you can't be part of it if you don't take action. Remember, I've missed opportunities by listening to the skeptical voices around me, so don't do that to yourself or to those who need your help. Since finishing this book, you now hold knowledge that most do not, and the truth is that other people's healing and fate are on the other side of you, saying, "It can wait."

When you focus on others instead of yourself, set aside your ego (which stands for "edging God out"), and allow yourself to be vulnerable and uncomfortable as you learn something new, you now hold the keys to unlock true healing. Don't keep them to yourself. Trust that divine guidance will lead you to meet needs you may not have even realized you were called to fulfill. You can achieve what feels like miracles, but you need a different perspective and a higher level of belief. This approach will not only transform your clients but also change your own life.

I hope this message encourages you and helps you see things from a new perspective for both your clients and yourself. I would love to hear about any healing testimonies that come from this experience. Please reach out to me at drlauren@healthrevivalcare.org and our team, because we are stronger together.

If you find yourself in a position where you want to learn more and take your passion to the next level without letting it fizzle out, you're in the right place. You don't want to spend the next forty years circling the same mountain. We offer board certification specifically designed for people like you: nurses, coaches, MDs, DOs, chiropractors, and more. We provide various paths tailored to different professionals, and we won't just help you become board certified so you can feel like the qualified professional you aspire to be; we'll also support you in growing your business. Our unique approach to practice growth is unlike anything else you'll find.

I want to share a personal experience: when I started my own business, I matched and surpassed my income as a nurse practitioner within just nine months, even while pregnant. It wasn't the ideal time, but I knew I needed that change. I didn't want to spend my time with my second baby working, the way I had with my first, so I made the decision to start my own practice. In doing so, I developed the Passive Clinic system that has revolutionized how providers assist their patients. It has transformed the way patients access the information they need to heal themselves and has also allowed providers to work less while still being effective. You don't have to work harder; you just need to work smarter.

To achieve this, it's essential to shift your perspective and change your business model from a one-to-one approach (trading time for money) to one that allows you to help more people at a higher volume with less direct interaction. I teach a variety of strategies that leverage your efforts so you can achieve more over time with the same amount of energy.

You can create a program that guides clients through a process. Once you build it correctly, you can simply share a link with various audiences. This allows you to leverage other people's audiences and adopt a one-to-many approach. By collaborating with others, you can build passive income just by developing one or two much-needed programs. The demand for these is extremely high right now. You are also entering this space at the right time. Functional medicine is not a passing trend; it has been used for centuries, and it works. But its impact on today's society is just getting started. It is transforming lives and is here to stay.

Business Practice Pearl

For our final "Practice Pearl," I want to give you the one thing that has probably helped me the most. Remember when I told you that you may have hesitation when it comes to charging a high amount, and you would be right? It is smart to have that hesitation if you don't know how to warm an audience up or have an LIA (Limitless Income Accelerator) system prior to inviting your clients to work with you. Unfortunately, "build it, and they will come" is a façade.

Getting clients in the door is often a lot of work, and start-up clinics do not often have the money to hire someone to do it for them and/or do not have time to spend doing it themselves (they need to be caring for patients). Fortunately, this is exactly the problem the LIA System was built to solve. LIA stands for Limitless Income Accelerator, and it's designed so you build it once, and then you can let it do the heavy lifting for you... on repeat. Instead of constantly recreating content, rewriting marketing, finding new audiences, or reinventing yourself every month, your LIA system becomes a living asset that attracts and warms up future patients automatically. It delivers real value, elevates understanding, and builds deep trust long before someone ever books a call. By the time a patient reaches out, they already feel that they know you, trust you, believe in your approach, and understand the transformation you offer. It eliminates convincing or chasing. You're not also having to become a salesperson; you're simply welcoming people who are already pre-aligned and ready to go.

The truth is that the first time I tried to sell a course and my expertise, *no one* bought. It was a steal of a deal at $150, and no one will ever see an offer like that again because I would not charge less than $18,000 for the same service today. Others missed out, but it wasn't their fault —*it was my fault* because I didn't know how to demonstrate the value they were getting. You can build yours on your own and guess what works, or you can learn directly from me what actually works in an opportunity you can only find here.

It took years to build this system by doing market research. To do this right, I firmly believe it is vital to immerse yourself in a community of like-minded individuals who are also growing their functional medicine practices and learning in real time. The functional medicine field is expanding rapidly, with increasing interest due to the successful outcomes that patients are experiencing. This success is shared widely, making it hard to overlook. Despite this growth, some pushback still exists, so it's essential to cultivate the right mindset within your practice every day. Personally, I invest time in listening to mentors who inspire and guide me, people who have already achieved what I aim to do. This investment significantly impacts my overall process and product.

Remember, if you burn out or allow yourself to get stuck in a negative mindset, you'll be unable to help the many people who rely on your guidance. Do *not* doubt that you have a calling in this. I know from experience that if you have a desire to heal, there are people out there with an equal and opposite energy who need your help. That is why your desire formed. It's not a selfish thing; it's a calling. But remember: other people's faith is on the other side of you, saying it can wait.

And don't let comparison stop you. Just because someone else is in year two or more and looks more polished and professional, that does not mean you are not meant to start. Because here is the thing: your people are not other people's people. In John 10:27 (ESV), the Lord says, *"My sheep hear My voice,"* and I think of that as a reflection of our passion and calling. Just as we follow our mission, there are others who need the purpose that you, and you alone, bring into life. The passion you possess is directly related to the needs of those people who seek your assistance.

So, if you are ready to answer that call and prefer not to reinvent the wheel and instead want to use a proven system designed for busy individuals, just for completing this book, I want to give you a special opportunity that is perfect for you. Just scan the QR code below, and you can explore further or take advantage of all our free training, as well as check out our Skool group, free for 7 days. That's right; it's a free course in addition to several other courses and community in Skool!

You can also learn about our full Functional Board Certification Course, where we dive even deeper into the topics here, in addition to specific detoxification protocols, social determinants of health, spiritual healing, advanced training in functional med labs, mitochondrial dysfunction, weight loss, cardiovascular disease, diabetes, perimenopause and postmenopause, gut-brain axis, nephrology, urology, respiratory and infectious disease, dermatology, oncology, legal support, telemedicine, and HIPAA compliance. You'll also get real, live support, where you can work directly with me and/or some of our leading professors. We are fully accredited for you to qualify for board certification in functional medicine and in mental health functional medicine, as well as approved for forty-eight continuing education hours.

Lastly, I want to thank you for reading this book and congratulate you on finishing! Most people start a book but never finish, so you are already among the 1%. If you want what the 1% has, you must do what 99% won't. You are already halfway there by showing perseverance. Do not stop now.

Congratulations on this achievement; thank you for your dedication, and I hope to meet you one day as an active student!

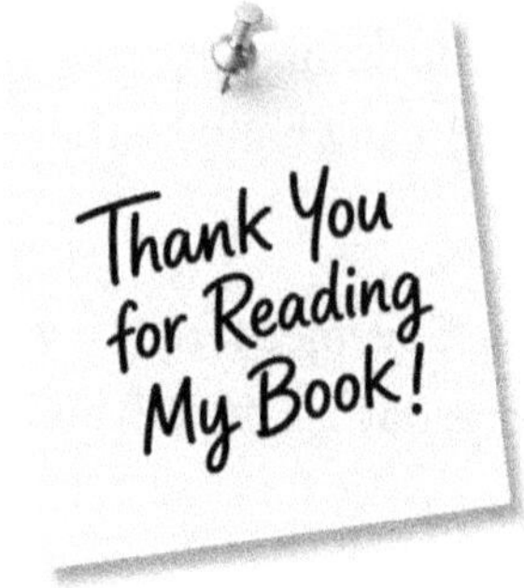

I'd love to connect and stay in touch!

SCAN ME

Your support means so much to me. I hope you enjoyed reading this book! If you have a moment, I would be grateful if you shared your thoughts by leaving a review on Amazon. Your review not only helps future readers, but also helps shape future editions.

References

1. Grand View Research. Complementary and alternative medicine market summary. Published 2023. https://www.grandviewresearch.com/industry-analysis/complementary-alternative-medicine-market
2. National Institute of Mental Health. (2023). Major depression. U.S. Department of Health and Human Services. https://www.nimh.nih.gov/health/statistics/major-depression
3. Alzheimer's Association. (2025). 2025 Alzheimer's disease facts and figures. Alzheimer's & Dementia, 21(4). https://doi.org/10.1002/alz.70235
4. Yu EL, Schwimmer JB. Epidemiology of pediatric nonalcoholic fatty liver disease. *Clinical Liver Disease (Hoboken)*. 2021;17(3):196-99. doi:10.1002/cld.1027
5. U.S. Department of Health and Human Services. 'Autism epidemic runs rampant,' new data shows 1 in 31 children afflicted [news release]. Published April 15, 2025. Accessed March 5, 2026. https://www.hhs.gov/press-room/autism-epidemic-runs-rampant-new-data-shows-grants.html
6. Pahwa R, Goyal A, Jialal I. Chronic inflammation. In: *StatPearls* [Internet]. StatPearls Publishing; Updated August 7, 2023.
7. Aronica L, Ordovas JM, Volkov A, et al. Genetic biomarkers of metabolic detoxification for personalized lifestyle medicine. *Nutrients*. 2022;14(4):768. doi:10.3390/nu14040768
8. Potocka N, Skrzypa M, Zadarko-Domaradzka M, et al. Effects of the Trp64Arg polymorphism in the ADRB3 gene on body composition, cardiorespiratory fitness, and physical activity in healthy adults. *Genes*. 2023;14(8):1541. doi:10.3390/genes14081541
9. Aboud F, et al. Nutrition in pediatrics. In: *NCBI Bookshelf* [Internet]. 2023. https://www.ncbi.nlm.nih.gov/books/NBK532999/
10. Zhang Y, Kutateladze TG. Epigenetic mechanisms and environmental exposures: Implications for human health. *Genes & Diseases*. 2024;11(5):1234-1248. doi:10.1016/j.gendis.2023.11.012
11. Camilleri M. Leaky gut: Mechanisms, measurement and clinical implications in humans. *Gut*. 2019;68(8):1516-26. doi:10.1136/gutjnl-2019-318427
12. Gillespie KM, Kemps E, White MJ, Bartlett SE. The impact of free sugar on human health—a narrative review. *Nutrients*. 2023;15(4):889.
13. Texas Institute for Neurological Disorders. Welcome to Texas Institute for Neurolog-

ical Disorders. Accessed March 5, 2026. https://www.texasinstituteforneurologicaldisorders.com/

14. Li F, et al. The impact of high-sugar diets on central nervous system function and metabolic health. *Nutrients*. 2025;17(2):245. doi:10.3390/nu17020245
15. Bays DJ, Savage HP. Candida albicans gastrointestinal colonization resistance: A host-microbiome balancing act. *Infect Immun*. 2025;93:e00610-24. doi:10.1128/iai.00610-24
16. Zmora N, Suez J, Elinav E. You are what you eat: Diet, health and the gut microbiota. *Nat Rev Gastroenterol Hepatol*. 2019;16(1):35-56. doi:10.1038/s41575-018-0061-2
17. Marraudino M, Bonaldo B, Farinetti A, Panzica G, Ponti G, Gotti S. Metabolism disrupting chemicals and alteration of neuroendocrine circuits controlling food intake and energy metabolism. *Front Endocrinol (Lausanne)*. 2019;9:766. doi:10.3389/fendo.2018.00766
18. Zuo M, Ye M, Lin H, et al. Mitochondrial dysfunction in environmental toxicology: Mechanisms, impacts, and health implications. *Chem Res Toxicol*. 2024;37(11):1794-1806. doi:10.1021/acs.chemrestox.4c00328
19. Ortega, et al. 2024. doi:10.1186/s40779-024-00577-w
20. Bjornevik K, Cortese M, Healy BC, et al. Longitudinal analysis reveals high prevalence of Epstein-Barr virus associated with multiple sclerosis. *Science*. 2022;375(6578):296-301. doi:10.1126/science.abj8222
21. Sadek AM, Mahmoud RH. From parasite-induced immune activation to neuroinflammation and behavioral dysfunction: Convergent mechanisms across protozoa and helminths: A review. *J Neuroinflammation*. 2026;23(1):129. doi:10.1186/s12974-026-03804-4
22. Moling O, Gandini L. Sugar and the mosaic of autoimmunity. *Am J Case Rep*. 2019;20:1364-1368. doi:10.12659/AJCR.915703
23. Chang M. *Mitochondrial Dysfunction: A Functional Medicine Approach to Diagnosis and Treatment*. Formatted Books; 2019.
24. Ahmad K, Manongi NJ, Rajapandian R, et al. Effectiveness of coenzyme Q10 supplementation in statin-induced myopathy: A systematic review. *Cureus*. 2024;16(8):e68316. doi:10.7759/cureus.68316
25. Biondi B, Cappola AR. Subclinical hypothyroidism in older individuals. *Lancet Diabetes Endocrinol*. 2021;9(8):539-549. doi:10.1016/S2213-8587(21)00133
26. Yaribeygi H, Panahi Y, Sahraei H, Johnston TP, Sahebkar A. The impact of stress on body function: A review. *EXCLI Journal*. 2017;16:1057-72. doi:10.17179/excli2017-480
27. Hackett RA, Steptoe A. Type 2 diabetes mellitus and psychological stress—a modifiable risk factor. *Nat Rev Endocrinol*. 2020;13(9):547-560. doi:10.1038/s41574-017-0002-3

28. Chen LK. Sarcopenia in the era of precision health: Toward personalized interventions for healthy longevity. *J Chin Med Assoc*. 2024;87(11):980-987.

29. Wilding JPH, Batterham RL, Calanna S, et al. Once-weekly semaglutide in adults with overweight or obesity. *N Engl J Med*. 2021;384(11):989-1002. doi:10.1056/NEJMoa2032183

30. Srikanthan P, Karlamangla AS. Muscle mass index as a predictor of longevity in older adults. *Am J Med*. 2020;133(10):1139-1145. doi:10.1016/j.amjmed.2020.03.012

31. Zhang Y, Jiang Y, Jin Z. Vitamin D and risk of type 1 diabetes: A systematic review and meta-analysis. *Nutrients*. 2022;14(7):1509. doi:10.3390/nu14071509

32. Wimalawansa SJ. Vitamin D's impact on cancer incidence and mortality: A systematic review. *Nutrients*. 2025;17(14):2333. doi:10.3390/nu17142333

33. Genovia Diagnostics. Microbiome. Published 2025. https://www.gdx.net/gut-health

34. Gingras BA, Maggiore JA. Performance of a new molecular assay for the detection of gastrointestinal pathogens. *Access Microbiology*. 2020;2(10):acmi000160. doi:10.1099/acmi.0.000160

35. Bryant. Secretory IgA: Understanding high and low levels, causes, and treatment options. Rupa Health. Published 2024. https://www.rupahealth.com/post/secretory-iga-understanding-high-and-low-levels-causes-and-treatment-options

36. Mosaic Diagnostics. Organic Acids Test (OAT). Mosaic Diagnostics. Accessed July 2025. https://mosaicdxinternational.com/products/organic-acids-test-oat

37. Guidi J, Lucente M, Sonino N, Fava GA. Allostatic load and its impact on health: A systematic review. *Psychother Psychosom*. 2021;90(1):11-27. doi:10.1159/000510696

38. Esteban M, Castaño A. Non-invasive matrices in human biomonitoring: A review. *Environ Int*. 2021;146:106170. doi:10.1016/j.envint.2020.106170

39. Eskandari, Sadighara, Bekheir. Investigating the impact of polycyclic aromatic hydrocarbons (PAHs) and their health impact. *Journal of research in environmental health*. 2025;11(1):98-100. doi:10.22038/jreh.2025.26106

40. Tang J, Shan S, Li F, Yun P. Effects of vitamin D supplementation on autoantibodies and thyroid function in patients with Hashimoto's thyroiditis: A systematic review and meta-analysis. *Medicine*. 2023;102(52):e36759.

41. Joseph A, Shahani P, Pradhan M. Improvement of gastrointestinal, metabolic, and thyroid biomarkers through advanced diagnostic techniques and functional nutrition approach in 40-year-old female: A case report. *Integrative Medicine: A Clinician's Journal*. 2025;24(3).

42. Lavine E. Blood testing for sensitivity, allergy or intolerance to food. *CMAJ*. 2012;184(6):666-668. doi:10.1503/cmaj.110026

43. Rentzos G, Weisheit A, Ekerljung L, van Odijk J. Measurement of diamine oxidase (DAO) during low-histamine or ordinary diet in patients with histamine intolerance. *Eur J Clin Nutr*. 2024;78(8):726-731.

44. Orlando A, Chimienti G, Pesce V, Fracasso F, Lezza AMS, Russo F. An In Vitro Study on Mitochondrial Compensatory Response Induced by Gliadin Peptides in Caco-2 Cells. Int J Mol Sci. 2019 Apr 15;20(8):1862. doi: 10.3390/ijms20081862. PMID: 30991726; PMCID: PMC6514596.

45. Chen L, Jiang Y. Association study of MTHFR C677T polymorphism with homocysteine level and coronary heart disease in elderly patients. *Cardiology Research and Practice*. 2025;2025(1):6246458.

46. Takeuchi T, Ohno H. IgA in human health and diseases: Potential regulator of commensal microbiota. *Front Immunol*. 2022;13:1024330.

47. Gillespie et al. Congenital hyperinsulinism workup. Medscape. Updated 2025. https://emedicine.medscape.com/article/923538-workup

48. Horner et al. [Title not provided in source]. Thieme Connect. 2023. doi:10.1055/a-1998-6889

49. Ollerman L. What are the behavioral effects of artificial dyes on children in the US? Psychology Student Publications, University of North Dakota. Published April 30, 2024. Accessed March 6, 2026. https://commons.und.edu/psych-stu/37/

50. Austin W, Mueller R. Forever chemicals: Challenges and opportunities for researchers. *Review of Environmental Economics and Policy*. 2025;19(1):118-130.

51. EWG. EWG's dirty dozen guide to food chemicals: Top 12 to avoid. Environmental Working Group. 2025. https://www.ewg.org/consumer-guides/ewgs-dirty-dozen-guide-food-chemicals-top-12-avoid

52. El-Sawaf EA, Shawky NO. The effect of sodium benzoate on the cerebellum of the adult male albino rats and the ameliorative effect of its withdrawal and zinc administration: Histological and immunohistochemical study. *Ain Shams Medical Journal*. 2025;76(1):40-54.

53. Hejazi L, Mahboubi-Rabbani M, Mahdavi V, Alemi M, Khanniri E, Bayanati M. A critical review on sodium benzoate from health effects to analytical methods. *Results in Chemistry*. 2024;11:101798.

54. Woodling KA, Chitranshi P, Jacob CC, et al. Toxicological evaluation of brominated vegetable oil in Sprague Dawley rats. *Food Chem Toxicol*. 2022;165:113137.

55. Carroll JE, Norris BJ, Villadiego A, Wheeler SD. Brominated vegetable oil myopathy: Inhibition at multiple sites. *Muscle Nerve*. 1984;7(8):642-646. doi:10.1002/mus.880070808

56. American Institute for Cancer Research. Processed meat research. American Institute for Cancer Research. Updated March 31, 2021. Accessed March 6, 2026. https://www.aicr.org/cancer-prevention/food-facts/processed-meat/

57. Valdes-Devesa V, Sanz-Rosa D, Thuissard-Vasallo IJ, Andreu-Vázquez C, Sainz de la Cuesta R. Xenoestrogen concentration in women with endometriosis or leiomyomas: A case-control study. *PLoS One*. 2024;19(6):e0304766.

58. Chmielewski J, Łuszczki J, Czarny-Działak M, et al. Environmental exposition to xenoestrogens and related health effects. *Journal of Elementology*. 2021;26(3):717-730.

59. Chen J, Wang Z, Zhou Y, Zhou Z, Yan W. Association between body mass index and sex hormones among men: Evidence from cross-sectional and Mendelian randomization studies. *Obes Res Clin Pract*. 2024;18(4):293-300.

60. Hager E, Chen J, Zhao L. Minireview: Parabens exposure and breast cancer. *Int J Environ Res Public Health*. 2022;19(3):1873. doi:10.3390/ijerph19031873

61. Abdulhameed AAR, Lim V, Bahari H, et al. Adverse effects of bisphenol A on the liver and its underlying mechanisms: Evidence from in vivo and in vitro studies. *Biomed Res Int*. 2022;2022:8227314. doi:10.1155/2022/8227314

62. Zhang J, Zhu S, Sun J, Liu Y. Bisphenol S promotes the transfer of antibiotic resistance genes via transformation. *Int J Mol Sci*. 2024;25(18):9819. doi:10.3390/ijms25189819

63. Karramass T, Sol C, Kannan K, Trasande L, Jaddoe V, Duijts L. Bisphenol and phthalate exposure during pregnancy and the development of childhood lung function and asthma: The Generation R Study. *Environ Pollut*. 2023;332:121853.

64. Wu M, Wang S, Weng Q, et al. Prenatal and postnatal exposure to bisphenol A and asthma: A systemic review and meta-analysis. *J Thorac Dis*. 2021;13(3):1684.

65. Harvey NE, Mercer GV, Stapleton D, et al. Maternal exposure to polystyrene nanoplastics impacts developmental milestones and brain structure in mouse offspring. *Environmental Science: Advances*. 2023;2(4):622-628.

66. Wang X, Wu L, Tao J, et al. A lipidomic approach to bisphenol F-induced non-alcoholic fatty liver disease-like changes: Altered lipid components in a murine model. *Environ Sci Pollut Res*. 2023;30(52):112644-112659.

67. Wisconsin Department of Health Services. PFAS chemicals and health. Wisconsin Department of Health Services. 2025. https://www.dhs.wisconsin.gov/chemical/pfas.htm

68. Säve-Söderbergh M, Gyllenhammar I, Schillemans T, et al. Fetal exposure to perfluoroalkyl substances (PFAS) in drinking water and congenital malformations: A nationwide register-based study on PFAS in drinking water. *Environ Int*. 2025;198:109381. doi:10.1016/j.envint.2025.109381

69. Pati S, Das D, Sinha A, Mahapatra P, Turuk J. Teflon flu: Is it a rising concern of only developed country? *Journal of Integrative Medicine and Research*. 2024;2(4):273-275.

70. Ren J, Li Z, Li X, et al. Exploring the mechanisms of the antioxidants BHA, BHT, and TBHQ in hepatotoxicity, nephrotoxicity, and neurotoxicity from the perspective of network toxicology. *Foods*. 2025;14(7):1095.

71. Petric D. Review on toxicity of food additives. ScienceOpen Preprints. 2021.

72. Bischoff NS, Bussi MR, Van Breda SG, et al. Food-grade titanium dioxide exposure between age groups and in global regions: A systematic review and meta-analysis. *Critical Reviews in Food Science and Nutrition*. 2025;65(31):7325-7335.

73. Al-Ishaq RK, Kubatka P, Büsselberg D. Sweeteners and the gut microbiome: Effects on gastrointestinal cancers. *Nutrients*. 2023;15(17):3675. doi:10.3390/nu15173675

74. Tsai YJ, Fan HY, Hsu SY, et al. Varied effects of sweeteners on pediatric hypertension: A multicenter study. *Clinical Nutrition*. 2025.

75. McIntyre RS, Alsuwaidan M, Baune BT, et al. Treatment-resistant depression: Definition, prevalence, detection, management, and investigational interventions. *World Psychiatry*. 2023;22(3):394-412. doi:10.1002/wps.21120

76. Palomar-Cros A, Straif K, Romaguera D, et al. Consumption of aspartame and other artificial sweeteners and risk of cancer in the Spanish multicase-control study (MCC-Spain). *Int J Cancer*. 2023;153(5):979-993.

77. Al-Askar AA, Al-Onazi MA, Al-Qahtani SM, et al. The progress on stevia (*Stevia rebaudiana* Bertoni): Chemical composition, pharmacokinetics, pharmacological effects, safety, applications, and biosynthesis. *Front Nutr*. 2026;13:1728578. doi:10.3389/fnut.2026.1728578

78. de Graaf L, Boulanger M, Bureau M, et al. Occupational pesticide exposure, cancer and chronic neurological disorders: A systematic review of epidemiological studies in greenspace workers. *Environ Res*. 2022;203:111822. doi:10.1016/j.envres.2021.111822

79. Panis C, Lemos B. Pesticide exposure and increased breast cancer risk in women population studies. *Sci Total Environ*. 2024;933:172988.

80. Shekhar C, Khosya R, Thakur K, et al. A systematic review of pesticide exposure, associated risks, and long-term human health impacts. *Toxicol Rep*. 2024;13:101840. doi:10.1016/j.toxrep.2024.101840

81. Fucic A, Duca RC, Galea KS, et al. Reproductive health risks associated with occupational and environmental exposure to pesticides. *Int J Environ Res Public Health*. 2021;18(12):6576.

82. Eakin CJ, Williams L, Moore J, et al. Examining bald eagle contaminant exposure and reproductive risk above and below dams on Great Lakes tributaries. *Arch Environ Contam Toxicol*. 2024;87(4):353-374.

83. United States Environmental Protection Agency. Proposed rule: Reconsideration of 2009 endangerment finding. Published July 29, 2025. https://www.epa.gov/regulations-emissions-vehicles-and-engines/proposed-rule-reconsideration-2009-endangerment-finding

84. Dhankhar N, Kumar J. Impact of increasing pesticides and fertilizers on human health: A review. *Materials Today: Proceedings*. 2023.

85. Mojtabai R, Olfson M. Trends in mental disorders in children and adolescents receiving treatment in the state mental health system. *J Am Acad Child Adolesc Psychiatry*. 2025;64(8):906-920.

86. Rehman H, Khan AHA, Rehman WU, Ahmad M, Iqbal M. Biochar for sustainable restoration of heavy metals contaminated soil: Performance, assessment, and mechanisms. *Advanced Sustainable Systems*. 2025;9(12):e00776.

87. Pongking T, Haonon O, Dangtakot R, et al. A combination of monosodium glutamate and high-fat and high-fructose diets increases the risk of kidney injury, gut dysbiosis and host-microbial co-metabolism. *PLoS One*. 2020;15(4):e0231237. doi:10.1371/journal.pone.0231237

88. Olabiyi O, Ajibewa A, Ajayi A. Analyzing the monosodium and dietary glutamate model of depression: A narrative review. *Annals of Psychophysiology*. 2025;12(2).

89. Urcar Gelen S, Ozkanlar S, Gedikli S, Atasever M. The investigation of the effects of monosodium glutamate on healthy rats and rats with STZ-induced diabetes. *J Biochem Mol Toxicol*. 2024;38(1):e23612.

90. Cakmakci S, Salik MA. Monosodium glutamate (MSG) as a food additive and comments on its use. In: *Proceedings of the 4th International Conference on Advanced Engineering Technologies*; September 2022:289-295.

91. Pu Z, Liu S, Guo Z, et al. Casein reactivates dopaminergic nerve injury and intestinal inflammation with disturbing intestinal microflora and fecal metabolites in a convalescent Parkinson's disease mouse model. *Neuroscience*. 2023;524:120-136.

92. Jeong H, Park YS, Yoon SS. A2 milk consumption and its health benefits: An update. *Food Sci Biotechnol*. 2024;33(3):491-503.

93. Bordoni A, Danesi F, Dardevet D, et al. Dairy products and inflammation: A review of the clinical evidence. *Critical Reviews in Food Science and Nutrition*. 2017;57(12):2497-2525. doi:10.1080/10408398.2014.967385

94. Kaskous S. Cow's milk consumption and risk of disease. *Emir J Food Agric*. 2021;33(1):1-11.

95. Bolat E, Eker F, Yılmaz S, et al. BCM-7: Opioid-like peptide with potential role in disease mechanisms. *Molecules*. 2024;29(9):2161. doi:10.3390/molecules29092161

96. Harris EM, et al. Alpha-lipoic acid supplementation increases mercury excretion and glutathione levels in humans: A randomized controlled trial. *Toxicol Appl Pharmacol*. 2022;437:115814.

97. Adegbola P, Aderibigbe I, Hammed W, Omotayo T. Antioxidant and anti-inflammatory medicinal plants have potential role in the treatment of cardiovascular disease: A review. *Am J Cardiovasc Dis*. 2017;7(2):19-32.

98. Gillespie KM, Kemps E, White MJ, Bartlett SE. The impact of free sugar on human health—a narrative review. *Nutrients*. 2023;15(4):889.

99. Taylor ZB, Stevenson RJ, Ehrenfeld L, Francis HM. The impact of saturated fat, added sugar and their combination on human hippocampal integrity and function: A systematic review and meta-analysis. *Neurosci Biobehav Rev*. 2021;130:91-106.

100. Sadeghpour Heravi F. Gut microbiota and autoimmune diseases: Mechanisms, treatment, challenges, and future recommendations. *Curr Clin Microbiol Rep*. 2024;11:18-33. doi:10.1007/s40588-023-00213-6

101. Rao M, Gershon MD. The bowel and beyond: The enteric nervous system in neurological disorders. *Nat Rev Gastroenterol Hepatol*. 2016;13(9):517-528. doi:10.1038/nrgastro.2016.107

102. Zimmermann P. The immunological interplay between vaccination and the intestinal microbiota. *npj Vaccines*. 2023;8(1):24.

103. Esfahani KS, Asri N, Mahmoudi Ghehsareh M, Rezaei-Tavirani M, Jahani-Sherafat S, Rostami-Nejad M. The role of gluten in the development of autoimmune thyroid diseases: A narrative review. *Int J Endocrinol Metab*. 2024;22(3):e153730. doi:10.5812/ijem-153730

104. Sharkey KA, Mawe GM. The enteric nervous system. *Physiol Rev*. 2023;103(2):1487-1564. doi:10.1152/physrev.00018.2022

105. Brookes Z, Teoh L, Cieplik F, Kumar P. Mouthwash effects on the oral microbiome: Are they good, bad, or balanced? *Int Dent J*. 2023;73:S74-S81.

106. Yen S, Johnson JS. Metagenomics: A path to understanding the gut microbiome. *Mamm Genome*. 2021;32(4):282-296.

107. Sung J, Rajendraprasad SS, Philbrick KL, et al. The human gut microbiome in critical illness: Disruptions, consequences, and therapeutic frontiers. *J Crit Care*. 2024;79:154436.

108. Letourneau J, Holmes ZC, Dallow EP, et al. Ecological memory of prior nutrient exposure in the human gut microbiome. *ISME J*. 2022;16(11):2479-2490. doi:10.1038/s41396-022-01292-x

109. Hwang YK, Oh JS. Interaction of the vagus nerve and serotonin in the gut-brain axis. *Int J Mol Sci*. 2025;26(3):1160.

110. Preiningerova JL, Jiraskova Zakostelska Z, Srinivasan A, et al. Multiple sclerosis and microbiome. *Biomolecules*. 2022;12(3):433.

111. Rew L, Harris MD, Goldie J. The ketogenic diet: Its impact on human gut microbiota and potential consequent health outcomes: A systematic literature review. *Gastroenterology and Hepatology from Bed to Bench*. 2022;15(4):326.

112. Mayer MH, Woldemariam S, Gisinger C, Dorner TE. Association of gut microbiome with muscle mass, muscle strength, and muscle performance in older adults: A systematic review. *Int J Environ Res Public Health*. 2024;21(9):1246.

113. Dyńka D, Kowalcze K, Paziewska A. The role of ketogenic diet in the treatment of neurological diseases. *Nutrients*. 2022;14(23):5003.

114. Borin JM, Liu R, Wang Y, et al. Fecal virome transplantation is sufficient to alter fecal microbiota and drive lean and obese body phenotypes in mice. *Gut Microbes*. 2023;15(1):2236750.

115. Perlmutter D, Loberg K. *Brain Maker: The Power of Gut Microbes to Heal and Protect Your Brain—for Life*. Little, Brown and Company; 2015.

116. Davis BT IV, Han H, Islam MB, et al. Short-chain fatty acid supplementation after traumatic brain injury attenuates neurologic injury via the gut-brain-microglia axis. *Shock*. 2026;65(2):329-341.

117. Fung J. *The Obesity Code: Unlocking the Secrets of Weight Loss*. Greystone Books; 2016.

118. Brown GC, Camacho M, Williams-Gray CH. The endotoxin hypothesis of Parkinson's disease. *Mov Disord*. 2023;38(7):1143-1155.

119. Saji N, Saito Y, Yamashita T, et al. Relationship between plasma lipopolysaccharides, gut microbiota, and dementia: A cross-sectional study. *J Alzheimers Dis*. 2022;86(4):1947-1957.

120. Wan Y, Zhou T, Slevin E, et al. Liver-specific deletion of microRNA-34a alleviates ductular reaction and liver fibrosis during experimental cholestasis. *FASEB J*. 2023;37(2):e22731.

121. Woodford KB. Casomorphins and gliadorphins have diverse systemic effects spanning gut, brain and internal organs. *Int J Environ Res Public Health*. 2021;18(15):7911.

122. Greenblatt J. Integrative medicine for anxiety. Psychiatry Redefined continuing education. 2023. https://www.courses.psychiatryredefined.org/courses/integrative-medicine-for-anxiety

123. Cárdenas-Torres FI, Cabrera-Chávez F, Figueroa-Salcido OG, Ontiveros N. Non-celiac gluten sensitivity: An update. *Medicina*. 2021;57(6):526.

124. Wicha K, Pokarowska A. Influence of gluten-free diet on mood disorders and symptoms of depression. *Journal of Education, Health and Sport*. 2022;12(10):281-285.

125. Khakham C. Unraveling the gluten puzzle: Exploring the divergent gluten sensitivity patterns between the US and Europe. Rupa Health. Published June 12, 2023. https://www.rupahealth.com/post/unraveling-the-gluten-puzzle-exploring-the-divergent-gluten-sensitivity-patterns-between-the-us-and-europe

126. Sakkas H, Bozidis P, Touzios C, et al. Nutritional status and the influence of the vegan diet on the gut microbiota and human health. *Medicina (Kaunas, Lithuania)*. 2020;56(2):88. doi:10.3390/medicina56020088

127. Sahin K, Orhan C, Karatoprak S, et al. Therapeutic effects of a novel form of biotin on propionic acid-induced autistic features in rats. *Nutrients*. 2022;14(6):1280.

128. Arthritis Foundation. Dairy and inflammation. Arthritis Foundation. 2025. https://www.arthritis.org/health-wellness/healthy-living/nutrition/healthy-eating/dairy-and-inflammation

129. Al Alawi Z, Majzoub RA, Zakaria OM. Formula modification and clinical outcomes in infants with atopic dermatitis and suspected non-IgE-mediated cow's milk protein allergy: A real-world comparative cohort study. *Allergies*. 2026;6(2):15.

130. Nieman KM, Anderson BD, Cifelli CJ. The effects of dairy product and dairy protein intake on inflammation: A systematic review of the literature. *J Am Coll Nutr*. 2021;40(6):571-582.

131. Wang P, Chen X, Na M, et al. Long-term consumption of ultraprocessed foods and prodromal features of Parkinson disease. *Neurology*. 2025;104(11):e213562.

132. d'Angelo M, Brandolini L, Catanesi M, et al. Differential effects of nonsteroidal anti-inflammatory drugs in an in vitro model of human leaky gut. *Cells*. 2023;12(5):728.

133. Tawam D, Baladi M, Jungsuwadee P, Earl G, Han J. The positive association between proton pump inhibitors and Clostridium difficile infection. *Innovations in Pharmacy*. 2021;12(1):10-24926.

134. Sarker SA, Ahmed T, Brüssow H. Hunger and microbiology: Is a low gastric acid-induced bacterial overgrowth in the small intestine a contributor to malnutrition in developing countries? *Microb Biotechnol*. 2017;10(5):1025-1030. doi:10.1111/1751-7915.12780

135. Tian L, Huang C, Fu W, et al. Proton pump inhibitors may enhance the risk of digestive diseases by regulating intestinal microbiota. *Front Pharmacol*. 2023;14:1217306. doi:10.3389/fphar.2023.1217306

136. Lazzerini PE, Cartocci A, Qu YS, et al. Proton pump inhibitors directly block hERG-potassium channel and independently increase the risk of QTc prolongation in a large cohort of US veterans. *Circ Arrhythm Electrophysiol*. 2021;14(7):e010042.

137. Morisaki H, Yamamoto S, Morita Y, Kotake Y, Ochiai R, Takeda J. Hypermagnesemia-induced cardiopulmonary arrest before induction of anesthesia for emergency cesarean section. *J Clin Anesth*. 2000;12(3):224-226. doi:10.1016/s0952-8180(00)00142-2

138. Hatfield J, Saad S, Housewright C. Dietary supplements and bleeding. *Proc (Bayl Univ Med Cent)*. 2022;35(6):802-807. doi:10.1080/08998280.2022.2121575

139. Wood JM, Sbar E. Jarisch-Herxheimer reaction. In: *StatPearls* [Internet]. StatPearls Publishing; 2025.

140. Ma J, Mahfuz S, Wang J, Piao X. Effect of dietary supplementation with mixed organic acids on immune function, antioxidative characteristics, digestive enzymes activity, and intestinal health in broiler chickens. *Front Nutr*. 2021;8:673316.

141. Cleveland Clinic. Hypochlorhydria. Cleveland Clinic. Published 2025. https://my.clevelandclinic.org/health/diseases/23392-hypochlorhydria

142. Hsu M, Safadi AO, Lui F. Physiology, stomach. In: *StatPearls* [Internet]. StatPearls Publishing; 2023. https://www.ncbi.nlm.nih.gov/books/NBK535425/

143. Fagnant HS, Isidean SD, Wilson L, et al. Orally ingested probiotic, prebiotic, and synbiotic interventions as countermeasures for gastrointestinal tract infections in nonelderly adults: A systematic review and meta-analysis. *Adv Nutr*. 2023;14(3):539-554.

144. Leeming ER, Johnson AJ, Spector TD, Le Roy CI. Effect of diet on the gut microbiota: Rethinking intervention duration. *Nutrients*. 2019;11(12):2862. doi:10.3390/nu11122862

145. Zhang H, Su Q. Low-FODMAP diet for irritable bowel syndrome: Insights from microbiome. *Nutrients*. 2025;17(3):544.

146. Pimentel M, Lin HC, Enayati P, et al. Lower frequency of MMC is found in IBS subjects with abnormal lactulose breath test, suggesting bacterial overgrowth. *Dig Dis Sci*. 2002;47(12):2639-2643.

147. Hilpert K, Mikut R. Is there a connection between gut microbiome dysbiosis occurring in COVID-19 patients and post-COVID-19 symptoms? *Front Microbiol.* 2021;12:732838. doi:10.3389/fmicb.2021.732838

148. Saadi M, McCallum RW. Rifaximin in irritable bowel syndrome: Rationale, evidence and clinical use. *Ther Adv Chronic Dis*. 2013;4(2):71-75. doi:10.1177/2040622312472008

149. Cleveland Clinic. Leaky gut syndrome: Symptoms, diet, tests & treatment. Cleveland Clinic. Published April 6, 2022. https://my.clevelandclinic.org/health/diseases/22724-leaky-gut-syndrome

150. Knez E, Kadac-Czapska K, Grembecka M. The importance of food quality, gut motility, and microbiome in SIBO development and treatment. *Nutrition*. 2024:112464.

151. Ruscio M, Guard G, O'Dwyer D, et al. Biofilm disruption enhances antimicrobial therapy for small intestinal bacterial overgrowth and intestinal methanogen overgrowth. *Cureus*. 2025;17(12).

152. Capuano E, Del Gaudio A, Nista EC, et al. Unraveling the complexities of small intestinal bacterial overgrowth. *Medicina*. 2026;62(3):485.

153. Marasco G, Savarino EV, Barbara G. The IBS and SIBO dilemma: Here we go again. *Dig Liver Dis*. 2024;56(12):2025-2026.

154. Triantafyllou K, Chang C, Pimentel M. Methanogens, methane and gastrointestinal motility. *J Neurogastroenterol Motil*. 2014;20(1):31-40. doi:10.5056/jnm.2014.20.1.31

155. Villanueva-Millan MJ, Leite G, Wang J, et al. Methanogens and hydrogen sulfide producing bacteria guide distinct gut microbe profiles and irritable bowel syndrome subtypes. *Am J Gastroenterol*. 2022;117(12):2055-2066. doi:10.14309/ajg.0000000000001997

156. Perez-Diaz-Del-Campo N, Castelnuovo G, Ribaldone DG, Caviglia GP. Fecal and circulating biomarkers for the non-invasive assessment of intestinal permeability. *Diagnostics (Basel)*. 2023;13(11):1976. doi:10.3390/diagnostics13111976

157. Mariamenatu AH, Abdu EM. Overconsumption of omega-6 polyunsaturated fatty acids (PUFAs) versus omega-3 PUFAs in modern-day diets: The disturbing factor for their imbalance. *J Lipids*. 2021;2021:8848161. doi:10.1155/2021/8848161

158. Christovich A, Luo J. Dietary fatty acids and cardiometabolic health: Balancing omega-6 and omega-3 fatty acids. *Nutrients*. 2022;14(18):3789. doi:10.3390/nu14183789

159. Nogoy KMC, Sun B, Shin S, et al. Fatty acid composition of grain- and grass-fed beef and their nutritional value and health implication. *Food Science of Animal Resources*. 2022;42(1):18-33. doi:10.5851/kosfa.2021.e73

160. Arboleda RN, Schneider BG, Bravo LE, et al. Use of the noninvasive Entero-test in the detection of Helicobacter pylori in children in an endemic area in Colombia. *J Pediatr Gastroenterol Nutr*. 2013;57(2):192-196. doi:10.1097/mpg.0b013e318293e1e1

161. Fasano A. All disease begins in the (leaky) gut: Role of zonulin-mediated gut permeability in the pathogenesis of some chronic inflammatory diseases. *F1000Research*. 2020;9:69. doi:10.1088/f1000research.20510.1

162. Qaisar R, Iqbal MS, Ahmad F, Karim A. Oral butyrate improves postural balance by repairing leaky gut in geriatric adults. *Gait Posture*. 2025;121:370-376. doi:10.1016/j.-gaitpost.2025.06.016

163. Marwaha K, Cain R, Asmis K, et al. Exploring the complex relationship between psychosocial stress and the gut microbiome: Implications for inflammation and immune modulation. *J Appl Physiol*. 2025;138(2):518-535. https://journals.physiol ogy.org/doi/abs/10.1152/japplphysiol.00652.2024

164. Bahrudin M, Al Fauzi A, Sugianto P. Development of atherosclerotic model through margarine diet induction in Wistar rats. Trop J Pharm Res. 2025;24(6):787-793. doi:10.4314/tjpr.v24i6.5

165. Singh MK, Aggarwal A, Dhyani P, Basumatary S, Das C. A2 milk: Status, technology, and limitations. *Trends in Animal-Based Foods*. 2025:45-54. doi: 10.1007/978-3-032-00575-5_3

166. Helal F. Hetta, Nizar Sirag, Hassabelrasoul Elfadil, Ayman Salama, Sara F. Aljadrawi, Amani J. Alfaifi, Asma N. Alwabisi, Bothinah M. AbuAlhasan, Layan S. Alanazi, Yara A. Aljohani, Yasmin N. Ramadan, Noura H. Abd Ellah, Abdelazeem M. Algammal. Artificial sweeteners: A double-edged sword for gut microbiome. *Diseases*. 2025;13(4):115. doi: 10.3390/diseases13040115

167. Teng ML, Ng CH, Huang DQ, et al. Global incidence and prevalence of nonalcoholic fatty liver disease. *Clin Mol Hepatol*. 2023;29(Suppl):S32-S42. doi:10.3350/cmh.2022.0365

168. Romero-Mascarell C, Fernández-Esparrach G, Rodríguez-De Miguel C, et al. Fecal calprotectin for small bowel Crohn's disease: Is it a cutoff issue? *Diagnostics (Basel)*. 2022;12(9):2226. doi:10.3390/diagnostics12092226

169. Wani AL, Bhat SA, Ara A. Omega-3 fatty acids and the treatment of depression: A review of scientific evidence. *Integr Med Res*. 2015;4(3):132-141. doi:10.1016/j.imr.2015.07.003

170. Li Z, et al. Blue light at night produces stress-evoked heightened aggression by enhancing brain-derived neurotrophic factor in the basolateral amygdala. *Neurobiol Stress*. 2023;28:100600. doi:10.1016/j.ynstr.2023.100600

171. Silvani MI, Werder R, Perret C. The influence of blue light on sleep, performance and wellbeing in young adults: A systematic review. *Front Physiol*. 2022;13:943108. doi:10.3389/fphys.2022.943108

172. Lopes LS, Valentini JP, Monteiro TH, et al. Problematic social media use and its relationship with depression or anxiety: A systematic review. *Cyberpsychol Behav Soc Netw*. 2022;25(11):691-702.

173. Chua KP, Volerman A, Zhang J, Hua J, Conti RM. Antidepressant dispensing to US adolescents and young adults: 2016-2022. *Pediatrics*. 2024;153(3):e2023064245. doi:10.1542/peds.2023-064245

174. Shaw KA. Prevalence and early identification of autism spectrum disorder among children aged 4 and 8 years—Autism and Developmental Disabilities Monitoring Network, 16 sites, United States, 2022. *MMWR Surveill Summ*. 2025;74.

175. Centers for Disease Control and Prevention. Mental health. Centers for Disease Control and Prevention. Published 2024. https://www.cdc.gov/healthy-youth/mental-health/index.html

176. Boreham ID, Schutte NS. The relationship between purpose in life and depression and anxiety: A meta-analysis. *J Clin Psychol*. 2023;79(12). doi:10.1002/jclp.23576

177. Al-Harbi KS. Treatment-resistant depression: Therapeutic trends, challenges, and future directions. *Patient Prefer Adherence*. 2012;6:369-388. doi:10.2147/PPA.S29716

178. Orsolini L, Pompili S, Tempia Valenta S, Salvi V, Volpe U. C-reactive protein as a biomarker for major depressive disorder? *Int J Mol Sci*. 2022;23(3):1616. doi:10.3390/ijms23031616

179. Bleibel L, Sokołowska P, Henrykowska G, Owczarek J, Wiktorowska-Owczarek A. Unveiling the anti-inflammatory effects of antidepressants: A systematic review of human studies over the last decade. *Pharmaceuticals (Basel, Switzerland)*. 2025;18(6):867. doi:10.3390/ph18060867

180. Correia AS, Vale N. Tryptophan metabolism in depression: A narrative review with a focus on serotonin and kynurenine pathways. *Int J Mol Sci*. 2022;23(15):8493. doi:10.3390/ijms23158493

181. Kezai AM, Badiane PY, Hennart B, Allorge D, Marion S, Hébert SS. MicroRNA-132 regulates quinolinic acid production in the brain during LPS-induced neuroinflammation. *Front Immunol*. 2025;16:1644783. doi:10.3389/fimmu.2025.1644783

182. Lee B, Kwon JT, Jeong Y, et al. Inflammatory and anti-inflammatory cytokines bidirectionally modulate amygdala circuits regulating anxiety. *Cell*. 2025;188(8):2190-2202. doi:10.1016/j.cell.2025.02.015

183. Passarino G, De Rango F, Montesanto A. Human longevity: Genetics or lifestyle? It takes two to tango. *Immunity & Aging*. 2016;13:12. doi:10.1186/s12979-016-0066-z

184. Krasko J, Intelisano S, Luhmann M. When happiness is both joy and purpose: The complexity of the pursuit of happiness and well-being is related to actual well-being. *Journal of Happiness Studies*. 2022;23(7):3233-3261.

185. Patton K, Oakes A. Despite behavioral health prescription volume growth, the behavioral health treatment gap has widened. Trilliant Health. Published April 16, 2026. https://www.trillianthealth.com/market-research/studies/bh-prescribing-volume-growth-bh-treatment-gap-widens

186. Abubaker S. Role of gut microbiota in the production and regulation of serotonin biosynthesis in the gastrointestinal tract [dissertation]. Université d'Ottawa/University of Ottawa; 2025.

187. Zhang Z, Kang W, Mi Y, Zhong X, He Y. The microbiota–gut–brain axis in autism: Associations, causal inference, and interventions—a narrative review. *Pathogens*. 2025;14(11):1145.

188. Pomeroy L. How gut microbes shape cognitive and mental health: Clinical applications from the GI-MAP. Diagnostic Solutions Laboratory. Published December 11, 2025. https://www.diagnosticsolutionslab.com/webinars/how-gut-microbes-shape-cognitive-and-mental-health

189. Diagnostics Solutions Laboratory. OAp: Organic Acids Profile™ interpretive guide. 2025. https://www.diagnosticsolutionslab.com/assets/documents/oap-organic-acids-interpretive-guide.pdf

190. Hey G, Nair N, Klann E, et al. Therapies for Parkinson's disease and the gut microbiome: Evidence for bidirectional connection. *Front Aging Neurosci*. 2023;15:1151850. doi:10.3389/fnagi.2023.1151850

191. Jung H, Lee D, You H, et al. LPS induces microglial activation and GABAergic synaptic deficits in the hippocampus accompanied by prolonged cognitive impairment. *Sci Rep*. 2023;13:6547. doi:10.1038/s41598-023-32798-9

192. Wieczorek, M., Swiergiel, A. H., Pournajafi-Nazarloo, H., & Dunn, A. J. (2005). Physiological and behavioral responses to interleukin-1beta and LPS in vagotomized mice. Physiology & behavior, 85(4), 500–511. https://doi.org/10.1016/j.physbeh.2005.05.012

193. Cárdenas-Torres FI, Cabrera-Chávez F, Figueroa-Salcido OG, Ontiveros N. Non-celiac gluten sensitivity: An update. *Medicina (Kaunas)*. 2021;57(6):526. doi:10.3390/medicina57060526

194. Mr, M. M. T. R. T., TAMIM, M. T. R., & Ahmed, R. (2025). The Gliadin and Casein Metabolism: Synthesis of Gliadomorphin and Casomorphin and Their Biological Consequences. RADINKA JOURNAL OF HEALTH SCIENCE, 3(2), 486-502.

195. Greenblatt J. Glutin in mental health: The missing link. Psychiatry Redefined. Published October 14, 2019. Updated May 23, 2025. https://www.psychiatryredefined.org/magnesium-mental-health/

196. Gao B, Li C, Qu Y, et al. Progress and trends of research on mineral elements for depression. *Heliyon*. 2024;10(15):e35469. doi:10.1016/j.heliyon.2024.e35469

197. American Academy of Neurology. Associations between ultra-processed food consumption and adverse brain health outcomes. AAN Online Learning Center. https://learning.aan.com/courses/126962

198. Gao Y, Song XN, Wen ZP, et al. The association of vitamin deficiency with depression risk in late-life depression: A review. *Front Nutr*. 2025;12:1551375. doi:10.3389/fnut.2025.1551375

199. Chu C, Tsuprykov O, Chen X, Elitok S, Krämer BK, Hocher B. Relationship between vitamin D and hormones important for human fertility in reproductive-aged women. *Front Endocrinol (Lausanne)*. 2021;12:666687. doi:10.3389/fendo.2021.666687

200. Jalili M, Vahedi H, Poustchi H, Hekmatdoost A. Effects of vitamin D supplementation in patients with irritable bowel syndrome: A randomized, double-blind, placebo-controlled clinical trial. *Int J Prev Med*. 2019;10:16. doi:10.4103/ijpvm.IJPVM_512_17

201. Greenblatt J. Magnesium in mental health: The missing link. Psychiatry Redefined. Published October 14, 2019. Updated May 23, 2025. https://www.psychiatryredefined.org/magnesium-mental-health/

202. Karunarathna I, Gunasena P, Gunawardana K, et al. Magnesium in clinical practice: A comprehensive review of indications, mechanisms, and toxicity for the interprofessional team. Uva Clinical Anaesthesia and Intensive Care. 2026. doi:10.5281/zenodo.20085416

203. Mori H, Tack J, Suzuki H. Magnesium oxide in constipation. *Nutrients*. 2021;13(2):421. doi:10.3390/nu13020421

204. Souza ACR, Vasconcelos AR, Dias DD, Komoni G, Name JJ. The integral role of magnesium in muscle integrity and aging: A comprehensive review. *Nutrients*. 2023;15(24):5127. doi:10.3390/nu15245127

205. Jhang WK, Lee YJ, Kim YA, Park SJ, Park YS. Severe hypermagnesemia presenting with abnormal electrocardiographic findings similar to those of hyperkalemia in a child undergoing peritoneal dialysis. *Korean J Pediatr*. 2013;56(7):308-311. doi:10.3345/kjp.2013.56.7.308

206. Magnesium for Joint Pain: How a Simple Mineral Can Give You Your Life Back. Rupa Health (blog). Published February 6, 2024; updated January 14, 2025. Medically reviewed by Dr. Jeannie Achuff, ND. https://www.rupahealth.com/post/magnesium-for-joint-pain-how-a-simple-mineral-can-give-you-your-life-back

207. Morales-Gutierrez J, Díaz-Cortés S, Montoya-Giraldo MA, Zuluaga AF. Toxicity induced by multiple high doses of vitamin B12 during pernicious anemia treatment: A case report. *Clin Toxicol (Phila)*. 2020;58(2):129-131. doi:10.1080/15563650.2019.1606432

208. Landress DP. The pellagra portraits. *JAMA*. 2024;331(5):375-377. doi:10.1001/jama.2023.27716

209. Robson MJ, Quinlan MA, Blakely RD. Immune system activation and depression: Roles of serotonin in the central nervous system and periphery. *ACS Chem Neurosci*. 2017;8(5):932-942. doi:10.1021/acschemneuro.6b00412

210. Baig A, Sial SA, Qasim M, et al. Harmful health impacts of heavy metals and behavioral changes in humans. *Indonesian Journal of Agriculture and Environmental Analytics*. 2024;3(2):77-90. doi:10.55927/ijaea.v3i2.9515

211. Tizabi Y, Bennani S, El Kouhen N, Getachew B, Aschner M. Interaction of heavy metal lead with gut microbiota: implications for autism spectrum disorder. *Biomolecules*. 2023;13(10):1549. doi:10.3390/biom13101549

212. Baik HW. Mental health and micronutrients: a narrative review. Ann Clin Nutr Metab. 2024;16(3):112-119. doi:10.15747/ACNM.2024.16.3.112

213. Mfem CC, Seriki SA, Oyama SE. Effects of heavy metal toxicity on anxiety disorder. *J Biomed Res Environ Sci*. 2021;2(8):660-668. doi:10.37871/jbres1294

214. Kandola AA. Associations of physical activity, sedentary behaviour, and physical fitness with common mental health symptoms in the population [dissertation]. University College London; 2022.

215. Wang X, He HJ, Xiong X, et al. NAD+ in Alzheimer's disease: molecular mechanisms and systematic therapeutic evidence obtained in vivo. *Front Cell Dev Biol*. 2021;9:668491. doi:10.3389/fcell.2021.668491

216. Hidese, S., Ogawa, S., Ota, M., Ishida, I., Yasukawa, Z., Ozeki, M., & Kunugi, H. (2019). Effects of L-Theanine Administration on Stress-Related Symptoms and Cognitive Functions in Healthy Adults: A Randomized Controlled Trial. Nutrients, 11(10), 2362. https://doi.org/10.3390/nu11102362

217. Moshfeghinia R, Sanaei E, Mostafavi S, Assadian K, Sanaei A, Ayano G. The effects of L-theanine supplementation on the outcomes of patients with mental disorders: a systematic review. *BMC Psychiatry*. 2024;24(1):886.

218. Llopis I, San-Miguel N, Serrano MÁ. The effects of psychobiotics and adaptogens on the human stress and anxiety response: a systematic review. *Applied Sciences*. 2025;15(8):4564.

219. Jung H, Lee D, You H, et al. LPS induces microglial activation and GABAergic synaptic deficits in the hippocampus accompanied by prolonged cognitive impairment. *Sci Rep*. 2023;13:6547. doi:10.1038/s41598-023-32798-9

220. Hamamah S, Aghazarian A, Nazaryan A, Hajnal A, Covasa M. Role of microbiota-gut-brain axis in regulating dopaminergic signaling. *Biomedicines*. 2022;10(2):436. doi:10.3390/biomedicines10020436

221. Avram OE, Bratu EA, Curis C, Moroianu LA, Drima E. Modifiable nutritional biomarkers in autism spectrum disorder: a systematic review and meta-analysis of vitamin D, B12, and homocysteine exposure spanning prenatal development through late adolescence. *Int J Mol Sci*. 2025;26(9):4410. doi:10.3390/ijms26094410

222. Zwierz M, Suprunowicz M, Mrozek K, Pietruszkiewicz J, Oracz AJ, Konarzewska B, Waszkiewicz N. Vitamin B12 and autism spectrum disorder: a review of current evidence. *Nutrients*. 2025;17(7):1220. doi:10.3390/nu17071220

223. Rossignol DA, Frye RE. The effectiveness of cobalamin (B12) treatment for autism spectrum disorder: a systematic review and meta-analysis. *J Pers Med*. 2021;11(8):784. doi:10.3390/jpm11080784

224. Xiao L, Yan J, Yang T, Zhu J, Li T, Wei H, Chen J. Fecal microbiome transplantation from children with autism spectrum disorder modulates tryptophan and serotonergic synapse metabolism and induces altered behaviors in germ-free mice. mSystems. 2021;6(2):e01343-20. doi:10.1128/msystems.01343-20

225. Sun W, Ma L, Feng X, Fan Y, Cai Y, Li X. Efficacy of gut microbiota-based therapy for autism spectrum disorder and attention deficit hyperactivity disorder: a systematic review and meta-analysis. *Psychology, Health & Medicine*. 2025:1-25.

226. Sahin K, Orhan C, Karatoprak S, et al. Therapeutic effects of a novel form of biotin on propionic acid-induced autistic features in rats. *Nutrients*. 2022;14(6):1280.

227. Li Y, Wang Y, Zhang T. Fecal microbiota transplantation in autism spectrum disorder. *Neuropsychiatr Dis Treat*. 2022;18:2905-2915. doi:10.2147/NDT.S382571

228. Otaru N, Ye K, Mujezinovic D, et al. GABA production by human intestinal Bacteroides spp.: prevalence, regulation, and role in acid stress tolerance. *Front Microbiol*. 2021;12:656895. doi:10.3389/fmicb.2021.656895

229. Kraljević Pavelić S, Saftić Martinović L, Simović Medica J, et al. Clinical evaluation of a defined zeolite-clinoptilolite supplementation effect on the selected blood parameters of patients. *Frontiers in Medicine*. 2022;9:851782.

230. Dorsey ER, Sherer T, Okun MS, Bloem BR. The emerging evidence of the Parkinson pandemic. *J Parkinsons Dis*. 2018;8(s1):S3-S8. doi:10.3233/JPD-181474

231. Tan AH, Lim SY, Lang AE. The microbiome-gut-brain axis in Parkinson disease - from basic research to the clinic. *Nat Rev Neurol*. 2022;18:476-495. doi:10.1038/s41582-022-00681-2

232. Muttalib Z, Aboukhalil D, Nwosu C, et al. Gluten and its relationship with inflammation and Parkinson's disease: a literature review. *AIMS Neurosci*. 2025;12(1):44-57. doi:10.3934/Neuroscience.2025004

233. Liu B, Fang F, Pedersen NL, et al. Vagotomy and Parkinson disease: a Swedish register-based matched-cohort study. *Neurology*. 2017;88(21):1996-2002. doi:10.1212/WNL.0000000000003961

234. Mendonça MD, Ferreira PC, Oliveira F, et al. Relative sparing of dopaminergic terminals in the caudate nucleus is a feature of rest tremor in Parkinson's disease. *npj Parkinson's Disease*. 2024;10(1):209.

235. Petrov VA, Saltykova IV, Zhukova IA, et al. Analysis of gut microbiota in patients with Parkinson's disease. *Bull Exp Biol Med*. 2017;162(6):734-737. doi:10.1007/s10517-017-3700-7

236. Jankovic J, Tan E. Parkinson's disease: etiopathogenesis and treatment. *J Neurol Neurosurg Psychiatry*. 2020;91:795-808.

237. Elsevier Ltd. Global, regional, and national burden of Alzheimer's disease and other dementias, 1990-2016: a systematic analysis for the Global Burden of Disease Study 2016. *Lancet Neurol*. 18(1):88-106. doi:10.1016/S1474-4422(18)30403-4

238. Brown GC, Heneka MT. The endotoxin hypothesis of Alzheimer's disease. *Mol Neurodegener*. 2024;19(1):30. doi:10.1186/s13024-024-00722-y

239. Wei BZ, Li L, Dong CW, Tan CC, Alzheimer's Disease Neuroimaging Initiative, Xu W. The relationship of omega-3 fatty acids with dementia and cognitive decline: evidence from prospective cohort studies of supplementation, dietary intake, and blood markers. *Am J Clin Nutr*. 2023;117(6):1096-1109. doi:10.1016/j.ajcnut.2023.04.001

240. Varga P, Lehoczki A, Fekete M, et al. The role of magnesium in depression, migraine, Alzheimer's disease, and cognitive health: a comprehensive review. *Nutrients*. 2025;17(13):2216. doi:10.3390/nu17132216

241. Zhang XX, Wang HR, Meng-Wei, et al. Association of vitamin D levels with risk of cognitive impairment and dementia: a systematic review and meta-analysis of prospective studies. *J Alzheimers Dis*. 2024;98(2):373-385. doi:10.3233/JAD-231381

242. Ramezani M, Fernando M, Eslick S, et al. Ketone bodies mediate alterations in brain energy metabolism and biomarkers of Alzheimer's disease. *Front Neurosci*. 2023;17:1297984. doi:10.3389/fnins.2023.1297984

243. Schöndorf DC, Ivanyuk D, Baden P, et al. The NAD+ precursor nicotinamide riboside rescues mitochondrial defects and neuronal loss in iPSC and fly models of Parkinson's disease. *Cell Rep*. 2018;23(10):2976-2988.

244. Paduraru E, Iacob D, Rarinca V, et al. Comprehensive review regarding mercury poisoning and its complex involvement in Alzheimer's disease. *Int J Mol Sci*. 2022;23(4):1992. doi:10.3390/ijms23041992

245. Mohan M, Okeoma CM, Sestak K. Dietary gluten and neurodegeneration: a case for preclinical studies. *Int J Mol Sci*. 2020;21(15):5407. doi:10.3390/ijms21155407

246. Ulaş AŞ, Çakır A, Erbaş O. Gluten and casein: their roles in psychiatric disorders. *Journal of Experimental and Basic Medical Sciences*. 2022;3(1):013-021.

247. Kelly D, Lee CM, Vyas G, et al. Randomized double blind inpatient study of a gluten-free diet in people with schizophrenia. 2025.

248. Longhitano C, Finlay S, Peachey I, et al. The effects of ketogenic metabolic therapy on mental health and metabolic outcomes in schizophrenia and bipolar disorder: a randomized controlled clinical trial protocol. *Front Nutr*. 2024;11:1444483. doi:10.3389/fnut.2024.1444483

249. Bai N. Pilot study shows ketogenic diet improves severe mental illness. Stanford Medicine. Published April 1, 2024. https://med.stanford.edu/news/all-news/2024/04/keto-diet-mental-illness.html?utm_source=chatgpt.com

250. Fuller-Thomson E, Methta R. Could a gene-environment interaction between NAPRT1 risk allele and pre-natal niacin deficiency explain 4 medical mysteries of schizophrenia research? *Schizophr Res*. 2019. doi:10.1016/j.schres.2019.11.049

251. Brown HE, Roffman JL. Vitamin supplementation in the treatment of schizophrenia. *CNS Drugs*. 2014;28(7):611-622. doi:10.1007/s40263-014-0172-4

252. Blom JD. Hallucinations and vitamin B12 deficiency: a systematic review. *Psychopathology*. 2024;57:492-503. doi:10.1159/000540003

253. Sajid M, Ilyas M. PTFE-coated non-stick cookware and toxicity concerns: a perspective. *Environ Sci Pollut Res Int*. 2017;24(30):23436-23440. doi:10.1007/s11356-017-0095-y

254. Zellner T, Prasa D, Färber E, Hoffmann-Walbeck P, Genser D, Eyer F. The use of activated charcoal to treat intoxications. *Dtsch Arztebl Int*. 2019;116(18):311-317. doi:10.3238/arztebl.2019.0311

255. Kuan WH, Chen YL, Liu CL. Excretion of Ni, Pb, Cu, As, and Hg in sweat under two sweating conditions. *Int J Environ Res Public Health*. 2022;19(7):4323. doi:10.3390/ijerph19074323

256. Morén C, et al. Mitochondrial oxidative phosphorylation system dysfunction in schizophrenia: evidence for compromised brain metabolism and oxidative stress. *Int J Mol Sci*. 2025;26(9):4415. doi:10.3390/ijms26094415

257. Precision Analytical Inc. DUTCH Test. Accessed May 9, 2026. https://dutchtest.com/

258. Al-Shami K, Awadi S, Khamees A, et al. Estrogens and the risk of breast cancer: a narrative review of literature. *Heliyon*. 2023;9(9):e20224. doi:10.1016/j.heliyon.2023.e20224

259. Brighten J. SHBG hormone levels: what high and low levels mean. Dr. Jolene Brighten. Accessed May 9, 2026. https://drbrighten.com/shbg-hormone-levels/

260. Rupa Health. Integrative medicine approach to estrogen excess: testing, diagnoses & treatment. Rupa Health. Published 2023. Accessed May 9, 2026. https://www.rupahealth.com/post/integrative-medicine-approach-to-estrogen-excess-testing-diagnoses-treatment

261. Jasuja R, Pencina KM, Peng L, Bhasin S. Accurate measurement and harmonized reference ranges for total and free testosterone levels. *Endocrinol Metab Clin North Am*. 2022;51(1):63-75.

262. Samuels MH, Bernstein LJ. Brain fog in hypothyroidism: what is it, how is it measured, and what can be done about it. *Thyroid*. 2022;32(7):752-763. doi:10.1089/thy.2022.0139

263. Shekhar S, Hall JE, Klubo-Gwiezdzinska J. The hypothalamic pituitary thyroid axis and sleep. *Curr Opin Endocr Metab Res*. 2021;17:8-14. doi:10.1016/j.coemr.2020.10.002

264. Persani L, Lania A, Beck-Peccoz P. Thyrotropin-secreting pituitary adenomas. In: Feingold KR, Adler RA, Ahmed SF, et al., eds. *Endotext* [Internet]. MDText.com, Inc.; Updated July 3, 2025. https://www.ncbi.nlm.nih.gov/books/NBK278978/

265. Hatch-McChesney A, Lieberman HR. Iodine and iodine deficiency: a comprehensive review of a re-emerging issue. *Nutrients*. 2022;14(17):3474. doi:10.3390/nu14173474

266. Alkahlout L, Hamran S, Darwish N, Dweidri Y, Babu GR, Al Saady RM. The association between estrogen-containing oral contraceptive pills and hypothyroidism. *Int J Endocrinol*. 2025;2025:5978558. doi:10.1155/ije/5978558

267. Refetoff S. Thyroid hormone serum transport proteins. In: Feingold KR, Ahmed SF, Anawalt B, et al., eds. *Endotext* [Internet]. MDText.com, Inc.; Updated March 10, 2023. https://www.ncbi.nlm.nih.gov/books/NBK285566/

268. Bowden SA, Goldis M. Congenital hypothyroidism. In: *StatPearls* [Internet]. Stat-

Pearls Publishing; Updated June 5, 2023. https://www.ncbi.nlm.nih.gov/books/NBK558913/

269. Ülker MT, Çolak GA, Baş M, Erdem MG. Evaluation of the effect of gluten-free diet and Mediterranean diet on autoimmune system in patients with Hashimoto's thyroiditis. *Food Sci Nutr*. 2023;12(2):1180-1188. doi:10.1002/fsn3.3833

270. Minxuri D, Mitre A, Kostrista E, Bino S, Hysaj K. A cohort study on diet and role of different food groups in Hashimoto thyroiditis. *Journal of Hygienic Engineering & Design*. 2022;38.

271. Gao Y, Liu Y, Ma T, et al. Fermented dairy products as precision modulators of gut microbiota and host health: mechanistic insights, clinical evidence, and future directions. *Foods*. 2025;14(11):1946. doi:10.3390/foods14111946

272. Vincenzi F, Smirne C, Tonello S, Sainaghi PP. The role of vitamin D in autoimmune diseases. *Int J Mol Sci*. 2026;27(1):555.

273. Koulouri O, Moran C, Halsall D, Chatterjee K, Gurnell M. Pitfalls in the measurement and interpretation of thyroid function tests. *Best Pract Res Clin Endocrinol Metab*. 2013;27(6):745-762.

274. Mancini A, Di Segni C, Raimondo S, et al. Thyroid hormones, oxidative stress, and inflammation. *Mediators Inflamm*. 2016;2016:6757154. doi:10.1155/2016/6757154

275. Gazzinelli-Guimaraes PH, Jones SM, Voehringer D, Mayer-Barber KD, Samarasinghe AE. Eosinophils as modulators of host defense during parasitic, fungal, bacterial, and viral infections. *J Leukoc Biol*. 2024;116(6):1301-1323.

276. Singh S, Pal N, Shubham S, et al. Polycystic ovary syndrome: etiology, current management, and future therapeutics. *J Clin Med*. 2023;12(4):1454. doi:10.3390/jcm12041454

277. Yılmaz SK, Eskici G, Mertoğlu C, Ayaz A. Effect of different protein diets on weight loss, inflammatory markers, and cardiometabolic risk factors in obese women. *J Res Med Sci*. 2021;26:28. doi:10.4103/jrms.JRMS_611_20

278. Javaheri, F. S. H., Ostadrahimi, A. R., Nematy, M., Arabi, S. M., & Amini, M. (2023). The effects of low calorie, high protein diet on body composition, duration and sleep quality on obese adults: A randomized clinical trial. Health science reports, 6(11), e1699. https://doi.org/10.1002/hsr2.1699

279. Minihane AM. Omega-3 fatty acids, brain health and the menopause. *Post Reproductive Health*. 2025;31(2):97-104. doi:10.1177/20533691251341701

280. Chambers P. Candida, the gut microbiome, and the epidemic levels of cancer and autoimmune disease in young women, dementia, and obesity. *J Biomed Res Environ Sci*. 2025;6(9):1210-1221.

281. Tang J, Krushelnycky L, Shaqo A, Cho CE. A comprehensive review of nutritional influences on the serotonergic system. *Adv Nutr*. 2025;16(11):100524. doi:10.1016/j.advnut.2025.100524

282. Rybaczyk LA, Bashaw MJ, Pathak DR, Moody SM, Gilders RM, Holzschu DL. An overlooked connection: Serotonergic mediation of estrogen-related physiology and pathology. *BMC Womens Health*. 2005;5:12. doi:10.1186/1472-6874-5-12

283. Niu Z, Duan L, Du Y, et al. Effect of zinc intake on association between fluoride exposure and abnormal sex steroid hormones among US pubertal males: NHANES, 2013-2016. *Environ Sci Pollut Res Int*. 2024;31(2):2759-2772. doi:10.1007/s11356-023-31135-x

284. Alagawany M, Elnesr SS, Farag MR, et al. Omega-3 and omega-6 fatty acids in poultry nutrition: Effect on production performance and health. *Animals (Basel)*. 2019;9(8):573. doi:10.3390/ani9080573

285. Beal T, Manohar S, Miachon L, Fanzo J. Nutrient-dense foods and diverse diets are important for ensuring adequate nutrition across the life course. *Proc Natl Acad Sci U S A*. 2024;121(50):e2319007121.

286. Demarquoy J. Revisiting the role of carnitine in heart disease through the lens of the gut microbiota. *Nutrients*. 2024;16(23):4244. doi:10.3390/nu16234244

287. Lim MT, Pan BJ, Toh DWK, Sutanto CN, Kim JE. Animal protein versus plant protein in supporting lean mass and muscle strength: A systematic review and meta-analysis of randomized controlled trials. *Nutrients*. 2021;13(2):661. doi:10.3390/nu13020661

288. Larnder AH, Manges AR, Murphy RA. The estrobolome: Estrogen-metabolizing pathways of the gut microbiome and their relation to breast cancer. *Int J Cancer*. 2025;157(4):599-613. doi:10.1002/ijc.35427

289. Chiu K, Warner G, Nowak RA, Flaws JA, Mei W. The impact of environmental chemicals on the gut microbiome. *Toxicol Sci*. 2020;176(2):253-284.

290. Pedersen HK, et al. Human gut microbes impact host serum metabolome and insulin sensitivity. *Nature*. 2016;535(7612):376-381. doi:10.1038/nature18646

291. Takeuchi T, et al. Gut microbial carbohydrate metabolism contributes to insulin resistance. *Nature*. 2023;621(7978):389-395. doi:10.1038/s41586-023-06466-x

292. Turnbaugh PJ, Ley RE, Mahowald MA, Magrini V, Mardis ER, Gordon JI. An obesity-associated gut microbiome with increased capacity for energy harvest. *Nature*. 2006;444(7122):1027-1031. doi:10.1038/nature05414

293. Ridaura VK, Faith JJ, Rey FE, et al. Gut microbiota from twins discordant for obesity modulate metabolism in mice. *Science*. 2013;341(6150):1241214. doi:10.1126/science.1241214

294. Domínguez-López I, Yago-Aragón M, Salas-Huetos A, Tresserra-Rimbau A, Hurtado-Barroso S. Effects of dietary phytoestrogens on hormones throughout a human lifespan: A review. Nutrients. 2020;12(8):2456. doi:10.3390/nu12082456

295. Szukiewicz D. Insight into the potential mechanisms of endocrine disruption by dietary phytoestrogens in the context of the etiopathogenesis of endometriosis. *Int J Mol Sci*. 2023;24(15):12195. doi:10.3390/ijms241512195

296. Abrams SA, Albin JL, Landrigan PJ. Use of genetically modified organism (GMO)-

containing food products in children. *Pediatrics*. 2024;153(1):e2023064774. doi:10.1542/peds.2023-064774

297. Taheri H, Mesgari-Abbasi M, Khordadmehr M, Rahimi Mamaghani A, Abbasalizad-Farhangi M. Effect of genetically modified soybean oil consumption on biochemical and histological changes of liver and kidney in rats. *International Journal of Drug Research in Clinics*. 2024;2:e11.

298. Zhang L, Rana I, Shaffer RM, Taioli E, Sheppard L. Exposure to glyphosate-based herbicides and risk for non-Hodgkin lymphoma: A meta-analysis and supporting evidence. *Mutat Res Rev Mutat Res*. 2019;781:186-206. doi:10.1016/j.mrrev.2019.02.001

299. Dagostin Ferraz S, Kuyunga L, Rech P, et al. Sexual dysfunction associated with selective serotonin reuptake inhibitors in adults with depression: A systematic review and meta-analysis. *Eur J Clin Pharmacol*. 2026;82(3):82. doi:10.1007/s00228-026-04011-z

300. Schooling CM, Au Yeung SL, Freeman G, Cowling BJ. The effect of statins on testosterone in men and women: A systematic review and meta-analysis of randomized controlled trials. *BMC Med*. 2013;11:57. doi:10.1186/1741-7015-11-57

301. Yasir M, Goyal A, Bansal P, Sonthalia S. Corticosteroid adverse effects. In: *StatPearls* [Internet]. StatPearls Publishing; 2023. Accessed May 9, 2026. https://www.ncbi.nlm.nih.gov/books/NBK531462/

302. Rubello D, Sonino N, Casara D, Girelli ME, Busnardo B, Boscaro M. Acute and chronic effects of high glucocorticoid levels on hypothalamic-pituitary-thyroid axis in man. *J Endocrinol Invest*. 1992;15(6):437-441. doi:10.1007/BF03348767

303. Ko DT, Hebert PR, Coffey CS, Sedrakyan A, Curtis JP, Krumholz HM. Beta-blocker therapy and symptoms of depression, fatigue, and sexual dysfunction. *JAMA*. 2002;288(3):351-357. doi:10.1001/jama.288.3.351

304. Corradetti, S., Gallo, G., Correale, M., Piepoli, M., Badagliacca, R., Nodari, S., Agostoni, P., & Magrì, D. (2022). β-Blockers and Erectile Dysfunction in Heart Failure. Between Myth and Reality. Reviews in cardiovascular medicine, 23(5), 173. https://doi.org/10.31083/j.rcm2305173

305. Ashfaq M, Khan Q, Haroon MZ, Abid SMA, Sharif MJH, Alkahraman YM. Long-term proton pump inhibitor therapy and its effect on endocrine hormones in selected patient population. *Horm Metab Res*. 2023;55(3):205-211.

306. Shulhai AM, Rotondo R, Petraroli M, et al. The role of nutrition on thyroid function. *Nutrients*. 2024;16(15):2496. doi:10.3390/nu16152496

307. Ward HA, Karakatsani A, Vermeulen R, et al. Catechol-O-methyltransferase (COMT) genotype modifies associations of circulating sex hormones with breast cancer risk in postmenopausal women. *Breast Cancer Res*. 2019;21(1):123.

308. Li X, Gong Y, Zhao Y, et al. Association of folate metabolism-related enzymes (MTHFR, MYD88, and TP53) and their single nucleotide polymorphisms with breast cancer susceptibility in women from Southwest China: A Bayesian network approach. *Front Oncol.* 2025;15:1560776.

309. Hassamal S. Chronic stress, neuroinflammation, and depression: An overview of pathophysiological mechanisms and emerging anti-inflammatories. *Front Psychiatry.* 2023;14:1130989.

310. Patani A, Balram D, Yadav VK, Lian KY, Patel A, Sahoo DK. Harnessing the power of nutritional antioxidants against adrenal hormone imbalance-associated oxidative stress. *Front Endocrinol (Lausanne).* 2023;14:1271521. doi:10.3389/fendo.2023.1271521

311. Dumesic DA, Oberfield SE, Stener-Victorin E, Marshall JC, Laven JS, Legro RS. Scientific statement on the diagnostic criteria, epidemiology, pathophysiology, and molecular genetics of PCOS. *Endocr Rev.* 2015;36(5):487-525.

312. Tsogbayar T, Korecky P. Can extremely low LDL levels cause health problems? SiPhox Health. Published June 18, 2025. https://siphoxhealth.com/articles/is-very-low-ldl-cholesterol-healthy

313. Chen C, Zhai H, Huang G, et al. Is lower low-density lipoprotein cholesterol associated with lower androgen and erectile dysfunction in men? *Nutr Metab Cardiovasc Dis.* 2018;28(12):1304-1310. doi:10.1016/j.numecd.2018.08.006

314. Balkrishna A, Sharma N, Diwakar S, et al. Integrated management of cortisol: A multidimensional perspective. *Future Integr Med.* 2026;5(1):27-49. doi:10.14218/FIM.2025.00062

315. Mandlik Ingawale DS, Namdeo AG. Pharmacological evaluation of Ashwagandha highlighting its healthcare claims, safety, and toxicity aspects. *J Diet Suppl.* 2021;18(2):183-226. doi:10.1080/19390211.2020.1741484

316. Eugene AR, Masiak J. The neuroprotective aspects of sleep. *MEDtube Science.* 2015;3(1):35-40.

317. Zaffanello M, Pietrobelli A, Cavarzere P, Guzzo A, Antoniazzi F. Complex relationship between growth hormone and sleep in children: Insights, discrepancies, and implications. Frontiers in Endocrinology. 2024;14:1332114. doi:10.3389/fendo.2023.1332114

318. Vijayashankar U, Ramashetty R, Rajeshekara M, et al. Leptin and ghrelin dynamics: Unraveling their influence on food intake, energy balance, and the pathophysiology of type 2 diabetes mellitus. Journal of Diabetes and Metabolic Disorders. 2024;23(1):427-440. doi:10.1007/s40200-024-01418-2

319. Addanki S, Patel K, Patel L, et al. Thyroid function and sleep patterns: A systematic review. *Cureus.* 2024;16(6):e63447. doi:10.7759/cureus.63447

320. Naghii MR, Mofid M, Asgari AR, Hedayati M, Daneshpour MS. Comparative effects of daily and weekly boron supplementation on plasma steroid hormones and proinflammatory cytokines. *J Trace Elem Med Biol.* 2011;25(1):54-58. doi:10.1016/j.jtemb.2010.10.001

321. Miller FW. The increasing prevalence of autoimmunity and autoimmune diseases: An urgent call to action for improved understanding, diagnosis, treatment, and prevention. *Curr Opin Immunol.* 2023;80:102266. doi:10.1016/j.coi.2022.102266

322. Singh JA, Wells GA, Christensen R, et al. Adverse effects of biologics: A network meta-analysis and Cochrane overview. *Cochrane Database Syst Rev.* 2011;2011(2):CD008794. doi:10.1002/14651858.CD008794.pub2

323. Altanam SY, Darwish N, Bakillah A. Exploring the interplay of antioxidants, inflammation, and oxidative stress: Mechanisms, therapeutic potential, and clinical implications. *Diseases.* 2025;13(9):309. doi:10.3390/diseases1309030

324. Rentzos G, Weisheit A, Ekerljung L, van Odijk J. Measurement of diamine oxidase (DAO) during low-histamine or ordinary diet in patients with histamine intolerance. *Eur J Clin Nutr.* 2024;78(8):726-731. doi:10.1038/s41430-024-01448-2

325. Cleveland Clinic. Histamine intolerance: Causes, symptoms & treatment. Cleveland Clinic. Published August 27, 2024. https://my.clevelandclinic.org/health/diseases/histamine-intolerance

326. Hsu TW, Bai YM, Tsai SJ, Chen TJ, Chen MH, Liang CS. Risk of autoimmune diseases after post-traumatic stress disorder: A nationwide cohort study. European Archives of Psychiatry and Clinical Neuroscience. 2024;274(3):487-495. doi:10.1007/s00406-023-01639-1

327. Goodrich JK, Waters JL, Poole AC, et al. Human genetics shape the gut microbiome. *Cell.* 2014;159(4):789-799. doi:10.1016/j.cell.2014.09.053

328. Abend AH, et al. Estimation of prevalence of autoimmune diseases in the United States using electronic health record data. *J Clin Invest.* 2025;135(4):e178722. doi:10.1172/JCI178722

329. Moulton VR. Sex hormones in acquired immunity and autoimmune disease. Frontiers in Immunology. 2018;9:2279. doi:10.3389/fimmu.2018.02279

330. Williams WV. Hormonal contraception and the development of autoimmunity: A review of the literature. *Linacre Q.* 2017;84(3):275-295. doi:10.1080/00243639.2017.1360065

331. Chen P, Li B, Ou-Yang L. Role of estrogen receptors in health and disease. Frontiers in Endocrinology. 2022;13:839005. doi:10.3389/fendo.2022.839005

332. Aryan L, Younessi D, Zargari M, et al. The role of estrogen receptors in cardiovascular disease. *Int J Mol Sci.* 2020;21(12):4314. doi:10.3390/ijms21124314

333. Tebbens M, Heijboer AC, T'Sjoen G, Bisschop PH, den Heijer M. The role of estrone in feminizing hormone treatment. *J Clin Endocrinol Metab.* 2022;107(2):e458-e466. doi:10.1210/clinem/dgab741

334. Graham JD, Roman SD, McGowan E, Sutherland RL, Clarke CL. Preferential stimulation of human progesterone receptor B expression by estrogen in T-47D human breast cancer cells. *J Biol Chem.* 1995;270(51):30693-30700. doi:10.1074/jbc.270.51.30693

335. Behlam I, Sudershan A, Priya I, et al. Association between ESR1 polymorphisms (XbaI & PvuII) and breast cancer risk: A comprehensive meta-analysis of case-control studies. *Breast Cancer Res Treat*. 2025;214(2):131-148.

336. Santana-Sánchez P, Vaquero-García R, Legorreta-Haquet MV, Chávez-Sánchez L, Chávez-Rueda AK. Hormones and B-cell development in health and autoimmunity. Frontiers in Immunology. 2024;15:1385501. doi:10.3389/fimmu.2024.1385501

337. Das P, Ingole N. Lipoproteins and their effects on the cardiovascular system. *Cureus*. 2023;15(11):e48865. doi:10.7759/cureus.48865

338. Sinha RA, Singh BK, Yen PM. Direct effects of thyroid hormones on hepatic lipid metabolism. *Nat Rev Endocrinol*. 2018;14(5):259-269. doi:10.1038/nrendo.2018.10

339. Scott DA, Ponir C, Shapiro MD, Chevli PA. Associations between insulin resistance indices and subclinical atherosclerosis: A contemporary review. American Journal of Preventive Cardiology. 2024;18:100676.

340. MacLeod C, Hadoke PWF, Nixon M. Glucocorticoids: Fuelling the fire of atherosclerosis or therapeutic extinguishers? *Int J Mol Sci*. 2021;22(14):7622. doi:10.3390/ijms22147622

341. Gaudet D, Larouche M, Raal FJ, Catapano AL. New and emerging therapeutic targets for ApoB-containing particles lowering. *Circ Res*. 2026;138(12):e327270.

342. Rupa Health. Cortisol only (4-point cortisol) by Sanesco. Rupa Health. Accessed May 9, 2026. https://www.rupahealth.com/lab-tests/sanesco-neurolab-cortisol-only-4-point-cortisol

343. Pellegrino A, Coppola G, Santopaolo F, Gasbarrini A, Ponziani FR. Role of Akkermansia in human diseases: From causation to therapeutic properties. *Nutrients*. 2023;15(8):1815. doi:10.3390/nu15081815

344. Mathew A, Fernandes D, Andreyev HJN. What is the significance of a faecal elastase-1 level between 200 and 500µg/g? Frontline Gastroenterology. 2023;14(5):371-376. doi:10.1136/flgastro-2022-102271

345. Vanga RR, Tansel A, Sidiq S, El-Serag HB, Othman MO. Diagnostic performance of measurement of fecal elastase-1 in detection of exocrine pancreatic insufficiency: Systematic review and meta-analysis. *Clin Gastroenterol Hepatol*. 2018;16(8):1220-1228.e4. doi:10.1016/j.cgh.2018.01.027

346. de la Iglesia D, Agudo-Castillo B, Galego-Fernández M, Rama-Fernández A, Domínguez-Muñoz JE. Diagnostic accuracy of fecal elastase-1 test for pancreatic exocrine insufficiency: A systematic review and meta-analysis. United European Gastroenterology Journal. 2025;13(8):1571-1582.

347. Madison AA, Bailey MT. Stressed to the core: Inflammation and intestinal permeability link stress-related gut microbiota shifts to mental health outcomes. *Biol Psychiatry*. 2024;95(4):339-347.

348. Knol EF, van Neerven RJJ. IgE versus IgG and IgA: Differential roles of allergenspecific antibodies in sensitization, tolerization, and treatment of allergies. *Immunol Rev*. 2024;328(1):314-333. doi:10.1111/imr.13386

349. Baarsma ME, Hovius JW. Persistent symptoms after Lyme disease: Clinical characteristics, predictors, and classification. *J Infect Dis*. 2024;230(Suppl 1):S62-S69. doi:10.1093/infdis/jiae203

350. Kraft S, Buchenauer L, Polte T. Mold, mycotoxins and a dysregulated immune system: A combination of concern? *Int J Mol Sci*. 2021;22(22):12269. doi:10.3390/ijms222212269

351. Ehsanifar, M., Rajati, R., Gholami, A., & Reiss, J. P. (2023). Mold and mycotoxin exposure and brain disorders. Journal of Integrative Neuroscience, 22(6), 137.

352. Park Compounding Pharmacy. Cholestyramine uses. Accessed May 9, 2026. https://www.parkcompounding.com/cholestyramine-uses/

353. Sochacka M, Kózka B, Kurek E, Giebułtowicz J. Spirulina and Chlorella dietary supplements—are they a source solely of valuable nutrients? Int J Mol Sci. 2025;26(21):10468. doi:10.3390/ijms262110468

354. Nair A, Sharma P, Tiwary MK. Glutathione deficiency in COVID19 illness-does supplementation help? Saudi J Anaesth. 2021;15(4):458-460.

355. Wimalawansa SJ. Physiological basis for using vitamin D to improve health. Biomedicines. 2023;11(6):1542. doi:10.3390/biomedicines11061542

356. Brenner M, Laragione T, Gulko PS. Short-term low-magnesium diet reduces autoimmune arthritis severity and synovial tissue gene expression. Physiol Genomics. 2017;49(4):238-242. doi:10.1152/physiolgenomics.00003.2017

357. Chen L, Yan C, Huang C, et al. Higher dietary zinc intake increases the risk of autoimmune thyroiditis. Postgrad Med J. 2025;101(1197):644-652. doi:10.1093/postmj/qgae202

358. Díez SC, de Las Cuevas Allende R, García EC. Anemia of inflammation and iron metabolism in chronic diseases. Revista Clínica Española (English Edition). 2024;224(9):598-608.

359. Takaoka K, Cyril AC, Jinesh S, Radhakrishnan R. Mechanisms of pain in sickle cell disease. Br J Pain. 2021;15(2):213-220. doi:10.1177/2049463720920682

360. LIV Hospital. Can stress cause high cholesterol? The scary link. Accessed May 9, 2026. https://int.livhospital.com/can-stress-cause-high-cholesterol-scary-link/

361. Xu W, Liu A, Gong Z, Xiao W. L-theanine prevents ulcerative colitis by regulating the CD4+ T cell immune response through the gut microbiota and its metabolites. J Nutr Biochem. 2025;139:109845. doi:10.1016/j.jnutbio.2025.109845

362. Yang W, Yu T, Cong Y. CD4+ T cell metabolism, gut microbiota, and autoimmune diseases: Implication in precision medicine of autoimmune diseases. Precision Clinical Medicine. 2022;5(3):pbac018. doi:10.1093/pcmedi/pbac018

363. Nehls S, Losse E, Armin M, Habel U, Chechko N. Progesterone-associated adjustments in brain structure during menstruation and the periovulatory phase—an MRI study. EBioMedicine. 2026;125:106184. doi:10.1016/j.ebiom.2026.106184

364. Banerjee S, Kong D, Wang Z, Bao B, Hillman GG, Sarkar FH. Attenuation of multi-targeted proliferation-linked signaling by 3,3'-diindolylmethane (DIM): From bench to clinic. Mutat Res. 2011;728(1-2):47-66. doi:10.1016/j.mrrev.2011.06.001

365. Rajoria S, Suriano R, Parmar PS, et al. 3,3'-diindolylmethane modulates estrogen metabolism in patients with thyroid proliferative disease: A pilot study. Thyroid. 2011;21(3):299-304. doi:10.1089/thy.2010.0245

366. Neelab, Zeb A, Jamil M. Milk thistle protects against non-alcoholic fatty liver disease induced by dietary thermally oxidized tallow. Heliyon. 2024;10(10):e31445. doi:10.1016/j.heliyon.2024.e31445

367. Herrera Vielma F, Quiñones San Martin M, Muñoz-Carrasco N, Berrocal-Navarrete F, González DR, Zúñiga-Hernández J. The role of dandelion (Taraxacum officinale) in liver health and hepatoprotective properties. Pharmaceuticals (Basel). 2025;18(7):990. doi:10.3390/ph18070990

368. Alpha lipoic acid. In: *LiverTox: Clinical and Research Information on Drug-Induced Liver Injury* [Internet]. National Institute of Diabetes and Digestive and Kidney Diseases; Updated May 3, 2023. https://www.ncbi.nlm.nih.gov/books/NBK591554/

369. Oliveira ALB, Monteiro VVS, Navegantes-Lima KC, et al. Resveratrol role in autoimmune disease-a mini-review. Nutrients. 2017;9(12):1306. doi:10.3390/nu9121306

370. Nandan A, Haritha J, Maniscalco D, et al. Hepatotoxicity from disease-modifying anti-rheumatic drugs (DMARDs) and association with metabolic syndrome in rheumatoid arthritis. Cureus. 2025;17(2):e78626. doi:10.7759/cureus.78626

371. Zhang Y, Lin J, You Z, et al. Cancer risks in rheumatoid arthritis patients who received immunosuppressive therapies: Will immunosuppressants work? Front Immunol. 2022;13:1050876. doi:10.3389/fimmu.2022.1050876

372. Davis JS, Ferreira D, Paige E, Gedye C, Boyle M. Infectious complications of biological and small molecule targeted immunomodulatory therapies. Clin Microbiol Rev. 2020;33(3):e00035-19. doi:10.1128/CMR.00035-19

373. Leiber KK, Parker RW. Therapeutic uses and efficacy of low-dose naltrexone: A scoping review. Cureus. 2025;17(3):e81086. doi:10.7759/cureus.81086

374. Malik A, Ye A, Chung M. Low dose naltrexone for refractory cancer pain: Case series of initial safety and effectiveness. J Pain Symptom Manage. 2025;70(6):e492-e497. doi:10.1016/j.jpainsymman.2025.08.015

375. de Carvalho JF, Skare T. Low-dose naltrexone in rheumatological diseases. Mediterr J Rheumatol. 2023;34(1):1-6. doi:10.31138/mjr.34.1.1

376. Parkitny L, Younger J. Reduced pro-inflammatory cytokines after eight weeks of low-dose naltrexone for fibromyalgia. Biomedicines. 2017;5(2):16. doi:10.3390/biomedicines5020016

377. de Carvalho JF, Skare T. Low-dose naltrexone in rheumatological diseases. Mediterr J Rheumatol. 2023;34(1):1-6. doi:10.31138/mjr.34.1.1

378. Younger J, Parkitny L, McLain D. The use of low-dose naltrexone (LDN) as a novel anti-inflammatory treatment for chronic pain. Clin Rheumatol. 2014;33:451-459. doi:10.1007/s10067-014-2517-2

379. American Fibromyalgia Syndrome Association. Low-dose naltrexone (LDN) for treating fibro. Accessed August 20, 2026. American Fibromyalgia Syndrome Association

380. Aalto H, Paul S, McEwen V. Real-world effectiveness and tolerability of low dose naltrexone to treat chronic pain: A retrospective cohort study of one pain physician's practice. J Pain Res. 2025;18:6637-6649.

381. Lerner A, Benzvi C, Vojdani A. Gluten is a proinflammatory inducer of autoimmunity. J Transl Gastroenterol. 2024;2(2):109-124. doi:10.14218/JTG.2023.00060

382. Wahls TL. *The Wahls Protocol: A Radical New Way to Treat All Chronic Autoimmune Conditions Using Paleo Principles*. Updated and expanded ed. Avery; 2020.

383. Moudgil KD, Venkatesha SH. The anti-inflammatory and immunomodulatory activities of natural products to control autoimmune inflammation. Int J Mol Sci. 2022;24(1):95. doi:10.3390/ijms24010095

384. Samuel CG, Singh P, Abdullahi H, Ibrahim I. Unlocking the therapeutic potential: Selenium and myo-inositol supplementation in thyroid disorders-efficacy and future directions. Life. 2025;15(10):1500.

385. Mashauri HL. Covid-19 histamine theory: Why antihistamines should be incorporated as the basic component in Covid-19 management? Health Sci Rep. 2023;6(2):e1109. doi:10.1002/hsr2.1109

386. Greenhalgh T, Sivan M, Perlowski A, Nikolich JŽ. Long COVID: A clinical update. Lancet. 2024;404(10453):707-724.

387. Youssef M, Ahmed HY, Zongo A, et al. Probiotic supplements: Their strategies in the therapeutic and prophylactic of human life-threatening diseases. Int J Mol Sci. 2021;22(20):11290.

388. Mouchati C, Durieux JC, Zisis SN, et al. Increase in gut permeability and oxidized LDL is associated with post-acute sequelae of SARS-CoV-2. *Front Immunol.* 2023;14:1182544.

389. British Dietetic Association. The ultimate guide to supporting your child with histamine intolerance. Accessed May 9, 2026. https://www.bda.uk.com/resource/the-ultimate-guide-to-supporting-your-child-with-histamine-intolerance.html

390. Silk E, Hedges DW, Farrer TJ. Medication effects: The cognitive impact of drug classes, polypharmacy, and drug interactions. In: *Reversible Causes of Cognitive Impairment and Dementia*. 2025:52-73.

391. Schnedl WJ, Enko D. Histamine intolerance originates in the gut. *Nutrients.* 2021;13(4):1262.

392. Boccatonda A, Campello E, Simion C, Simioni P. Long-term hypercoagulability, endotheliopathy and inflammation following acute SARS-CoV-2 infection. *Expert Rev Hematol*. 2023;16(12):1035-1048.

393. Spolarich AE, Andrews L. An examination of the bleeding complications associated with herbal supplements, antiplatelet and anticoagulant medications. *J Dent Hyg*. 2007;81(3):67.

394. Jha P, Brown PE, Ansumana R. Counting the global COVID-19 dead. *Lancet*. 2022;399(10339):1937-1938.

395. Molnar T, Lehoczki A, Fekete M, et al. Mitochondrial dysfunction in long COVID: Mechanisms, consequences, and potential therapeutic approaches. *GeroScience*. 2024;46:5267-5286. doi:10.1007/s11357-024-01165-5

396. Sumantri S, et al. Immunological dysfunction and mast cell activation syndrome in long COVID. *Front Immunol*. 2023;14:1198048.

397. Sola D, Tonello S, Casciaro GF, et al. Higher serum monolaurin is associated with a lower risk of COVID-19: Results from a prospective observational cohort study. *Int J Mol Sci*. 2025;26(6):2452. doi:10.3390/ijms26062452

398. Karosanidze I, Kiladze U, Kirtadze N, et al. Efficacy of adaptogens in patients with long COVID-19: A randomized, quadruple-blind, placebo-controlled trial. *Pharmaceuticals*. 2022;15(3):345.

399. Lee YF, Arusa G, Powell P, Qi S. Antiviral effects of English grape pomace extracts against respiratory viruses. Preprint. SSRN 5670814.

400. Nikolaidis A, Kramer R, Ostojic S. Nitric oxide: The missing factor in COVID-19 severity? *Medical Sciences (Basel, Switzerland)*. 2021;10(1):3. doi:10.3390/medsci10010003

401. Das A, Balakrishnan P. Mechanisms and clinical applications of palmitoylethanolamide (PEA) in the treatment of neuropathic pain. *Inflammopharmacology*. 2025;33(1):121-133. doi:10.1007/s10787-024-01623-8

402. Shareef J, Sridhar SB, Al Naqbi SH, Bakshi AI. Beyond pain relief: A cross-sectional study on NSAID prescribing, polypharmacy, and drug interaction risks in community pharmacies. *Healthcare (Basel, Switzerland)*. 2025;13(24):3264. doi:10.3390/healthcare13243264

403. Li R, Wu H, Xu Y, et al. Underlying mechanisms and treatment of acetaminophen-induced liver injury (Review). *Mol Med Rep*. 2025;31(4):106. doi:10.3892/mmr.2025.13471

404. Zaiss MM, Joyce Wu HJ, Mauro D, Schett G, Ciccia F. The gut-joint axis in rheumatoid arthritis. *Nat Rev Rheumatol*. 2021;17(4):224-237.

405. Longo UG, Lalli A, Bandini B, et al. Role of the gut microbiota in osteoarthritis, rheumatoid arthritis, and spondylarthritis: An update on the gut-joint axis. *Int J Mol Sci*. 2024;25(6):3242. doi:10.3390/ijms25063242

406. Echeverria-Villalobos M, Tortorici V, Brito BE, Ryskamp D, Uribe A, Weaver T. The role of neuroinflammation in the transition of acute to chronic pain and the opioid-induced hyperalgesia and tolerance. *Front Pharmacol.* 2023;14:1297931.

407. Sebba A. Pain: A review of interleukin-6 and its roles in the pain of rheumatoid arthritis. *Open Access Rheumatology: Research and Reviews.* 2021;31-43.

408. Rikard SM, Strahan AE, Schmit KM, Guy GP Jr. Chronic pain among adults—United States, 2019-2021. *MMWR Morb Mortal Wkly Rep.* 2023;72(15):379-385. doi:10.15585/mmwr.mm7215a1

409. Schleicher E, Didangelos T, Kotzakioulafi E, Cegan A, Peter A, Kantartzis K. Clinical pathobiochemistry of vitamin B12 deficiency: Improving our understanding by exploring novel mechanisms with a focus on diabetic neuropathy. *Nutrients.* 2023;15(11):2597.

410. Lombardo M, Feraco A, Ottaviani M, et al. The efficacy of vitamin D supplementation in the treatment of fibromyalgia syndrome and chronic musculoskeletal pain. *Nutrients.* 2022;14(15):3010.

411. Liguori S, Moretti A, Paoletta M, Gimigliano F, Iolascon G. Role of magnesium in skeletal muscle health and neuromuscular diseases: A scoping review. *Int J Mol Sci.* 2024;25(20):11220.

412. McDermott GC, Choufani M, Monshizadeh A, Ermann J. HLA-B27 testing in clinical practice: A retrospective analysis of testing indications and rheumatology referral patterns. *J Rheumatol.* 2025;52(10):1021-1027.

413. Polli A, Hendrix J, Ickmans K, et al. Genetic and epigenetic regulation of catechol-O-methyltransferase in relation to inflammation in chronic fatigue syndrome and fibromyalgia. *J Transl Med.* 2022;20. doi:10.1186/s12967-022-03662-7

414. Alshahrani AA, Saini RS, Okshah A, et al. The association between genetic factors and temporomandibular disorders: A systematic literature review. *Arch Oral Biol.* 2024;166:106032.

415. Gerra M, Dallabona C, Manfredini M, et al. The polymorphism Val158Met in the COMT gene: Disrupted dopamine system in fibromyalgia patients? *Pain.* 2024;165:e184-e189. doi:10.1097/j.pain.0000000000003313

416. Gleason B, Chisari E, Parvizi J. Osteoarthritis can also start in the gut: The gut-joint axis. *Indian J Orthop.* 2022;56(7):1150-1155.

417. Fariduddin MM, Haq N, Bansal N. Hypothyroid myopathy. In: *StatPearls* [Internet]. Treasure Island, FL: StatPearls Publishing; Updated June 7, 2024. https://www.ncbi.nlm.nih.gov/books/NBK519513/

418. Xia F, Li Q, Luo X, Wu J. Identification for heavy metals exposure on osteoarthritis among aging people and machine learning for prediction: A study based on NHANES 2011-2020. *Front Public Health.* 2022;10:906774.

419. Haddad R, Elbeialy A, El Sawy S, Elzomor H. Impact of heavy metals on serum vitamin D3 and PTH in fibromyalgia and rheumatoid arthritis and their correlation to disease activity. Research Square. Preprint. Posted 2024. doi:10.21203/rs.3.rs-4596002/v1

420. Shepherd J, Rogers A, Garey L, et al. Tobacco use severity in relation to opioid misuse and dependence among adult tobacco users with chronic pain: The moderating role of pain-related anxiety. *Addict Behav*. 2021;117:106844. doi:10.1016/j.addbeh.2021.106844

421. Chittrakul J, Sapbamrer R, Sirikul W. Pesticide exposure and risk of rheumatoid arthritis: A systematic review and meta-analysis. *Toxics*. 2022;10(5):207.

422. Saravanan P, Saravanan V, Rajeshkannan R, et al. Comprehensive review on toxic heavy metals in the aquatic system: Sources, identification, treatment strategies, and health risk assessment. *Environ Res*. 2024;258:119440. doi:10.1016/j.envres.2024.119440

423. Gochfeld M, Burger J. Mercury interactions with selenium and sulfur and the relevance of the Se: Hg molar ratio to fish consumption advice. *Environ Sci Pollut Res Int*. 2021;28(15):18407-18420.

424. Alende-Castro V, González-Quintela A. Response: Re: C-reactive protein versus erythrocyte sedimentation rate: Implications among patients with no known inflammatory conditions. *J Am Board Fam Med*. 2022;35:209. doi:10.3122/jabfm.2022.01.210423

425. McCrone J, Pignanelli C, Lydiate G, et al. The effects of body hydration on perceptual responses during blood flow restriction exercise. *Physiol Rep*. 2025;13. doi:10.14814/phy2.70343

426. Palsson TS, Rubio-Peirotén A, Doménech-García V. Sleep deprivation increases pain sensitivity following acute muscle soreness. *Sleep Med*. 2023;109:75-81.

427. Kuldeyev E, Seitzhanova M, Tanirbergenova S, et al. Modifying natural zeolites to improve heavy metal adsorption. *Water*. 2023. doi:10.3390/w15122215

428. Zhang S, Ning Y, Yang Y, et al. Decoding pain chronification: Mechanisms of the acute-to-chronic transition. *Front Mol Neurosci*. 2025;18:1596367.

429. Takeda M, Sashide Y. Pain management with natural products: Neurophysiological insights. *Int J Mol Sci*. 2025;26. doi:10.3390/ijms26136305

430. Majumdar A, Prasad M, Gandavarapu S, et al. Efficacy and safety evaluation of Boswellia serrata and Curcuma longa extract combination in the management of chronic lower back pain: A randomised, double-blind, placebo-controlled clinical study. *Explore*. 2024;21(1):103099. doi:10.1016/j.explore.2024.103099

431. Pérez-Piñero S, Muñoz-Carrillo JC, Echepare-Taberna J, et al. Dietary supplementation with plant extracts for amelioration of persistent myofascial discomfort in the cervical and back regions: A randomized double-blind controlled study. *Front Nutr*. 2024;11:1403108.

432. Farsani HA, Heidari-Soureshjani S, Sherwin CM, Tafrishinejad A, Azadegan-

Dehkordi Z. The analgesic effect of ginger on postoperative pain: A systematic review of clinical trials. *The Natural Products Journal*. 2024;14(2):81-89.

433. Du Z, Chen H, Cai Y, Zhou Z. Pharmacological use of gamma-aminobutyric acid derivatives in osteoarthritis pain management: A systematic review. *BMC Rheumatol*. 2022;6(1):28.

434. Paschke-Dahl L, Klinger R. Open-label-placebos can reduce pain, but not indigestion during gluten challenge in chronic pain patients. *Front Psychol*. 2025;16. doi:10.3389/fpsyg.2025.1572761

435. Hadjivassiliou M, Trott N, Hoggard N, Sanders D. Sensory symptoms without structural pathology in patients with gluten sensitivity. *Nutrients*. 2024;16. doi:10.3390/nu16081209

436. Buosi JAO, Nogueira SA, Sousa MP, et al. Gluten-free diet reduces pain in women with myofascial pain in masticatory muscles: A preliminary randomized controlled trial. *J Oral Facial Pain Headache*. 2021;35(3):199-207.

437. Zhang C, Zhu M. Activation of NF-κB signaling by a high-fat and high-sugar diet enhances macrophage polarization and aggravates postoperative pain and inflammatory responses. *Immunol Invest*. 2025:1-15.

www.ingramcontent.com/pod-product-compliance
Lightning Source LLC
LaVergne TN
LVHW021735071126
851857LV00040B/1140
* 9 7 9 8 9 0 1 5 8 0 8 4 4 *